S'WEN SHAH

GW00818421

Manual of
Practical Medicine

Preface to the First Edition

Medicine is an everchanging science. The vast clinical experience, the technological advancement in the field of investigatory modalities, tremendous explosion in the invention and addition of newer drugs in the field of pharmacology, and a wide variety of interventional therapeutic advancements have contributed to the voluminous growth of medical literature.

Human brain cannot remember all the facts. It is impossible to learn, register, remember and to recall all the medical facts in the course of time bound undergraduate and postgraduate medical education. It is the realization of these difficulties that prompted me to write this manual. Hence, an earnest attempt has been made to merge the clinical methods and the principles of internal medicine and to present both in a condensed form. To keep the size of the volume compact and small, only certain important clinical topics are included in this manual. Even references are not included since high-tech reference system is available in all the good libraries.

The manual will be of practical value to the medical students and practising physicians with an emphasis not only on clinical methods, clinical features, various essential investigations, but also on the management of various important clinical disorders.

I am deeply indebted to three of my postgraduate students Dr K Narayanasamy MD, Dr Rajesh Bajaj MD, and Dr S Sujatha MD who have helped me in preparation of the manuscript, computer and laser printing and upto the stage of submission to the publishers. But for their untiring efforts and hardwork, the timely publication of this manual would not have been possible.

I wish to acknowledge the contribution of my associates and colleagues in securing the clinical photographs, echocardiograms, X-rays, CT films, nuclear imaging photographs and computer line diagrams for this manual: C Lakshmikanthan, R Alagesan, P Thirumalai, K Kannan (Madurai), CU Velmurugendran, SG Krishnamoorthy, S Sethuraman, P Raja Sambandam, MA Muthusethupathy, P Soundarrajan, AS Natrajan, D Sivagnanasundaram, C Panchapakesa Rajendran, KR Suresh Bapu, Thirumoorthy and Hari Ramesh.

I wish to thank my postgraduate students who did the proofreading of the entire manual.

Last, but by no means the least, I wish to acknowledge the help and encouragement provided by the editorial department and the editorial staff of the Jaypee Brothers Medical Publishers for their kind cooperation in bringing out this manual.

I do wish that this manual will be a good guide and primer to the internal medicine students and practising physicians.

R Alagappan

Contents

1. Introduction to Internal Medicine   *1*

2. Nutrition   *52*

3. Cardiovascular System   *75*

4. Respiratory System   *190*

5. Abdomen   *254*

6. Hematology   *318*

7. Nephrology   *366*

8. Nervous System   *395*

9. Endocrine and Metabolic Disorders   *566*

10. Connective Tissue Disorders   *648*

11. Oncology   *672*

12. Geriatric Medicine   *706*

13. Substance Abuse   *713*

14. Imaging Modalities in Internal Medicine   *723*

15. Procedures   *743*

Laboratory Reference Values   *760*

Index   *763*

CHAPTER 1

Introduction to Internal Medicine

THE HISTORY

NAME
AGE (Date of birth)
SEX
ADDRESS
SOURCE OF HISTORY

PRESENTING COMPLAINTS
(in chronological order)

HISTORY OF PRESENTING
COMPLAINTS
Duration/Severity
Mode of onset
Progression
Agg./Relieving factors
Associated symptoms

PAST ILLNESS
H/o past medical/
surgical illness

PERSONAL HISTORY
H/o smoking/alcohol use
H/o illicit drug use
Pre/extramarital contact

OCCUPATIONAL HISTORY

MARITAL STATUS

LIVING CIRCUMSTANCES

IN CHILDREN,
Prenatal/natal
Postnatal history
Developmental history
Immunisation history

DIET HISTORY

MENSTRUAL HISTORY

FAMILY HISTORY

DRUGS AND ALLERGIES

SUMMARY

THE PHYSICAL EXAMINATION

GENERAL EXAMINATION
Consciousness
Mental state
General appearance
Face and body habitus
Skin/Hair/Nails
Eyes-pallor
    Icterus
Oral cavity
    Dental hygiene
    Hydration
    Odour of breath
    Cyanosis
    Tongue
Clubbing
Pedal oedema
Lymph node enlargement

VITAL SIGNS
Temperature
Pulse
Respiration
Blood pressure

ANTHROPOMETRY
Height and weight
BMI
In children,
MAC and HC

SYSTEM EXAMINATION
(prioritise the system
which is involved)
Cardiovascular sys.
Respiratory sys.
Gastrointestinal sys.
Nervous sys.

WORKING DIAGNOSIS

INVESTIGATIONS

EXPLANATION TO
THE PATIENT

TREATMENT/FUTURE PLAN

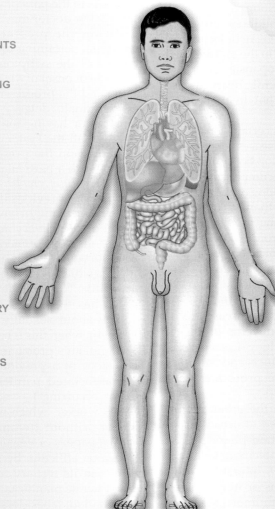

History Taking

History taking is an art, which forms a vital part in approaching the patient's problem, and arriving at a diagnosis. History taking helps to form a healthy doctor-patient relationship. It also builds up the patient's confidence and trust in his doctor.

Even before going into the patient's complaints, important facts can be gleaned from the following data, asked as a routine from every patient, helping the consulting doctor to arrive at a most probable conclusion to the patient's problems.

1. **Name:** Gives a clue to the country, state, and religion to which the patient may belong.

2. **Age:** Problems setting in at childhood are probably congenital in origin. Degenerative, neoplastic, and vascular disorders are more common in the middle aged or elderly. In women beyond the menopausal age group, the incidence of problems like ischaemic heart disease increases in equal proportion as that in their male counterparts.

3. **Sex:** Males are prone to inherit certain conditions transmitted as X-linked recessive diseases, e.g. hemophilia. They are more prone to develop conditions like IHD, bronchogenic carcinoma and decompensated liver disease, as they are habituated to smoking and consumption of alcohol, in larger numbers than their female counterparts. Females are more prone for developing autoimmune disorders like SLE, thyroid disorders, etc.

4. **Religion:** Jews practice circumcision soon after birth, and so development of carcinoma of penis is rare in them. Muslims do not consume alcohol, and so are less prone to develop problems related to its consumption, e.g. decompensated liver disease. Sikhs do not smoke and are less likely to develop problems related to smoking, e.g. carcinoma of lung. Certain sects of Hindus do not consume meat products and consume a high fibre diet and are therefore protected from developing carcinoma of the colon.

5. **Address:** People hailing from the urban region are prone to develop problems related to urbanisation like exposure to constant stress and atmospheric pollutants (industrial and vehicular) and problems developing consequent to this, e.g. IHD, COPD, interstitial lung disease, etc. Inhabitants of mountains or hilly regions may develop problems like primary pulmonary hypertension, may have a persistent patent ductus arteriosus (from childhood) or may be goitrous secondary to iodine deficiency. The particular place from which the patient hails may be endemic for certain diseases, e.g. fluorosis prevalent in certain pockets in Andhra Pradesh.

After having obtained the above details, the patient should be approached as follows:

1. Greet the patient, preferably by his name and start off the consultation with some general questions such as, "What can I do for you?", or "How can I help you?", or "What is the problem?"

2. *The presenting of complaints:* Allow the patient to tell his complaints in his own words. Do not put leading questions to the patient. The current complaints and their duration should be noted in a chronological order.

3. *History of present illness:* Allow the patient to elaborate on the story of his illness from its onset to its present state. Take care so as not to put any leading questions to the patient which may distort the patient's history. The doctor may, however, interrupt the patient to ask for the presence of 'positive' or 'negative' symptoms pertaining to patient's current problems. In analysis of the symptoms, it is important to consider the mode of onset of the illness (acute, subacute, or insidious) and the progression of the illness to the present state (gradually deteriorating, getting better, remaining the same or having remissions and exacerbations). A review of all the systems can be made by questioning the patient on the presence or absence of symptoms pertaining to a particular system.

4. *History of previous illnesses:* This should include all important previous illnesses, operations, or injuries that the patient might have suffered from birth onwards. The mode of delivery and the timing of attainment of the various developmental milestones in infancy may be important in some cases. It is always wise to be cautious while accepting readymade diagnosis from the patient like 'Typhoid fever', 'Malaria', etc. unless the patient has records of the mentioned illness. Tactful enquiry about sexually transmitted diseases and its treatment, when this is considered of possible relevance to the patient's problem, should be made.

History of a previous single painless penile ulcer with associated painless masses over the inguinal regions, occurring 3-4 weeks after exposure to a commercial sex worker, which may have healed subsequently with or without treatment with the formation of a residual papery or velvety scar over the penis indicates a previous affliction by syphilis. This is important, as syphilis in its tertiary form, later in life, can present with systemic manifestations, e.g. aortic aneurysm and regurgitation, tabes dorsalis.

History of white discharge per urethrum with associated dysuria, 2-3 days after exposure to a commercial sex worker indicates gonorrhoea. This is important as gonorrhoea can later lead to gonococcal arthritis or urethral stricture.

5. *The menstrual history:* The following enquiries are made:

  (i) Age of menarche
  (ii) Duration of each cycle
  (iii) Regular or irregular cycles
  (iv) Approximate volume of blood loss in each menstrual cycle
  (v) Age of attainment of menopause
  (vi) Post-menopausal bleeding.

6. *Obstetric history:* The following enquiries are made:

  (i) Number of times the patient conceived
  (ii) Number of times pregnancy was carried to term
  (iii) Number of abortions (spontaneous or therapeutic)
  (iv) Number of living children, their ages and the age of the last child delivered.
  (v) The time interval between successive pregnancies/abortions.
  (vi) Mode of delivery (vaginal, forceps assisted, or caesarean).
  (vii) Development of edema legs, hypertension or seizures in the antenatal or postnatal period (seizure within 48 hrs of delivery is due to pregnancy induced hypertension, beyond 48 hrs may be due to cerebral sinus thrombosis).
  (viii) Presence of impaired glucose tolerance in the course of pregnancy or history of having given birth to a large baby may give a clue to the presence of diabetes mellitus in the patient.

7. *Treatment history:* This should include all previous medical and surgical treatment and also any medication that the patient may be continuing to take to the present date. Details of drugs taken, including analgesics, oral contraceptives, psychotropic drugs and of previous surgery and radiotherapy are particularly important. It is important to find out if the patient had been allergic or had experienced any untoward reactions to any medication that he may have consumed previously, so that the same medication can be avoided in the patient in future and the patient is also appraised of the same. Knowledge of any current therapy that the patient may be on is necessary in order to avoid adverse drug reactions, when new drugs are introduced by the consulting doctor.

8. *Family history:* Enquire about the presence of consanguinity in the patient's parents, any disease states in the patient's parents, brothers, sisters and close relatives (presence of disease states like HTN, DM, IHD in the above may make the patient more prone to develop a similar problem). It is prudent to record the state of health, important illnesses, the cause and age of death in any member of the patient's family (may give a clue to the presence of HOCM, or development of IHD). Presence of a hereditary disorder prevalent in the family should be enquired for. Marital status of the patient and the number of children that the patient has should also be enquired for (infertility in a patient may give a clue to the presence of immotile cilia syndrome, cystic fibrosis or Young's syndrome).

9. *Social history:* Enquire about the patient's family life style, daily habits, and diet; about the nature of the patient's work (hard work or sedentary), as this may help in rehabilitation of the patient; about the possibility of over crowding at home (over crowding aids in the spread of communicable diseases) and the sanitation in and around the house; about the presence of pets in the house; about the use of alcohol (number of days in a week and also the quantity consumed each day), tobacco (whether chewed or smoked) and betel nut.

An alcoholic consumes alcohol almost everyday and develops withdrawal symptoms on abstaining from alcohol.

Smoking: Enquire about the number of cigarettes/beedis smoked per day and the duration of smoking. This may be presented as:

Pack years: Duration of smoking in years × Number of packets of cigarettes smoked/day, e.g. two packs of cigarettes smoked per day for twenty years constitutes 40 pack years (Risk for development of bronchogenic carcinoma increases when pack years exceed 40).

Smoking index: It is the number of cigarettes or beedis smoked per day and its duration, e.g. the smoking index of a person smoking 20 cigarettes or beedis per day for 20 years is 400. Smoking index greater than 300 constitutes a risk factor for bronchogenic carcinoma.

Chewing betel nut or tobacco is a habit common with people living in the rural areas, and this increases the risk of developing oral malignancies.

Enquire about history of travel abroad or other places within the country, as it may give a clue to the import of a disease by the patient, endemic in the place visited.

10. *Occupational history:* Enquiry must be made on all previous and present occupation, as it may give a clue to the presence of an occupational disease in the patient and also to plan the rehabilitation, e.g.

  (i) Mesothelioma—exposure to asbestos
  (ii) Carcinoma of the urinary bladder—exposure to aromatic amines in dyestuff industry.
  (iii) Silicosis—occurs in mine workers.

On the other hand, the presence of a disease in an individual may make him unfit for his occupation by proving to be hazardous to him as well as to others, e.g.

(i) Salmonella infection or carrier state in food handlers.

(ii) Epilepsy in drivers of public transport vehicles.

General Examination

Examination of the Skin

Pigmentation of the skin varies from dark skinned to fair individuals, depending on the race to which they belong.

(a) Generalised absence of skin pigmentation occurs in albinism. Syndromes with features of albinism are:
  (i) Chédiak-Higashi syndrome (phagocyte deficiency disease)
  (ii) Phenylketonuria (inborn error of amino acid metabolism).

(b) Patchy absence of skin pigmentation may be due to vitiligo (Fig. 1.1). In the presence of vitiligo, suspect presence of DM or other autoimmune disorders in that patient.

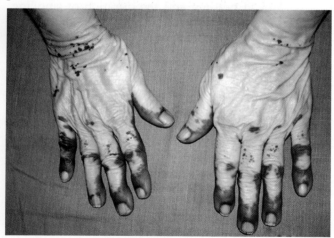

Fig. 1.1: Vitiligo

(c) Circumscribed hypopigmented lesions of the skin may occur in
  (i) Hansen's disease (Tuberculoid or Borderline Tuberculoid types).
  (ii) Tinea versicolor.

(d) Generalised hyperpigmentation of the skin is seen in
  (i) Haemochromatosis
  (ii) Endocrine disorders
    • Addison's disease
    • Cushing's syndrome
    • Ectopic ACTH production.

(e) Patchy hyperpigmentation of the skin is seen in
  (i) Pellagra (in parts exposed to sunlight)
  (ii) Porphyria Cutanea Tarda
  (iii) Scleroderma
  (iv) Café au lait spots* (Fig. 1.2)
  (v) Chloasma
  (vi) Butterfly rash over face in SLE
  (vii) Acanthosis nigricans
  (viii) Drugs—chlorpromazine, clofazimine, heavy metals like gold, bismuth
  (ix) Fixed drug eruptions.

(f) Yellow pigmentation of the skin:
  (i) Jaundice (there is yellowish discoloration of the skin, mucous membranes, and the sclera seen through the bulbar conjunctiva. This usually occurs when the total serum bilirubin value has exceeded 2 mg/dl).
  (ii) Carotenemia (this occurs due to excessive ingestion of carotene. There is a yellowish discoloration of the skin and the mucous membrane, but there is no yellow discoloration of the sclera.
  (iii) Lemon yellow discoloration of the skin can occur in long standing severe anemia.

(g) *Bluish discoloration:* Bluish discoloration of the skin, mucous membranes and sclera can occur in the presence of cyanosis. In peripheral cyanosis, the bluish discolo-

---

* Café au lait spots are macules, present in more than 90 % of patients with neurofibromatosis (both types I and II). They appear as light brown round to ovoid macules, with smooth borders, often located over nerve trunks, their long axis being parallel to the underlying cutaneous nerve. Its presence is significant when 6 or more of these macules, each more than 1.5 cm in diameter, are present. Café au lait macules with irregular borders are present over the midline of the body and are seen in McCune-Albright syndrome (fibrous dysplasia).

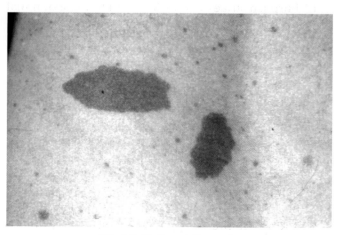

Fig. 1.2: Café au lait macule

Age	Arm span minus height (in cm)
a. 0–7 years	–3
b. 8–12 years	0
c. More than 12 years	+1 (in females) +4 (in males)

2. The relationship between upper segment measurement (from vertex to symphysis pubis) and lower segment measurement (from symphysis pubis to the heel) also varies with age as follows:

Age	Upper segment/lower segment
a. At birth	1.7
b. 3 years	1.4
c. 10 years	1.0
d. Adult	0.8

Stature > Arm Span

1. Adrenal cortex tumour
2. Precocious puberty.

This is because of early epiphyseal fusion.

Arm Span > Stature

1. Eunuchoidism
2. Hypogonadism
3. Marfan's syndrome
4. Homocystinuria
5. Klinefelter's syndrome.

This is because of delayed epiphyseal fusion. The difference in measurement must be greater than five centimeters to be significant.

Upper Segment > Lower Segment

1. Adrenal cortex tumour
2. Precocious puberty.

Lower Segment > Upper Segment

1. Eunuchoidism
2. Hypogonadism
3. Homocystinuria
4. Klinefelter's syndrome
5. Marfan's syndrome.

Marfan's Syndrome

It is a syndrome comprising of the following Tetrad:
1. Familial (autosomal dominant)
2. Lens dislocation (upward)

Marfan's syndrome	Homocystinuria
1. It is a connective tissue disorder	It is an inborn error of metabolism, due to lack of the enzyme cystathionine synthase, leading to an accumulation of homocystine and methionine and a deficiency of cystathionine and cystine
2. It is transmitted as an autosomal dominant trait	It is transmitted as an autosomal recessive trait
3. Mental faculty normal	Mental defect is present
4. Bones are normal	Osteoporosis is present
5. Mitral valve prolapse and dilatation of the aortic root and sinus of Valsalva may be present	Medial degeneration of the aorta and elastic arteries may be present
6. There is no predilection to development of thrombosis	Arterial and venous thrombosis can occur
7. Supero lateral subluxation of the lens.	Infero lateral subluxation of the lens.

3. Great vessel (aortic or pulmonary) dilatation or dissection
4. Long tubular bones.

Skeletal Defects

a. Stature—Tall and thin (asthenic)
b. Skull—Dolicocephalus
c. High arched palate
d. Chest and spine—Pectus carinatum, pectus excavatum, straight back syndrome, kyphosis, scoliosis
e. Limbs—Long thin limbs and long thin fingers (Arachnodactyly)
f. Joint hypermobility and ligament laxity
g. Feet—Pes planus, pes cavus, hallux valgus.

Wrist sign (Fig. 1.22): The patient with Marfan's syndrome is able to enclose his wrist with the thumb and little

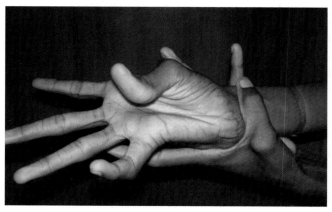

Fig. 1.22: Wrist sign

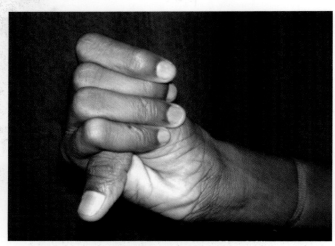

Fig. 1.23: Thumb sign

finger of the other hand, and the digits will overlap. The little finger overlaps the thumb by at least 1 cm.

Thumb sign (Fig. 1.23): In a patient with Marfan's syndrome, a part of the distal phalanx of the thumb is seen beyond the ulnar border of the hand, when a fist is formed with the thumb flexed, within the palm.

Height and arm span: The patient is tall, the lower segment being more than the upper segment by at least 5 cm. The arm span is more than the height of the patient by at least 5 cm.

Ocular Defects

a. Micro cornea
b. Ectopia lentis (Bilateral upward and outward dislocation)
c. Cataract
d. Strabismus
e. Myopia
f. Retinal detachment
g. Iridodonesis.

Cardiac Defects

a. Aneurysm of aorta
b. Dissection of aorta
c. Sinus of Valsalva aneurysm
d. Aortic regurgitation
e. Mitral or tricuspid valve prolapse syndrome
f. Atrial septal defect (ostium secundum)
g. Ventricular septal defect
h. Dilatation of the pulmonary artery.

Pulmonary Defects

a. Cystic bronchiectasis
b. Spontaneous pneumothorax.

Investigations

1. Slit-lamp examination of the eyes for detection of ectopia lentis
2. X-ray of the hands.

Metacarpal index (MCI): This is calculated by measuring the average length of the second, third, fourth and fifth metacarpals, and the average midwidth of the same.

$$MCI = \frac{\text{average length of the four metacarpals}}{\text{average midwidth of the four metacarpals}}$$

If MCI is > 8.4, it indicates presence of Marfan's syndrome (Normal MCI = 5.4 to 7.9).

Gigantism

Gigantism is said to be present in an individual, when his height exceeds six feet, six inches.

Types of Gigantism

1. *Hereditary:* Primary or genetic. In this type the body is perfectly proportioned. They are normal mentally, physically and sexually.
2. *Endocrine gigantism:* The following types are seen:
   a. *Hyperpituitary gigantism:* They are well-proportioned and have good physical and sexual development.
   b. *Eunuchoid gigantism:* They are tall, lanky and long limbed individuals with infantile sex organs, e.g. Klinefelter's syndrome.

Dwarfism

Dwarfism is said to be present when there is a marked, permanent shortness of stature, with predicted adult height less than 4 standard deviations from the mean. An adult may be called a dwarf, if his height is less than 4 feet.

Classification of Short Stature

I. *Normal variant*
   1. Familial short stature
   2. Constitutional growth delay
   3. Racial.
II. *Pathological*
   a. *Proportionate*
      i. *Prenatal*
         1. Intrauterine growth retardation
         2. Antenatal infection in mother (TORCH*, syphilis, AIDS)
         3. Antenatal consumption of alcohol, tobacco, heroin

---

* Toxoplasmosis, other infections Rubella, Cytomegalovirus, Herpes simplex.

4. Chromosomal disorders (Down's syndrome, Turner's syndrome).
  ii. *Postnatal*
    1. Malnutrition (Protein-energy malnutrition, anorexia nervosa)
    2. Endocrine disorders (growth hormone deficiency, hypothyroidism, congenital adrenal hyperplasia, precocious puberty)
    3. Cardiovascular disorders (cyanotic and acyanotic congenital heart disease, early onset rheumatic heart disease)
    4. Respiratory disorders (Kartagener's syndrome, cystic lung disease, childhood asthma)
    5. Renal disorders (renal tubular acidosis, renal rickets, nephrotic syndrome, chronic pyelonephritis)
    6. Blood disorders (chronic anemia like thalassemia or sickle cell anemia, leukemia)
    7. Psychosocial disorders (maternal deprivation).
b. *Disproportionate*
  1. Rickets
  2. Skeletal dysplasia (kyphosis, lordosis, scoliosis)
  3. Defective bone formation (osteopetrosis, osteogenesis imperfecta)
  4. Defective cartilage growth (achondroplasia, multiple cartilagenous exostosis)
  5. Defective bone matrix (fibrous dysplasia)
  6. Inborn errors of metabolism (mucopolysaccharidosis)
  7. Calcium and phosphorus metabolism defects (hyperphosphatemic rickets)
  8. Mineral metabolism defects (Wilson's disease, zinc deficiency).

Short Stature—Causes

1.	Hereditary	Constitutionally small
2.	Genetic	Down's syndrome, Turner's syndrome, Achondroplasia
3.	Nutritional	Intrauterine growth retardation, protein and energy deprivation, Rickets
4.	Endocrine	Cretinism, Hypopituitarism, Craniopharyngioma
5.	Alimentary	Malabsorption syndromes, Crohn's disease, Cystic fibrosis
6.	Cardio-respiratory	Congenital heart disease, suppurative lung disease
7.	Locomotor	Severe scoliosis
8.	Miscellaneous	Chronic wasting diseases including renal failure and biliary diseases

State of Nutrition

The state of nutrition depends mainly on the distribution of adipose tissue in the body. On this basis individuals can be classified as normal, overweight (fat or obese) and underweight.

The state of nutrition can be assessed in the following ways:
1. Ideal body weight (IBW) = $22.5 \times$ (height in metres)^2
   In women, the ideal body weight is calculated as follows $0.94 \times 22.5 \times$ (height in metres)^2
   If the body weight > 10% of IBW, the individual is overweight
   If the body weight > 20% of IBW, the individual is obese.
2. Body mass index (BMI) is calculated as follows:
   BMI = weight in kg/(height in metres)^2
   The normal range of BMI is 19–25
   In males, it is 20–25
   In females, it is 18–23
   If BMI is between 25 and 30, the individual is over weight.
   If BMI > 30, the individual is obese.

   Grading of Obesity
   Grade I   if BMI 25–30 (over weight)
   Grade II   if BMI 30–40 (obese)
   Grade III if BMI > 40 (very obese)
3. The amount of subcutaneous fat can be estimated by measuring the skinfold thickness over the triceps, biceps, subscapular region and suprailiac region, by using a special pair of calipers. Equations and nomograms are available for conversion of skin fold thickness to body fat. (Normal triceps skin fold thickness: Adult males—12.5 mm; Adult females—16.5 mm).
4. Rough calculation of body weight (Broca's index) can be done provided the height of the individual is > 100 cm, and so is possible in adults only.
   Height in cm − 100 = desired body weight (in kg).
   Height in inches = body weight (in kg).

Obesity

A person is said to be obese, if his body weight > 20 % of IBW and his BMI > 30.

Types of Obesity

1. *Generalised obesity:* There is excess fat deposition uniformly throughout the body. Over eating is the most common cause. It is characterised by the presence of a 'double chin'.

2. *Android obesity (Fig. 1.24):* It is a type of obesity, which is characterised by excess deposition of fat over the region of the waist.
3. *Gynoid obesity (Fig. 1.24):* It is a type of obesity, which is characterised by excess deposition of fat over the region of the hips and thighs.
4. *Superior or central type of obesity:* In this type there is excess fat deposition over face, neck and upper part of the trunk and the arms are thin. This is seen in Cushing's syndrome.

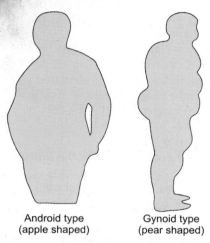

Android type
(apple shaped)

Gynoid type
(pear shaped)

Fig. 1.24: Pattern of obesity

Recent evidence suggests that regional distribution of fat may be of greater prognostic significance than absolute degree of obesity. This is assessed by measuring the hip : waist ratio.

The hip measurement is taken by measuring at a level that gives the maximal measurement of the hip, over the buttocks.

The waist is measured by taking a circumference that gives the narrowest measurement between the ribcage and the iliac crest.

Waist–hip ratio	Type of obesity	Prognosis
1. 0.8 or less	Pear-shaped obesity	Good
2. 0.9 or greater	Apple-shaped obesity	Greater risk of developing complications of obesity

Under Weight

Adults are significantly under weight if their BMI is 18 or less. Causes for weight loss:
(i) Malnutrition
(ii) Grief or depression
(iii) Thyrotoxicosis
(iv) Diabetes mellitus
(v) Addison's disease
(vi) Tuberculosis
(vii) HIV infection
(viii) Chronic bronchitis
(ix) CCF
(x) Malignancy
(xi) Malabsorption syndromes
(xii) Anorexia Nervosa (This is diagnosed when the weight of the patient is < 25 % of his IBW).

Posture

The position or attitude constantly assumed by a patient at rest or in motion is referred to as posture. The posture of a patient, when viewed from the side, may be characteristic enough to suggest a diagnosis.

The various postures seen in clinical practice are:
1. Postures seen when the patient is standing/sitting.
   a. Vertical line seen in standing posture, when viewed from the side, is a good posture.
   b. Standing posture, when it assumes a S-shaped curve, when viewed from the side, is a poor posture.
   c. *Asthenic posture:* The normal curves of the spine are exaggerated. Seen in debility, wasting and in senility.
   d. *Parkinsonian posture:* Universally flexed posture.
   e. *Lordotic posture:* There is an exaggerated lumbar lordosis. Seen in muscular dystrophy, due to proximal muscle weakness. It is also seen in bilateral hip problems.
   f. *Cerebellar posture:* In lesions of the cerebellum or its connections, the patient stands with his feet wide apart, and is unable to maintain a steady posture when standing with both his feet placed close together. Patient is ataxic on sitting (truncal ataxia) when the vermis of the cerebellum is involved.
   g. *Posture in ankylosing spondylitis:* There is loss of the lumbar lordosis, with an exaggeration of the upper thoracic kyphosis.
   h. *Catatonic posture:* In this the patient maintains a particular posture of the body and limb for hours together. This is seen in schizophrenia.
2. Postures seen when the patient is lying down:
   a. *Decerebrate posture:* Extension of elbows and wrists, with pronation of the arms is seen. It suggests that the lesion is at the brainstem level, disconnecting the cerebral hemispheres from the brainstem.
   b. *Decorticate posture:* Flexion of elbows and wrists, with supination of the arms is seen. It suggests severe bilateral hemispherical damage above the midbrain.

c. *Hemiplegic posture:* The patient lies on his back, with the cheek on the affected side blowing out with each expiration. The affected upper limb lies flaccidly by his side, and the affected lower limb is externally rotated. This picture is seen immediately after the onset of hemiplegia. In long standing hemiplegia, there may be loss of naso-labial fold of the face on the side of the paresis, with the affected upper limb in a flexed posture and the affected lower limb in an extended posture.

d. *Opisthotonus:* In this posture the patient is arched up like a bow, with his heel and occiput in contact with the bed. This posture is seen in patients with tetanus and strychnine poisoning.

e. Lateral decubitus posture with curled up limbs to minimise the stretching of the meninges, is seen with meningitis or meningism.

f. Patient lying up with a back rest or cardiac rest suggests a possibility of the patient having CCF or COPD.

g. Patient sitting up and holding on to a support before him, in order to fix his shoulders, and having dyspnoea, suggests a diagnosis of bronchial asthma.

h. Patient lying down still and
   (i) Clutching his chest—anginal chest pain
   (ii) Shallow breathing, with minimal or no movement of the anterior abdominal wall—peritonitis.

i. Patient rolling about in the bed from side to side and
   (i) Clutching his chest—Myocardial infarction.
   (ii) Holding his upper abdomen—Biliary colic.

j. Patient sitting up and bending forwards, may be seen in
   (i) Pericarditis
   (ii) Pancreatitis
   as the pain caused by both these conditions is relieved by assuming this posture.

k. *Prone posture:* Patient preferring to lie in the prone position than in the supine position may be due to the presence of an abdominal aortic aneurysm which may erode on the vertebra in the supine posture and cause back pain. On lying prone the aorta falls forward from the vertebra and the pain subsides.

Hands and Fingers

Hands

(i) *Cretinism:* Square palm, short, fat and blunt fingers and short radius.

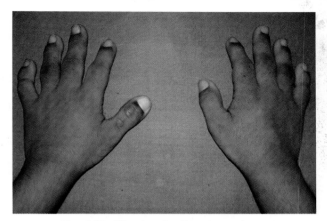

Fig. 1.25: Clinodactyly—Down's syndrome

(ii) *Down's syndrome:* Short and thick hand. Short thumb arising at a level lower than normal from the palm with incurving of the distal phalanx of the little finger (clinodactyly) (Figs 1.25 and 1.26) and a single palmar crease is seen over the palm (Fig. 1.27).

(iii) *Acromegalic hand (Fig. 1.28):* This is known as the 'Paw hand'. It is a massive hand with fat, cylindrical, spatulate fingers with blunt tips and broad and square nails.

(iv) *Eunuchoidal hand:* The hand is long and narrow and thin skinned, with delicate and tapering fingers.

(v) *Marfan's syndrome:* The hand is long with tapering, spidery fingers (arachnodactyly).

(vi) *Pseudohypoparathyroidism:* Short fourth and fifth metacarpals producing a 'dimpling sign' (knuckle-knuckle-dimple-dimple sign).

(vii) *Holt-Oram syndrome:* The thumb is hypoplastic and in the same plane as the rest of the fingers. Thumb may be triphalangeal. Fifth finger may be missing.

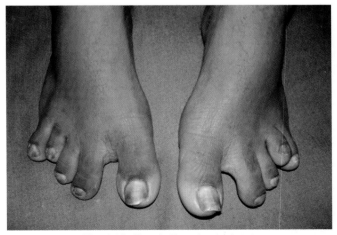

Fig. 1.26: Foot in Down's syndrome

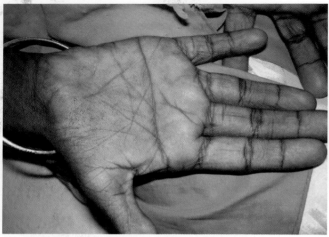

Fig. 1.27: Simian crease

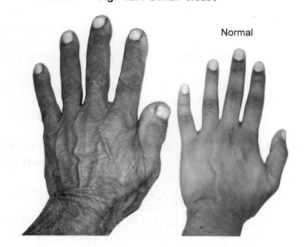

Fig. 1.28: Acromegalic hand

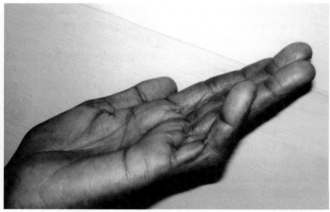

Fig. 1.29: Dupuytren's contracture

Causes
(a) Congenital
(b) Familial
(c) Associated with VSD
(d) Laurence-Moon-Biedl syndrome
(e) Turner's syndrome.

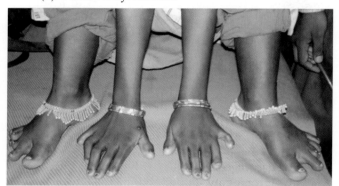

Fig. 1.30: Polydactyly

There may be radio-ulnar synostosis. The radius may be absent.

(viii) *Dupuytren's contracture (Fig. 1.29):* This occurs due to fibrositis commonly involving the ulnar side of palmar aponeurosis. This causes thickening and contraction of the aponeurosis. This initially affects the proximal and middle phalanx of the ring finger and later the little finger may be affected.

It is seen in the following conditions
a. Idiopathic
b. Cirrhosis liver
c. Phenytoin therapy
d. People working with machines producing vibration
e. Intake of oral contraceptive pills.

Fingers

(i) *Polydactyly (Fig. 1.30):* Supernumerary fingers

(ii) *Syndactyly (Fig. 1.31):* Webbed fingers. May occur in normal individuals or in those with, certain

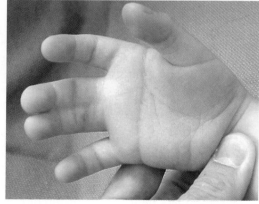

Fig. 1.31: Syndactyly

congenital abnormalities. It is seen in Poland's syndrome (absent unilateral pectoralis major muscle with TOF).

(iii) *Arachnodactyly (Fig. 1.32):* Spider fingers. These are long and thin fingers.

Causes
(a) Marfan's syndrome
(b) Hypogonadism
(c) Hypopituitarism
(d) Homocystinuria
(e) Normal individuals.

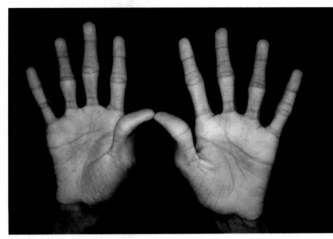

Fig. 1.32: Arachnodactyly

(iv) *Absence of digits (Fig. 1.33):* Absence of one or more fingers may be congenital. Thumb may be absent in Fanconi's congenital aplastic anemia.

(v) *Sausage fingers:* Thick and fleshy fingers seen in
(a) Acromegaly

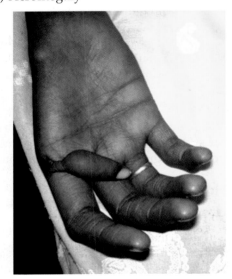

Fig. 1.33: Hypoplastic thumb—Fanconi's anaemia

(b) Myxoedema
(c) Psoriatic arthropathy.

Feet and Toes

Genu Varum (bow legs)

Causes
(a) Rickets
(b) Osteomalacia
(c) Osteitis deformans (Paget's disease)
(d) Achondroplasia.

Genu Valgum (knock knees)

Causes
(a) Congenital
(b) Rickets.

Large Feet

It is seen in acromegaly.

Short and Broad Feet

It is seen in achondroplasia.

"Rocker Bottom" Feet (Fig. 1.34)

This is a severe type of flat foot with a protuberant heel. Seen in Trisomy-18 (Edward's syndrome, which may be associated with PDA).

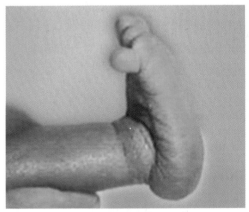

Fig. 1.34: Rocker-Bottom foot

Pes Cavus (Claw Foot) (Fig. 1.35)

Causes
(a) Familial
(b) Peroneal muscular atrophy
(c) Friedreich's ataxia
(d) Syringomyelia
(e) Spina bifida occulta
(f) Anterior poliomyelitis.

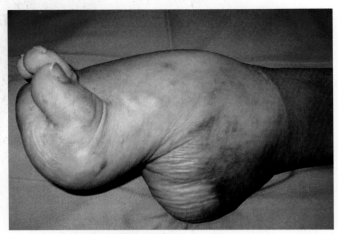

Fig. 1.35: Pes cavus

Clawed Toes

It is seen in
(a) Friedreich's ataxia
(b) Peroneal muscular atrophy.

Heel Pad Thickness

It is the distance measured in a X-ray film of the patient's foot taken laterally from the lower most point of the calcaneum to the lower most point of the heel pad soft tissue shadow.

Heel pad thickness is said to be increased when
   (i) It is more than 23 mm in males
   (ii) It is more than 21 mm in females.

Causes of Increased Heel Pad Thickness

(a) Acromegaly
(b) Myxoedema
(c) Obesity
(d) Peripheral edema
(e) Infection or injury to heel
(f) Eptoin therapy.

The Skin in Clinical Medicine

The skin has three layers (Fig. 1.36). The epidermis forms the outer layer which consists of avascular epithelium. The tough fibroelastic dermis forms the middle layer which contains blood vessels, nerves, sebaceous and sweat glands and hair follicles. The hypodermis containing loose connective tissue and fat forms the inner layer.

90% of the epidermal cells are keratinocytes. They synthesize insoluble proteins, keratins. Keratins form the main component of impervious surface of the epidermis. The pigment melanin is synthesized from

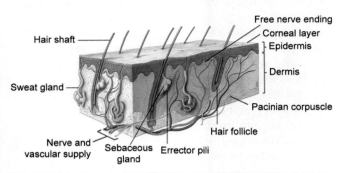

Fig. 1.36: Structure of skin

phenylalanine by melanocytes which are present in the basal layer of the epidermis.

The skin is the largest organ of the human body. It weighs about 4 kg and it covers an area of 2m². The brown or black colour of the skin is due to melanin. The amount of melanin present is decided by hereditary factors and the environmental factors like exposure or withdrawal from ultraviolet light.

Functions of the Skin

1. *Protection:* Physical, Chemical, Infection
2. *Thermoregulation:* Blood vessels and Eccrine sweat glands
3. *Homeostasis* of water, electrolytes and protein
4. *Lubrication and waterproofing:* Sebum secreted by sebaceous glands
5. *Sensations* – specialized nerve endings
6. *Immunological:* Lymphocytes, macrophages, Langerhans cells
7. *Synthesis* of vitamin D by keratinocytes
8. *Body odour:* Apocrine glands
9. *Protection and prising:* Nails
10. *Calorie reserve:* Subcutaneous fat
11. *Psychosocial :* Cosmetic –skin, lips, hair, nails.

Primary Skin Lesions

Universal and symmetrical skin lesions favor the diagnosis of systemic disorder and focal asymmetrical lesions favor the diagnosis of local infection or allergy.

Terminology of Skin Lesions

Macule – Altered colour
Papule (Fig. 1.37) – Elevated skin lesion -<0.5 cm
Plaque – Palpable skin lesion - >2 cm
Nodule – Solid palpable lesion ->0.5 cm
Vesicle (Fig. 1.38) – Fluid filled blister -<0.5 cm

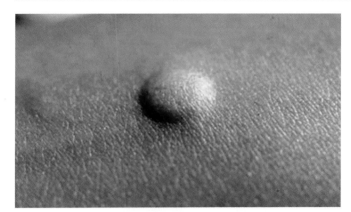

Fig. 1.37: Papule

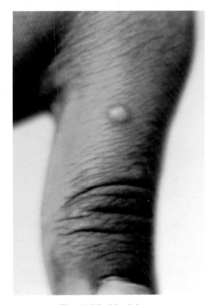

Fig. 1.38: Vesicle

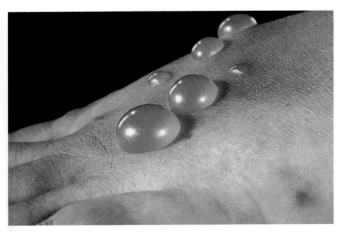

Fig. 1.39: Bullae

Bulla (Fig. 1.39) – Large fluid filled blister –>0.5 cm
Pustule – Blister filled with pus
Papilloma – Pedunculated projecting lesion
Wheal – Elevated central white lesion with red margin
Telangiectasia – Dilated small cutaneous blood vessel
Petechiae (Fig. 1.40) – Pinhead size macule of blood in the skin.

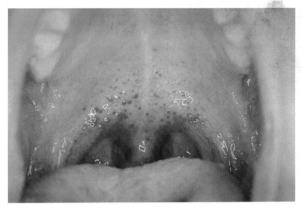

Fig. 1.40: Petechiae

Purpura – Larger petechiae –which do not blanch on pressure
Ecchymosis (Fig. 1.41)– Large extravasation of blood into the skin

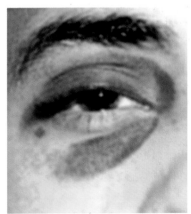

Fig. 1.41: Ecchymosis

Haematoma – Swelling due to bleeding –collection of blood
Erythema – Redness of the skin.

Distribution and Site of Skin Lesions

Centrifugal – Smallpox, Erythema multiforme, Erythema nodosum
Centripetal – Chickenpox, Pityriasis rosea

jaundice, paralytic ileus, gallstones, and shock. There is profound elevation of amylase levels.

Biliary Colic

Acute distention of gallbladder causes pain in the right hypochondrium with radiation to the right, posterior region of thorax or to the tip of right scapula.

Distention of common bile duct (CBD) causes pain in the epigastrium radiating to upper part of lumbar region.

Murphy's sign: In acute cholecystitis, the patient is asked to breathe in deeply and gallbladder is palpated in the usual way. At the height of inspiration, the breath is arrested with a gasp as the mass is felt.

Pain of Peritonitis

It is a steady and aching pain located directly over inflamed area. The pain is accentuated by pressure or changes in tension of the peritoneum and hence the patient lies still. There is associated tonic muscle spasm. The intensity of pain is dependent on the type and amount of foreign substance to which the peritoneal surfaces are exposed.

If the peritonitis is due to perforation of a hollow abdominal viscera, liver dullness is obliterated.

Superior Mesenteric Artery Occlusion

It is a mild, continuous, diffuse pain present for 2 to 3 days before vascular collapse or peritonitis sets in. There is no tenderness or rigidity. Bloody diarrhoea may be present.

In chronic mesenteric artery insufficiency, abdominal pain occurs after intake of food (abdominal angina).

Pain Referred to Abdomen

Possibility of intrathoracic disease must be considered in every patient with abdominal pain. Apparent abdominal muscle spasm caused by referred pain will diminish during inspiration whereas it is persistent throughout respiratory phases, if it is of abdominal origin.

Pain of diaphragmatic pleuritis is felt at right upper quadrant of abdomen.

Referred pain from spine is characteristically intensified by certain motions like coughing, sneezing or straining and is associated with hyperaesthesia over involved dermatomes.

Pain referred from testicles or seminal vesicles is accentuated by slightest pressure on either of these organs. The abdominal discomfort is of dull aching character and is poorly localized.

Abdominal Wall Pain

It is a constant, aching pain, aggravated by movement, prolonged standing and pressure. When muscles of other parts of the body are also involved, myositis should be considered.

Metabolic Causes of Abdominal Pain

Whenever the cause of abdominal pain is obscure, one of the following metabolic causes must be considered.
1. Diabetic ketoacidosis
2. Porphyria
3. Uremia
4. Lead colic
5. Hyperlipidemia
6. C1 esterase deficiency.

Neurogenic Abdominal Pain

Causalgic pain is of burning character and is limited to the distribution of peripheral nerve. Normal stimuli like touch can evoke this type of pain. There is no muscle spasm or change with respiration or food intake.

Pain from spinal nerves or roots is of lancinating type. It may be caused by herpes zoster, arthritis, tumors, herniated nucleus pulposus, diabetes, syphilis. Pain is aggravated by movement of spine and is usually confined to a few dermatomes. Hyperaesthesia is common.

Psychogenic Abdominal Pain

There is no relation to meals. Onset is usually at nights. There is no nausea or vomiting. There is no abdominal muscle spasm; even if present does not persist. There is no change with respiration. But restriction of depth of respiration occurs as a part of anxiety state.

Renal Pain

Pain due to obstruction of urinary bladder causes a dull suprapubic pain of low intensity.

Pain due to ureteric obstruction (intravesical portion) is characterized by severe suprapubic and flank pain which radiates to genitalia and upper part of thigh.

Obstruction of ureteropelvic junction causes pain at costovertebral angle, whereas obstruction of the remainder of the ureter is associated with flank pain which radiates from loin to groin.

Peripheral Vascular Pain

Arterial Occlusion

Intermittent Claudication

Patient often complains that after walking a distance (claudication distance), the pain starts and on continued walking the pain is aggravated and compels the patient to take rest. Pain disappears when the exercise stops.

Rest Pain

This pain is continuous and aching in nature. This is due to ischemic changes in the somatic nerves (cry of the dying nerves).

Venous Pain

Venous pain may be due to:

Varicose Veins

Pain felt in lower leg or whole of the leg according to the site of varicosities. Pain gets worse when the patient stands up for a long time and is relieved when he lies down. Pain of varicocele of testes is of similar character.

Venous Thrombosis

Patient may have pain and swelling of leg (around ankle).

Homan's sign: Dorsiflexion of foot elicits pain in the calf.

Moses's sign: Squeezing of calf muscle from side to side elicits pain.

In superficial thrombophlebitis, there is pain and tenderness over superficial inflamed veins.

The above manoeuvres may dislodge the thrombus resulting in pulmonary embolism.

Neurogenic Claudication

Symptoms of dysfunction of cauda equina appear on walking or prolonged standing and are relieved by rest. This is due to lumbar canal stenosis which is made worse in middle age due to degenerative changes especially between L_4 and L_5 vertebrae.

There is march of pain with paresthesia and absent ankle jerk after exercise. Symptoms take 5–10 minutes to fade.

Edema

Edema is a collection of excess fluid in the body interstitium, from the intravascular compartment.

Ascites	Pathological collection of fluid in the peritoneal cavity
Hydrothorax	Pathological collection of fluid in the pleural cavity

Normal Body Fluid Compartments

Compartment	Volume (in litres)	Percentage lean body weight
1. Total body water	42	60
2. Extracellular water	14	20
- Plasma	3–4	4–5
- Interstitial	11	16
3. Intracellular water	28	40

Anasarca	Generalised edema
Pericardial effusion	Pathological collection of fluid in the pericardial cavity.

Etiology and Types of Edema

Generalised Edema

1. Cardiac edema
2. Renal edema
3. Hepatic edema
4. Nutritional edema
5. Cyclic-premenstrual
6. Idiopathic.

Localised Edema

1. Venous edema
2. Lymphatic edema
3. Inflammatory edema
4. Allergic.

Fast Edema

This indicates edema occurring in conditions causing hypoalbuminemia. The edema pits on pressure application but disappears within 40 seconds of its application.

Slow Edema (Fig. 1.59)

This indicates edema occurring in conditions causing congestion (CCF). The edema pits on pressure application but lasts for more than 1 minute.

Pathophysiology of Edema (Fig. 1.60)

Normal hydrostatic pressure at the arteriolar end of the capillary bed = 35 mm Hg.

Normal hydrostatic pressure at the venular end of the capillary bed = 12-15 mm Hg.

Oncotic pressure of plasma = 20-25 mm Hg.

Normally, fluid volume in different compartments of the body is maintained by the normal Starling's forces, mentioned above.

1. Hydrostatic pressure at the arteriolar end of the capillary tends to push the intravascular fluid into the interstitium.

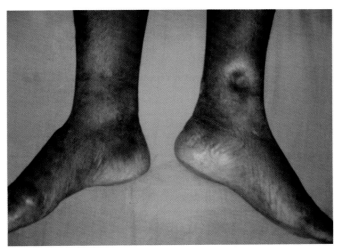

Fig. 1.59: Pitting pedal edema

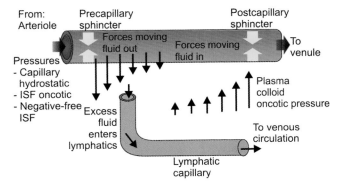

Fig. 1.60: Pathophysiology of edema

2. The oncotic pressure at the venous end of the capillary, maintained chiefly by body albumin, tends to remove fluid from the interstitium into the vascular compartment.

The normal lymphatic flow carries the albumin, extruded from the intravascular compartment into the interstitium, back into the intravascular compartment, to maintain the normal oncotic pressure.

Edema may result when there is:
1. Increase in hydrostatic pressure
2. Decrease in oncotic pressure
3. Obstruction to veins/lymphatic flow
4. Vascular wall injury (mechanical, thermal, chemical).

Characteristic Features of Edema of Various Etiologies

Cardiac Edema

The pathophysiology of this edema is:

(a) Increased back pressure on the venous side of circulation leading to transudation of fluid into the interstitium.
(b) Decreased intravascular volume leading to decreased renal blood flow and thereby stimulation of the renin-angiotensin mechanism.
(c) Decreased intravascular volume leads to hyperosmolality of the blood, which in turn stimulates the osmoreceptors in the posterior pituitary to secrete antidiuretic hormone. This hormone stimulates the thirst mechanism and the patient consumes more water, which contributes to the edema formation.
(d) In left sided cardiac failure there is accumulation of fluid in the lung interstitium leading to development of pulmonary edema.

Cardiac edema is a dependent edema found over the ankles in ambulant patients, and over the sacrum in bed ridden patients.

Renal Edema

The pathophysiology of this edema is:
(a) Primary increase in sodium and water retention by the kidneys (as in AGN)
(b) Decrease in oncotic pressure due to increased loss of albumin in urine (as in nephrotic syndrome)
(c) However, in CRF, edema need not be present initially. In the last stage of CRF, edema develops due to retention of sodium and water.

Renal edema characteristically involves the loose connective tissues, especially over the periorbital region, more prominent when the patient wakes up in the early morning, as the patient with renal edema are able to lie down flat (comfortably).

Edema Seen in Liver Disease

The pathophysiology of this edema is that the collection of fluid occurs characteristically first in the peritoneal cavity (Ascites), because of the following:
(a) Increased portal venous pressure (Portal HTN).
(b) Obliteration of the lymphatic drainage of the liver.
(c) Hypoalbuminemia (Due to impaired synthesis of albumin by the decompensated liver).
(d) Decrease in the intravascular volume leading to activation of renin-angiotensin-aldosterone mechanism and retention of salt and water. Decreased metabolism of aldosterone by the decompensated liver leads to secondary hyperaldosteronism and increased retention of salt and water.
(e) Tense ascites leads to increased intra-abdominal pressure thereby decreasing venous return from the lower limbs and hence development of pedal edema.

Edema of Nutritional Origin

It is a generalised edema. Causes of nutritional edema are:
  (i) Decreased ingestion of proteins leading to hypo-albuminemia and therefore edema.
  (ii) Thiamine deficiency leading to beriberi. Edema in beriberi occurs because of the following:
      a. Due to lack of thiamine, glucose is incompletely metabolised and lactic and pyruvic acids accumulate, which causes peripheral vasodilatation and transudation of fluid through the capillaries.
      b. The resulting anemia also contributes to the development of edema.
      c. Development of high output cardiac failure results in edema.
  (iii) Edema can occur on refeeding after prolonged starvation due to:
      a. Increased salt intake.
      b. Increased release of insulin which acts directly on the renal tubules to increase sodium reabsorption.

Idiopathic Edema

Periodic episodes of edema occurring exclusively in women. Diurnal variation of weight occurs with orthostatic retention of salt and water. This suggests an increase in capillary permeability on erect posture.

Cyclical or Premenstrual Edema

This edema is due to sodium and water retention, secondary to excessive estrogen stimulation.

Other Causes of Edema

a. Myxoedema (edema typically located in pretibial region along with periorbital puffiness)
b. Pregnancy.

Less Common Causes of Facial Edema

a. Myxoedema
b. Allergic reaction
c. Trichinosis.

Localised Edema

  (i) *Venous edema*
      a. Deep vein thrombosis
      b. Thrombophlebitis
      c. Varicose veins
      d. SVC/IVC obstruction.
  (ii) *Lymphatic edema*
      a. Chronic lymphangitis

      b. Resection of regional lymph nodes
      c. Filariasis
      d. Radiotherapy
      e. Congenital (Milroy's disease—congenital absence of lymphatic tissue).
  (iii) *Inflammatory/allergic causes*
      a. Cellulitis
      b. Bee/wasp sting.

Drugs Causing Edema

1. Nonsteroidal anti-inflammatory drugs
2. Arteriolar vasodilators
   • Minoxidil
   • Hydralazine
   • Clonidine
   • Alpha-methyl dopa
   • Guanethedine
3. Calcium channel blockers
4. Alpha-blockers
5. Cyclosporin
6. Growth hormone
7. Steroidal hormones
   • Glucocorticoids
   • Anabolic steroids
   • Estrogens
   • Progestins
8. Immunotherapy
   • Interleukin-2
   • Monoclonal antibody
   • OKT-3

Shock

Shock may be defined as a state in which there is profound and widespread reduction in the effective delivery of oxygen and other nutrients to tissues leading to reversible, and if prolonged, to irreversible cellular injury.

Acute circulatory failure, shock, low cardiac output states are various terms used to describe a clinical syndrome of hypotension, peripheral vasoconstriction, oliguria and often impaired consciousness.

Control of Arterial Blood Pressure

Organ perfusion is dependent on an appropriate perfusion pressure which is determined by cardiac output and systemic vascular resistance. Cardiac output in turn is a product of stroke volume and heart rate. Stroke volume depends upon preload, afterload and myocardial contractility.

Control Mechanism

1. Release of vasodilator metabolites (adenosine)
2. Release from endothelium of substances which relax (EDRF or nitric oxide) vascular smooth muscle
3. Release from endothelium of substances which contract (endothelin) vascular smooth muscle
4. Autonomic nervous system (baroreceptor reflexes and vasomotor center in the brainstem)
5. Release of vasopressin
6. Renin angiotensin aldosterone system
7. Release of vasodilators (prostaglandins and kinins)
8. Fluid and electrolyte balance.

Classification

Cardiogenic Shock

Myopathic

a. Acute MI
b. Dilated cardiomyopathy
c. Myocardial depression in septic shock
d. Myocarditis.

Mechanical

MR, VSD following MI
Ventricular aneurysm
LV outflow obstruction (AS, HOCM).

Electrical

Arrhythmias
- Tachyarrhythmias (SVT, VT, VF)
- Bradyarrhythmias (complete heart block—Stokes-Adams attacks)
- Tachybradyarrhythmias (Sick sinus syndrome).

Extracardiac Obstructive Shock

Pericardial tamponade
Constrictive pericarditis
Acute massive pulmonary embolism
Severe pulmonary hypertension
Coarctation of the aorta.

Oligemic Shock

Fluid depletion (vomiting, diarrhoea, burns, sweating, fistulae, pancreatitis)
Haemorrhage
a. Internal: GIT perforation, splenic rupture, ectopic pregnancy
b. External: Trauma, fracture femur, etc.

Distributive Shock

Septic shock
Toxins
Anaphylaxis
Neurogenic shock
Endocrinologic shock.

Hypovolemic Shock

Because of decreased blood volume, there is inadequate ventricular filling, decreased preload and stroke volume.

Cardiogenic Shock

Systolic arterial pressure is < 80 mm Hg and cardiac index is < 1.8 L/min/m^2. LV filling pressure is elevated.

Common Causes

MI (> 40% of LV involvement), myocarditis, following cardiac arrest or prolonged cardiac surgery.

Cardiac Causes of Acute Circulatory Failure

Endocardial	Mitral valve disease
	Aortic valve disease
Myocardial	RV infarct
	LV infarct
	Cardiomyopathy
	Myocarditis
	Atrial arrhythmias
Pericardial	Tamponade
	Constrictive pericarditis
Great vessels	Aortic dissection
	Pulmonary embolism.

Extracardiac Obstructive Shock

There is inability of the ventricles to fill during diastole, markedly limiting stroke volume and ultimately the cardiac output.

Distributive Shock

There is profound decrease in peripheral vascular resistance by the release of histamine, kinins, prostaglandins, lipid A, endorphins, TNF, IL-1 and IL-2. Some prostaglandins and leukotrienes produce vasoconstriction.

Patient may suffer from more than one form of shock simultaneously.

Clinical Features

Patients have hypotension (mean arterial BP <60 mm Hg, systolic BP < 100 mm Hg), tachycardia (> 120/min),

Classification of Shock

Type of shock	Filling pressures	Cardiac output	Sys. vascular resistance	PCWP	Etiologies
Cardiogenic	↑	↓	↑	↑↑ ↑ or N ↓ or N	MI, cardiomyopathy, valvular heart disease, arrhythmias, acute VSD, MR RV infarct
Distributive (septic)	↓	↑	↓	↓	Sepsis, anaphylaxis, toxic shock syndrome
Hypovolemic	↓	↑↓	↑	↓	Hemorrhage, hypovolemia
Obstructive	↑ (Proximal) ↓ (Distal)	↓	↑	↑	Pulmonary embolism tamponade, tension pneumothorax

oliguria (< 30 ml/hr), altered sensorium, cold clammy extremities (not a characteristic of distributive shock).

Patients also have manifestations specific to the type of shock.

Investigations

- Complete blood count
- Serum electrolytes
- Serum creatinine
- Coagulation studies
- Blood grouping and typing
- ABG
- Examination of the stool and nasogastric contents for blood
- Culture of appropriate body fluids
- Chest X-ray
- ECG
- Right heart catheterization (gives clue as to the type of shock)
- Ventilation-perfusion lung scan
- Echocardiogram
- Endocrine studies.

Management

Shock is an emergency necessitating IMCU management.

Goals

1. To keep mean arterial pressure > 60 mm Hg or systolic BP > 100 mm Hg.
2. To maintain blood flow to organs which are vulnerable (kidneys, liver, brain and lungs).
3. To maintain arterial blood lactate < 22 mmol/L.

Treatment

1. Maintenance of airway and ventilation is essential.
2. Volume resuscitation should be done in all cases except in cardiogenic shock.

a. The pneumatic antishock garment (PASG) with sequential inflation of legs and abdominal compartments to 15–40 mm Hg may be useful in all types of shock except cardiogenic shock. It helps by increasing peripheral vascular resistance.
b. Trendelenburg's position to aid venous return and cardiac index.
c. Fluid resuscitation by giving 500 ml bolus of normal saline with further infusions depending on BP and other parameters. Fresh frozen plasma or packed cells may be needed.

3. Vasopressors
   (i) Dopamine is the pressor of first choice except in cyclic antidepressant and phenothiazine overdoses (5 µg/kg/min if renal perfusion is impaired or 10 µg/kg/min when renal perfusion is adequate).
   (ii) Norepinephrine given in a dose of 2-8 µg/minute causes peripheral vasoconstriction and lesser chronotropic and inotropic response.
   (iii) Dobutamine can be given in a dose of 1–10 µg/kg/minute to increase cardiac output in a low cardiac output state.
   (iv) Amrinone can be given by adding 500 mg to 150 ml of normal saline for a final volume of 250 ml. A loading dose of 0.75 mg/kg is given over 2–3 minutes, with infusion following at 5–10 µg/kg/minute.
   (v) Isoproterenol in a dose of 1–4 µg/minute can be tried only in atropine unresponsive bradycardia requiring pacemaker.

4. Sodium bicarbonate should be given when pH falls less than 7.2. Inappropriate bicarbonate use may cause CNS acidosis and diminish peripheral tissue oxygenation.

5. Antibiotics should be given empirically when sepsis is suspected, and glucocorticoids when adrenal insufficiency is suspected (after drawing blood for basal cortisol).

Cardiogenic Shock

1. Oxygen
2. Nitrates
3. Intra-aortic balloon counter pulsation for salvaging reversibly damaged myocardium
4. Thrombolytic therapy or CABG or PTCA to restore myocardial perfusion
5. Vasopressors like dopamine or dobutamine or both.

Cardiac Tamponade

1. Inotropic agents (norepinephrine, dopamine)
2. Pericardiocentesis.

Septic Shock

a. Infection must be treated (antimicrobials, surgical drainage of pus or both)
b. CVS monitoring and support
c. Interruption of pathogenic sequence by
   (i) Inhibition of endorphin receptors with naloxone
   (ii) Inhibition of arachidonic acid metabolites
   (iii) Human monoclonal antibody against lipid A, inhibitors of sepsis mediators like IL-1 and TNF-α.

Anaphylactic Shock

1. Maintenance of airway.
2. Epinephrine is the cornerstone of therapy. It is given in a dose of 0.3–0.5 mg (0.3–0.5 ml of 1:1,000 solution) SC and repeated twice at 20 minute intervals if necessary.
   It can be given intravenously (3–5 ml of 1:10,000 solution) or sublingually (0. 5 ml of 1 : 1,000 solution) or via endotracheal tube (3–5 ml of 1 : 10,000 solution).
3. Volume expansion by crystalloid or colloid.
4. Inhaled beta-agonists to treat bronchospasm.
5. Aminophylline is used as a second line drug.
6. General measures to delay the absorption of the offending antigen. For orally ingested antigens, activated charcoal (50–100 g) with 1–2 g/kg (maximum 150 g) of sorbitol or 300 ml of magnesium citrate can be given. Emesis is not indicated.
   For injected antigens, slight constriction and local epinephrine injection at the affected site may be useful.
7. Antihistamines may shorten the duration of the reaction. For recurrent symptoms, H$_2$ blockers may be useful.
8. Glucocorticoids (Hydrocortisone 100 mg IV every 6 hours) have no effect for 6–12 hours, but they may prevent recurrence or relapse of severe reactions.
9. Glucagon in a dose of 1 mg bolus followed by a drip of 1 mg/hour provides direct inotropic support for patients taking beta blockers.
10. Patients should be readmitted when there is relapse.
11. Patients requiring radiocontrast administration despite a previous reaction should receive prednisone, 50 mg PO q6h for 3–4 doses and diphenhydramine, 50 mg PO 1 hour before the procedure. Cardiac resuscitative measures should be available.

Fundamentals in Genetics

Introduction

Chromosomes are the carriers of inherent factors. They are situated in the nucleus of the cell. They are made up of double stranded Deoxyribonucleic acid (DNA).

DNA are found only in the chromosomes and are double stranded helical structures, bound together by hydrogen bonds. It is made up of nucleic acid, a complex substance composed of long chains of molecules called nucleotides. Each nucleotide is composed of:

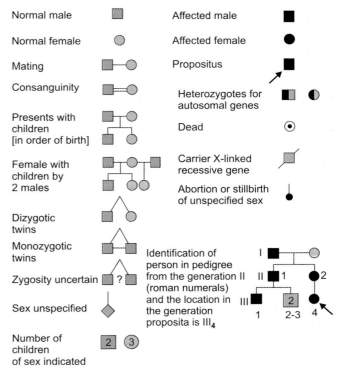

Fig. 1.61: Symbols used in pedigree chart

a. Nitrogenous bases
   Purines   Adenine (A) & Guanine (G)
   Pyrimidines   Cytosine (C) & Thymine (T)
b. Sugar moiety   Deoxyribose
c. Phosphate molecule.

Genes are made up of DNA. The function of the genes is to provide exact information for synthesis of specific amino acid sequence of the protein they control. The genetic code for this information is founded on triplet codons (the sequential nitrogenous bases for specific amino acids).

Ribonucleic acid or RNA are mainly found in the nucleolus and cytoplasm. They contain uracil instead of thymine as pyrimidine base, pairing with adenine. The sugar moiety is ribose and they are single stranded. They form a conduit in the formation of the polypeptide chain, as coded by the gene for the specific protein.

Normal Chromosome Number and Structure

There are 22 pairs of autosomes and 1 pair of sex chromosomes (XX in females and XY in males).

The arrangement of chromosomes in pairs in decreasing order of size, and numbered from 1 to 22 is known as *Karyotyping of chromosomes*. It represents the chromosomal constitution of a person.

The chromosomes are divided into 7 groups, from A to G depending upon their size and position of the centromere (nipped-in narrow portion, where the chromatids meet) of the chromosome.

Metacentric chromosome: The centromere is in the centre.

Acrocentric chromosome: The centromere is close to one end.

Submetacentric chromosome: The centromere is in intermediate position.

Each chromosome has a short arm called 'p' (petit) and a long arm called 'q'. These arms are divided into regions, bands and sub-bands, numerically, e.g. 7q 21.2 means long arm of chromosome 7, region 2, band 1 and sub-band 2.

The normal male has 46 XY chromosomal constitution.

The normal female has 46 XX chromosomal constitution.

Turner's syndrome: When a sex chromosome has been lost it may result in chromosomal constitution of 45 XO.

Klinefelter's syndrome: When a sex chromosome has been added it may result in chromosomal constitution of 47 XXY.

When a chromosome is added or deleted, a (+) or (−) sign is incorporated.

Example: Down's syndrome, in which an extra chromosome is added on chromosome 21, is indicated as 47, XY, +21.

If part of short arm is missing on chromosome 5, it is indicated as 46, XY, 5p− (Cri-du-chat syndrome).

Chromosomal Abnormalities

These can be divided into those which involve
a. Autosomes
b. Sex chromosomes,
   which may in turn be due to either numerical (addition or loss of one or more chromosomes) or due to structural abnormalities.

Numerical Chromosome Aberrations

Autosomal Aneuploidy

Aneuploidy means numerical gain or loss of one or few chromosomes.
a. *Monosomy:* It means loss of an autosome, and is incompatible with life as even one chromosome may carry many important genes.
b. *Trisomy:* It means addition of an autosome.
   Examples
   Trisomy 21 (Down's syndrome) 47, XY, +21
   Trisomy 18 (Edward's syndrome) 47, XY, + 18
   Trisomy 13 (Patau's syndrome) 47, XY, +13
c. *Polyploidy:* It means that the chromosome number is a multiple of 23, but exceeds the number 46. These are incompatible with life.
   Examples: Triploidy (69 chromosomes)
   Tetraploidy (92 chromosomes).

Sex Chromosome Aneuploidy

These are more common than autosomal aneuploidy, with the exception of trisomy 21. This occurs as a result of non-dysjunction (failure of homologous chromosomes to separate) during one of the meiotic divisions in oogenesis or spermatogenesis.

If the number of X chromosomes added is more, there are higher chances of the presence of mental retardation.

If the number of Y chromosomes added is more, the male is tall, aggressive in behaviour and often delinquent.

Structural Aberration of Chromosome

These arise from chromosomal breakage. The abnormalities that occur may be
a. *Deletion:* A segment of chromosome is lost after breakage, e.g. Cri-du-chat syndrome (deletion of short arm of chromosome 5) 46, XY, 5p−

b. *Translocation:* There is aberrant rejoining of the broken segments, occurring on two chromosomes. There is, therefore an exchange of segments between two non-homologous chromosomes, e.g. Down's syndrome occurring due to translocation between chromosomes 14 and 21. Philadelphia chromosome, an acquired translocation occurring between chromosomes 9 and 22, is seen in patients with CML.

Single Gene Disorders

These occur due to mutation (change in a gene) in either one or in a pair of homologous alleles at a single locus of the chromosome.

Allele   Gene at a given locus
Homologous chromosome   Paired chromosomes

If the locus is on one of the 22 autosomes, it called autosomal (dominant or recessive) and if on X or Y chromosome, then it is called sex-linked (dominant or recessive).

Autosomal Dominant Inheritance

Disorders inherited in this manner, manifest in a *heterozygous state* (i.e. people who have one normal and one mutant allele at the locus involved).
- It is characterised by vertical transmission to subsequent generations.
- Nearly always one parent is affected.
- If the affected individual does not have an affected parent, it may be due to:
  a. Illegitimacy
  b. New mutation occurring in the germ cell of the unaffected parent
  c. Mild affection, and so disorder not detected in parent.

Autosomal dominant traits may show variable expression (variation in severity of the same genetic disorder). Sometimes a gene may not express itself (non-penetrance) and this explains apparent skipped generations. Penetrance of a gene results in complete expression of the characteristics of the gene.
- There is 50% chance that the child of an affected parent will be affected.
  Examples:
  1. Achondroplasia
  2. Facioscapulohumeral muscular dystrophy
  3. Gilbert's syndrome
  4. Hereditary spherocytosis
  5. Huntington's chorea
  6. Hyperlipoproteinaemia type II
  7. Marfan's syndrome
  8. Myotonic dystrophy

9. Neurofibromatosis
10. Polycystic disease of the kidney
11. von Willebrand's disease
12. Porphyria.

Autosomal Recessive Inheritance

These disorders manifest in the *homozygous state* (i.e. people who have two mutant alleles, one on each of the homologous chromosomes, one from each parent).
- Heterozygous carriers of the single mutant allele are clinically normal.
- Mating between two heterozygotes have a 25% chance of producing affected homozygote, 50% chance of heterozygote (clinically normal) and 25% chance of normal homozygote.
- It is characterised by horizontal transmission with affected persons all in the same generation.
- If an affected individual mates with the heterozygote, then there is a 50% chance of producing an affected child and 50% chance of producing a heterozygous (clinically normal) child.
  Examples:
  1. Albinism
  2. Ataxia telangiectasia
  3. Cystic fibrosis
  4. Friedreich's ataxia
  5. Glycogen storage disorder
  6. Limb girdle muscular dystrophy
  7. Wilson's disease.

X-Linked Recessive Inheritance

In these disorders, the mutant gene is carried on the X-chromosome. These disorders manifest only in the male and not in the female children (as the mutant gene on one X-chromosome is counteracted by the normal gene on the other X-chromosome. The absence of another normal X-chromosome in a male makes the disorder manifest in them).
- A mother who is a carrier will have her daughters to be carriers and all her sons affected.
- Very rarely, a woman can exhibit a X-linked recessive disorder when
  a. She may have Turner's syndrome (45, XO)
  b. Testicular feminization syndrome (XY sex chromosome constitution)
  c. She may have had a mother as a carrier and an affected father
  d. Normal father in whom mutation occurred in the X-chromosome and a carrier mother
  e. Affected father and normal mother in whom mutation occurred in one transmitted X-chromosome.

T-cells bind and kill only infected cells that bear self class I antigens (MHC restriction).

Class II Antigens

MHC-II antigens are coded in the HLA-D region. These are characteristically confined to antigen presenting cells. They typically bind and present exogenous antigens to CD_4 T-cells (helper T-cells) and they also exhibit MHC restriction.

Class III Proteins

Some components of the complement system (C_2, C_4, Bf) and some cytokines (TNF-α and β) are encoded within the MHC cluster. These are not histocompatibility antigens.

Transplant Rejection

Hyperacute Rejection

When the recipient has been previously sensitized to antigens (following blood transfusion, previous pregnancy) in graft by developing antidonor IgM, IgG antibodies and complement, hyperacute rejection sets in immediately within one to two days, i.e. immediately after revascularisation.

Acute Rejection

It occurs within a few days after transplantation, after stopping immunosuppressive drugs.

Chronic Rejection

It occurs over months to years and is caused by several types of immune reaction.

Diseases Associated with HLA

HLA antigen	Diseases
HLA B27	Ankylosing Spondylitis
	Reiter's disease
DR2	Multiple sclerosis
A3	Hemochromatosis
B13	Psoriasis
B8, DR3, DR4	IDDM
B8, DR3	Addison's disease
	Thyrotoxicosis
	Myasthenia gravis
	Coeliac disease

Autoimmune Diseases

If an individual mounts a significant immune response against his/her own body constituents as a result of a defect in immunological tolerance, secondary to some exogenous factors, e.g. virus, autoimmune disorders occur.

Organ Specific Disorders

Hashimoto's thyroiditis
Primary myxoedema
Thyrotoxicosis
Pernicious anemia
Autoimmune atrophic gastritis
Autoimmune Addison's disease
Type I diabetes
Goodpasture's syndrome
Myasthenia gravis
Sympathetic ophthalmia
Autoimmune hemolytic anemia
Primary biliary cirrhosis
Chronic active hepatitis
Sjögren's syndrome.

Non-organ Specific Disorders

Rheumatoid arthritis
Dermatomyositis
Progressive systemic sclerosis
SLE.

Immunology and Malignancy

Tumor Antigens

These are present in malignant cells and induce immune response when the tumour is transplanted into syngenic animals. Such tumour specific antigens which induce rejection of tumour transplants in immunised hosts are termed 'tumour specific transplantation antigens' (TSTA).

Second type of antigens are fetal antigens. These are found in embryonic cells and malignant cells and not in normal adult cells, e.g. Alfafetoprotein in hepatoma, carcinoembryonic antigen in colonic cancers especially with metastasis. Occasionally found in alcoholic cirrhosis also.

Inefficiency of immunological surveillance mechanism, as a result of ageing, congenital or iatrogenic immunodeficiency may lead to increased incidence of cancer.

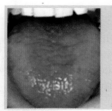

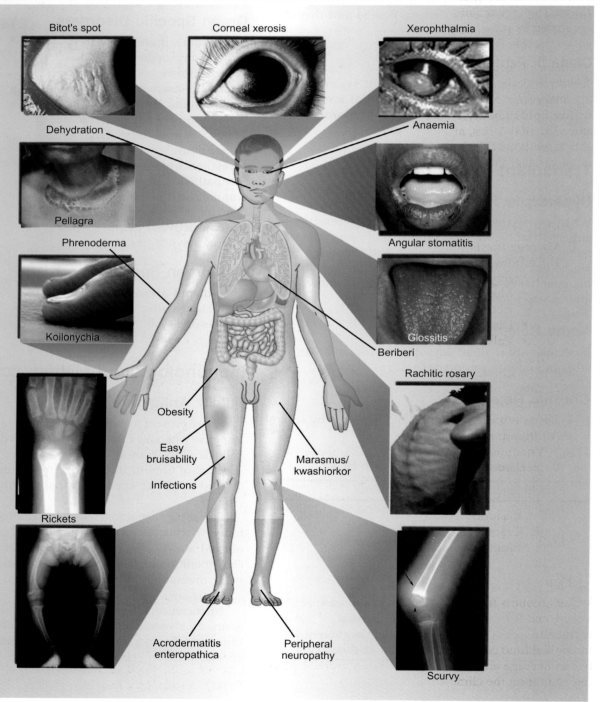

Bitot's spot

Corneal xerosis

Xerophthalmia

Dehydration

Anaemia

Pellagra

Angular stomatitis

Phrenoderma

Koilonychia

Glossitis

Beriberi

Rachitic rosary

Obesity

Easy bruisability

Infections

Marasmus/kwashiorkor

Rickets

Acrodermatitis enteropathica

Peripheral neuropathy

Scurvy

Balanced nutrition is essential to maintain health and to prevent diseases. We eat intermittently but the energy needs are continuous. Neurophysiologic mechanisms control appetite and eating behaviour. Energy needs of the body during feeding are met by the nutrients absorbed from gastrointestinal tract and at other times, body's needs are met by the release of energy from stores. The excess amino acids, fatty acids and glucose are stored as proteins, triglycerides and glycogen. The above process is under the control of insulin.

Nutrition plays a major role in causing certain systemic disorders:
Coronary heart disease, diabetes mellitus, hypertension (excess lipids, obesity, sodium intake) renal stones, gall-stones, dental caries, and carcinomas of stomach, liver and large bowel. Either excess or poor nutrition can cause disease and diseases can cause malnutrition.

Classification of Nutrients

I. *Water*
II. *Macro-nutrients*
   1. Carbohydrates.
      A. *Energy yielding*
         • Monosaccharides (glucose, fructose, ribose)
         • Disaccharides (lactose, maltose, sucrose)
         • Polysaccharides (starch)
      B. *Non-energy yielding*
         • Dietary fibres
   2. Fats
   3. Proteins
III. *Micro-nutrients*
   A. *Organic micro-nutrients*
      Vitamins (not synthesized in the body)
   B. *Inorganic micro-nutrients*
      i. Electrolytes (sodium, potassium, chloride)
      ii. Minerals (calcium, phosphorus, iron, magnesium)
      iii. Trace elements (Zinc, copper, iodine, selenium, chromium and manganese).

Water

Water accounts for 60 to 65% of the body weight (75% at birth and 50% in old age). Water is distributed between intracellular (40%) and extracellular (Plasma and interstitial fluid 20%) compartments. Daily water intake for an average adult will vary between 1 and 3 liters depending on the climate.

Energy Yielding Macro-nutrients
Carbohydrates

An average adult consumes 55 to 65% of calories as carbohydrates and they form the major source of energy. 200 gm of carbohydrate is required/day. 1gm of carbohydrate yields 4 kilocalories (1 kcal = 4.184 kilo joules). Ketosis is likely to occur when the intake is less than 100 gm/day.

Source of Carbohydrates
1. Available as sugars—Mono and disaccharides
   Intrinsic sugars—fruits and milk (good for health)
   Extrinsic sugars—cane sugar and beet-root sugar (dental caries)
2. Available as polysaccharides—Starch, glycogen
   Starch is available in cereals (wheat, rice, maize, etc.), roots (Potatoes and Cassava), plantains and legumes.

Glycaemic Index

Two hour plasma curve after 50 gm of carbohydrate in a given food divided by a curve of 50 gm glucose in water. Glycaemic index is high for glucose, bread, and potatoes and low for legumes and whole grain cereals. Carbohydrates with low glycaemic index are preferable for diabetic patients.

Non-energy Yielding Carbohydrates
Dietary Fibre

It is the natural packing of plant foods and not digested by human enzymes. They are of two types:

A. *Water Soluble Fibres*

Oat bran, beans, pectin and guar gum. They act in upper GIT and induce early satiety, flatten glucose tolerance curve and decrease serum cholesterol.

B. *Water Insoluble Fibres*

Wheat bran—hemicellulose of wheat because of increased water holding capacity increases the bulk of stool and prevents constipation, diverticulosis and cancer colon. Flatus formation is common with fibre diet.

Daily requirement is 15 to 20 gm/day.

Fats

An average adult consumes 30 to 40% of calories as fats. 1 gm of fat yields 9 kcal of energy. It is the cause for obesity in sedentary people.

There are three types of fats.
1. Saturated fats—Ghee, palmitic acid, myristic acids—They increase plasma LDL and total cholesterol. They predispose to CAD.
2. Monounsaturated fatty acids—Oleic acid,
3. Polyunsaturated fatty acids—Linoleic acid in plant seed oils and its derivatives—gamma linolenic acid, arachidonic acids are the essential fatty acids. They are precursors of prostaglandins, eicosanoids and they form part of the lipid membrane in all cells.

The omega 3 series of polyunsaturated fatty acids occur in fish oil.

By antagonizing thromboxane A-2, they inhibit thrombosis. Their use is advocated to prevent hyperlipidemia and CAD and to reduce triglycerides.

Stage I Diet

It is advocated to prevent hyperlipidemia and CAD. It consists of 10% of each type of fats with daily cholesterol less than 300 mg/day.

Stage II Diet

It is advocated in hyperlipidemia when stage I diet fails to achieve the goal.

It consists of 7% of each type of fat with daily intake of cholesterol less than 200 mg.

Proteins

Proteins form the basic building units of tissue. They play the major role in the formation of enzymes and hormones and also in the transport mechanisms. Unlike carbohydrates and fats, no proteins are stored in the body. The amino acids in excess proteins are transaminated and the non-nitrogenous portion is stored as glycogen or fat. Protein requirements are highest during growth spurts—infancy and adolescence. (Protein requirement during these stages—1.5 to 2 gm/kg/day).

There are 20 different amino acids of which 9 amino acids are essential—Tryptophan, threonine, histidine, leucine, isoleucine, lysine, methionine + cysteine, phenylalanine + tyrosine and valine.

They are essential for the synthesis of different proteins in the body.

Proteins of animal origin—eggs, milk, meat—have higher biological value than the proteins of vegetable origin.

An average adult requires 10 to 15% of total calories as proteins.

It is equivalent to 1gm/kg body weight.

Daily Energy Requirements

* Energy requirements depend on—Age, sex, body weight, lactation, climate, (lower calories for tropical climate and higher calories for colder climate).

Type of work	Males/kcals/d	Females/kcals/d
Rest	2000	1500
Light	2500	2000
Moderate	3000	2250
Heavy	3500	2500

Growing children, pregnant and lactating mother need more calories. Brain uses glucose at the rate 5 gm/hour (Preference for ketones when ketone levels are high).

Balanced Diet

Balanced diet contains carbohydrates, protein, fat, mineral, vitamins and trace elements in adequate quantum and proportion in order to maintain good health.

Classification of Nutritional Disorders

1. **Under-nutrition**
   Quantitative deficiency
   In children—Marasmus
   In adults—various forms of starvation, anorexia nervosa, bulimia, etc.
2. **Malnutrition**
   Qualitative deficiency
   Protein deficiency—PCM or PEM
   Vitamin D—rickets
   Vitamin C—scurvy, etc.
3. **Excess nutrition**
   Quantitative—Obesity
4. **Excess nutrition**
   Qualitative
      Excess cholesterol—hyperlipidemia
      Excess vitamins—hypervitaminosis A, D, etc.
5. **Effect of toxins in food**
   Migraine, urticaria, coeliac disease, lathyrism

Pathological Causes of Nutritional Disorders

I. *Defective intake*
   It can be due to:
   1. Poor economic status
   2. Loss of appetite—excess coffee, tea, alcohol, smoking
      Systemic disorders—renal failure, liver cell failure
      Psychiatric disorders—depression, anorexia nervosa

3. Persistent vomiting—organic obstruction, bulimia
4. Food faddism
5. Prolonged parenteral therapy.
II. *Defective digestion and absorption:*
 1. Hypo or achlorhydria
 2. Various types of malabsorption syndromes (steatorrhoea, GJ)
 3. Prolonged use of antimicrobials.
III. *Defective utilization:*
 1. End organ failure—cardiac failure, hepatic failure, renal failure
 2. Severe systemic infections
 3. Malignancy of various organs.
IV. *Excessive loss of nutrients:*
 Protein losing enteropathy, nephrotic syndrome, enteric fistulas.
V. *Altered metabolism:*
 Hyperthyroidism, diabetes mellitus, etc
 Trauma, prolonged fever, malignancy, burns, surgery.
VI. *Increased requirements:*
 1. Pregnancy and lactation
 2. Growth—infancy, childhood, adolescence.

Effects of Malnutrition

1. Reduced inflammatory response (cellular and humoral) to infection
2. Inability to cough due to muscle wasting, leading to pneumonia and bronchopneumonia
3. Impaired wound healing
4. Reduced haemopoiesis
5. Prolonged drug metabolism
6. Altered mental function
7. Inadequate water intake –dehydration
8. Bedsores and ulcers on pressure points.

Protein Energy Malnutrition (PEM)

It may be primary due to inadequate intake of protein (famine), or secondary due to defective intake, or digestion, or absorption, or altered metabolism and or increased demand. The commonly associated illnesses with secondary PEM are AIDS, CRF, inflammatory bowel disease, intestinal malabsorption, and malignancy.

PEM in Young Children

There are two types of malnutrition—Marasmus, kwashiorkor and a combined form—Marasmic-kwashiorkor.

Marasmus

Body weight is reduced below 60% of the WHO standard.

Early weaning from breastfeeding and poor diet low in energy, protein and essential nutrients are the causes. Poor hygiene leading to gastroenteritis and further malnutrition.

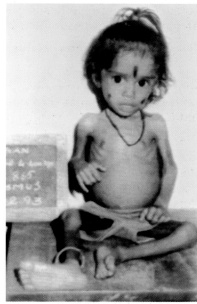

Fig. 2.1: Marasmus

Clinical Features

Child is wasted, with bone and skin with no subcutaneous fat and poor muscle mass (Fig. 2.1).

Gaseous distension of abdomen with diarrhoea can occur.

In contrast to kwashiorkor, there is no oedema, skin or hair changes. There is no anorexia.

Kwashiorkor

It is almost a pure form of protein malnutrition, occurring in the second year of life in a child weaned from breastfeeding on to a starchy diet with low protein.

Secondary infection like-malaria, AGE, measles, etc (increased protein requirement) further precipitate protein malnutrition.

Clinical Features (Fig. 2.2)

The child is apathetic, irritable and drowsy.
Fairly intact subcutaneous fat and pitting oedema.
The child is stunted and puberty is delayed.

- Finally, the teeth are lost
- Lassitude, anorexia and pain in limbs
- Epiphyseal separation is common
- Inward sinking of sternum with sharp elevation of costochondral junctions (scorbutic rosary)
- Purpura and echymoses may appear in the skin
- Painful joint swelling due to haemorrhage into the joint cavities.

Common sites of haemorrhages: Retrobulbar, subarachnoid and intracerebral.
Normocytic normochromic anaemia is common.

Adults

- Total body content of vitamin C is 1.5 gm
- Gum involvement occurs only in people with teeth
- Swollen, spongy gums with increased friability, bleeding, secondary infection and loosening of the teeth
- Perifollicular hyperkeratosis with haemorrhage
- Haemorrhage into the muscles of the arms and legs
- Haemorrhage into the joints and in the nail-beds
- Petechial haemorrhages in the viscera and echymoses
- Delayed wound healing
- Other clinical manifestations are icterus, oedema, fever, convulsions and hypotension
- Vitamin C deficiency causes normochromic normocytic anaemia
- Associated nutritional folate deficiency can result in macrocytic/megaloblastic anaemia.

Investigations

1. Low ascorbic acid level in platelets and plasma.
2. Elevated serum bilirubin value.
3. Abnormal capillary fragility.
4. Classical X-ray changes of bones.

Management

Scurvy is potentially fatal.

100 mg of vitamin C tid until a total dose of 4 gm has been administered and then followed by 100 mg od.

Hypervitaminosis C

Large doses interfere with the absorption of B_{12} resulting in anaemia.

Large amount of iron may be absorbed leading to haemochromatosis.

Excess amount of oxalate crystals is passed in the urine, which may precipitate oxalate stone formation.

Inorganic Nutrients

Fourteen minerals are essential for life. They are sodium, potassium, calcium, magnesium, iron, iodine, copper, zinc, cobalt, phosphorus, sulphur, chromium, selenium, and fluorine.

Sodium

It is the main electrolyte in extracellular fluid (Plasma and interstitial fluid). Along with chlorides it determines osmolality of extracellular fluid.

Source

Common salt—sodium chloride, small amounts in milk and vegetables.

Requirement

1 to 2 gm/day but average intake by Indians—10 to 12 gm/day.

Hyponatremia

Serum sodium level less than 130 mEq/L.

Causes

Extrarenal losses—vomiting, diarrhoea, sweating, pancreatitis, burns, peritonitis
Renal losses—Diuretics, salt losing nephropathy, ARF, CRF, Renal injury, renal tubular acidosis
Dilutional hyponatremia—increase in total body water content—nephrosis, cirrhosis and CCF
SIADH –syndrome of inappropriate ADH secretion
Addison's disease
Hypothyroidism.

Clinical Features

Confusion, anorexia, lethargy, cramps dehydration. When the sodium level falls below 120 mEq/L. seizures, hemiparesis, and coma.

Management

Hypovolemic patients—normal saline
Dilutional hyponatremia—water restriction
SIADH—Water restriction + demeclocycline.
Serum level below 120 mEq/L—Hypertonic saline infusion.

Hypernatremia

When the serum sodium is elevated above 150 mEq/L.

Causes

1. Primary aldosteronism
2. Cushing's syndrome
3. Congenital adrenal hyperplasia
4. Hypertonic saline infusion
5. Hypertonic haemodialysis/peritoneal dialysis
6. Haemoconcentration due to excessive fluid loss—vomiting, diarrhoea, diuretics, etc.
7. Diabetes insipidus (central type and nephrogenic).

Clinical Features

Altered mental status, twitching, seizures and coma. When serum level exceeds 160 mEq/L—it dehydrates cerebral vessels and causes ruptures of cerebral vessels—leading to permanent neurological deficit.

Management

Hypovolemic hypernatremia (haemoconcentration)
    — Normal saline followed by 0.45% saline
Hypervolemic hypernatremia
    — Loop diuretics, hypotonic fluids or dialysis
Central diabetes insipidus
    — Desmopressin

Potassium

Potassium is mainly present in the intracellular compartment. Oral intake and renal excretion maintain the extracellular potassium balance. Acidosis shifts potassium out of cells and alkalosis shifts potassium into the cell.

It maintains the intracellular osmotic pressure. Extracellular potassium level plays a major role in skeletal and cardiac muscle activities.

Normal serum value: 3.5 to 4.5 mEq/L.

Sources

Banana, orange, lime, apple, pineapple, almond, beans, dates, yam, potato, and tender coconut water. It maintains the intracellular osmotic pressure. Extracellular potassium level plays a major role in skeletal and cardiac muscle activities.

Daily Requirement

3 to 4 gm/day.

Hypokalemia

When the serum level falls below 3.5 mEq/L.

Causes

1. GIT—loss due to vomiting diarrhoea, fistulae
2. Renal—diuretics, metabolic alkalosis, renal tubular acidosis
3. Primary aldosteronism
4. Cushing's syndrome
5. Drugs—insulin and glucocorticoids.

Clinical Features

Muscle weakness, ileus, and polyuria.

ECG—'U' wave, prolonged Q-T interval, flat or inverted T- wave and premature beats. Hypokalemia predisposes to digitalis toxicity.

In severe hypokalemia—flaccid paralysis and cardiac arrest.

Management

1. Potassium rich dietary supplements or potassium chloride in liquid form.
2. In severe hypokalemia—IV KCl 20 to 40 mEq/hour with cardiac monitoring.

Hyperkalemia

When the serum level exceeds 5.5 mEq/L.

Causes

1. Acute and chronic renal failure
2. Addison's disease
3. Hypoaldosteronism
4. Shift of potassium from tissues—Acidosis, crush injuries, internal bleeding, blood transfusion.
5. Drugs—Potassium sparing diuretics, ACE inhibitors,
6. Pseudohyperkalemia—due to increased cell destruction—haemolysis, thrombocytosis, and leukocytosis.

Clinical Features

Conduction disturbances and various arrhythmias.

ECG—Peaked T waves in pre-cordial leads-absent P wave and wide QRS.

Management

1. Furosemide 40 mg IV
2. Calcium gluconate 10 ml 10% IV

3. Insulin + glucose to shift the potassium into the cells.
4. NaHCO$_3$ to correct acidosis.
5. Haemodialysis.

Calcium

The total calcium in human body is 1 to 1.5 kg, of which 99% is in bone and 1% is in extracellular fluid. The major quantum of calcium is used in the formation of bone and teeth. Calcium is essential for transmission of nerve impulses and muscle contraction. It serves as intra-cellular messenger of different hormones. It takes part in blood coagulation.

Normal serum value: 9 to 11 mg/dl.

Daily Requirements

Adults—500 mg
Pregnant and lactating women—1200 mg
Postmenopausal women—1200 to 1500 mg.

Dietary Sources

Milk, cheese, yogurt, eggs, fish eaten with bone, almonds and peanuts, leafy vegetables and dried fruits. 100 cc of milk contains 100 mg of calcium.

Calcium is absorbed actively from jejunum and passively from ileum. Acidic pH, vitamin D, and presence of protein enhances absorption of calcium. Eighty per cent of calcium taken is lost in stool and some amount is also lost in the urine, and that is the cause for negative balance when the calcium is consumed in small quantum. The metabolism of calcium is intimately related to vitamin D, parathyroid hormone and calcitonin.

Phosphorus

Total body phosphorus is about 1 gm. Similar to calcium 80% is present in bone and teeth and 10% in muscles. It plays a major role in the formation of bone, teeth, production of energy phosphate compounds such as ATP, CTP, GTP, DNA and RNA synthesis and acts as buffer system in blood.

Normal serum level: 3 to 4 mg/dl.

Dietary Sources

Milk, cheese, eggs, cereals, meat.

Eighty percent of ingested phosphorus is absorbed in jejunum and the serum level is controlled by the excretory function of the kidney. Fifteen percent is excreted in the urine and the remaining 85% are reabsorbed in the proximal tubule and so its level goes up in renal failure. Antacid aluminium hydroxide prevents its absorption.

Hypophosphataemia

It occurs in hyperparathyroidism and rickets.

It causes muscle weakness, anorexia, malaise and bone pains. Dietary deficiency is rare and hyper-phosphataemia does not produce any adverse symptoms. However, in the presence of hypercalcaemia, hyperphosphataemia can lead to metastatic calcification.

Iron

The total body iron content is 4 gm. Sixty per cent of that is present in haemoglobin. It is used in erythropoiesis.

Normal serum level: 80 to 120 μgm/dl.

Daily Requirement

For Males—1 mg
For Females—2 mg
Pregnant/lactating women—3 mg.

Only 10% of consumed iron are absorbed in duodenum and upper jejunum and so, the daily intake has to be 10, 20 and 30 mg respectively for the above categories.

Dietary Sources

Green leafy vegetables, fruits, onions, cereals, pulses, jaggery, grapes, dates, animal foods like meat, liver, fish, kidney, egg yolk. Food rich in vitamin C enhances absorption of iron.

Iron Deficiency

Iron deficiency causes microcytic hypochromic anaemia.

Iron Excess

Siderosis denotes excessive deposition of iron in various sites like liver, pancreas leading to cirrhosis, DM.

Iodine

It is required for the synthesis of thyroid hormones. Total body iodine content is 30 mg and 80% of it is in thyroid.

Normal serum level: 5 to 10 μgm/dl.

Daily Requirement

150 to 200 μgm/day.

Dietary Source

Seawater, salt, sea-fish, vegetables and milk. Iodine deficiency is common in mountainous terrains such as Alps and Himalayas—endemic thyroid goitres are common.

Prevention

Fortification of common salt with potassium iodide. Iodized poppy seed oil 1 to 2 ml IM injection will protect the individual against iodine deficiency for 5 years.

Zinc

It acts as a cofactor for a number of enzymes. It improves appetite, wound healing, and sense of wellbeing. Zinc deficiency causes thymic atrophy. Insulin in the stored form in beta cells of pancreas contains zinc but not when released.

Normal serum value: 100 µgm/dl.

Daily Requirement

5 to 10 mg/day.

Dietary Sources

Grains, beans, nuts, cheese, meat and shellfish. Plasma zinc is lowered in acute myocardial infarction, infections, and malignancies. Patients on prolonged IV alimentation (zinc free) may develop acute zinc deficiency leading to diarrhoea, mental apathy, and eczema around mouth and loss of hair (Fig. 2.8).

Chronic zinc deficiency leads to dwarfism and hypogonadism and ophthalmoplegia. Secondary zinc deficiency is seen in alcoholism and poorly controlled diabetes mellitus.

Fluorine

It plays a major role in the prevention of dental caries. The safe limit of fluorine is 1 part per million in water (1 PPM).

Source

Soft water contains no fluoride. Hard water contains fluoride and sometimes to the tune of toxic level—10 PPM. Sea-fish and tea when taken frequently can contribute as much as 3 mg/day. Fluoride level more than 2 PPM can cause loss of appetite, AGE, and loss of weight.

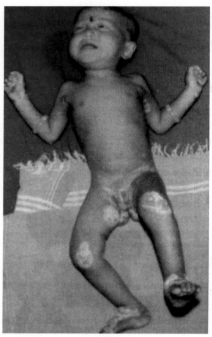

Fig. 2.8: Acrodermatitis enteropathica (zinc deficiency)

Fluoride level more than 5 PPM causes mottling of enamel and discolouration of teeth.

Fluoride level more than 10 PPM causes osteosclerosis, increase in bone density and calcification of ligaments (Fluorosis in certain endemic areas).

Prevention of Caries

When fluorine level is low, addition of traces of fluoride—1 PPM to the public waters supplies.

Magnesium

Total body magnesium is 20 gm and 75% of it is complexed with calcium in bone.

Normal serum level: 2 to 3 mg/dl.

Daily Requirement

300 mg/day.

Sources

Cereals, beans, leafy vegetables and fish.

It is an activator of many enzymes and deficiency causes neuromuscular irritability, tremors and carpopedal spasm. Chronic diarrhoea, chronic alcoholism and cirrhosis cause deficiency. Increased magnesium level causes renal damage.

Manganese (Mn)

Total body content is 15 mg and maximum quantum is in liver. It is an activator of many enzymes, stimulates bone growth and cholesterol synthesis and also takes part in glucose metabolism.

Source

Nuts and tealeaves.

Daily Requirement

5 mg/day.

Copper (Cu)

Total body copper is 100 mg and it is present in muscles, bone, liver, kidney, brain, heart and hair. It is present in many enzymes including cytochrome oxidase and ceruloplasmin.

Normal serum value: Ceruloplasmin 25 to 50 mg/dl and its equivalent amount of copper is 3 to 5 µgm.

Daily Requirement

2 to 3 mg/day

Source

Dairy products, cereals, meat, and nuts. Copper containing ceruloplasmin helps in iron transport and in the formation of haemoglobin.

Copper deficiency causes iron deficiency anaemia and low ceruloplasmin causes Wilson's hepatolenticular degeneration due to copper deposition.

Cobalt

Vitamin B_{12} contains cobalt. Cobalt stimulates production of erythropoietin.

Nickel

It is present in certain enzymes like arginase and carboxylases. Nickel content of the hair—male 1 PPM and female 4 PPM. Some chocolate preparations contain nickel.

Chromium

Total body content of chromium is 6 mg and this level decreases with age. Cooking in stainless steel containers improves the chromium of food.

Chromium deficiency causes glucose intolerance. Chromium improves receptor binding of insulin.

Tobacco contains large amount of chromium and the carcinogenic effect of tobacco is linked to chromium. (bronchogenic carcinoma).

Selenium

By its intracellular antioxidant effect, it protects tissues and cell membrane against peroxidation and because of this property, it is considered to have anticancer activity (? human cancer). Selenium deficiency causes cardiomyopathy, and myopathy.

Selenium excess causes alopecia, abnormal nails, emotional lability, and lassitude and garlic odor to breathe.

Dietary Modifications—Diet Therapy

Type of diet	Disorders
Low protein	Chronic renal failure, nephrotic syndrome, hepatic encephalopathy
High carbohydrate	70% of kcal—Athletes
Low simple sugar	Postgastrectomy state, lactose intolerance
Low energy	Obesity, hypertension
High energy	Undernourished
Small feedings	Gastroesophageal reflux
Low fat	Steatorrhoea, gastroesophageal reflux, acute hepatic, gallbladder or pancreatic disorders, colon, prostate and breast cancers
Low fat and Low cholesterol	Hyperlipidaemia and coronary heart disease
High fibre	Hyperlipidaemia, diabetes mellitus
Low fibre	Crohn's disease, regional enteritis, ulcerative colitis
Low sodium	Hypertension, congestive cardiac failure ascites, chronic renal failure
Low potassium	Chronic renal failure, hyperkalaemia
High potassium	Diuretic therapy, hypokalaemia
High calcium	Osteoporosis
Low phosphorus	Renal failure
Low oxalate	Renal stones
Gluten free	Coeliac disease

Obesity

As per the state of nutrition, the individuals can be classified as normal, overweight and underweight.

Vitamins and Trace Minerals – Requirement/day – Deficiency-induced Disorders

Nutrient	Intake/day	Deficiency-induced disorders	Evaluation
Vitamin A (Retinol)	5000 IU	Xerophthalmia, Bitot's spots, Night blindness, Keratomalacia, Follicular hyperkeratosis, Immune dysfunction,Impaired embryonic development	Serum retinol
Vitamin B_1 (Thiamine)	1-2 mg	Peripheral neuropathy, Beriberi, Cardiomegaly with or without failure, Fatigue, Ophthalmoplegia,Wernicke's encephalopathy	RBC transketolase activity
Vitamin B_2 (Riboflavin)	1-2 mg	Angular stomatitis, Sore tongue and mouth (Magenta tongue), Cheilosis, Seborrheic dermatitis, Eye irritation	RBC glutathione reductase activity
Vitamin B_3 (Niacin)	15-20 mg	Pellagra (dermatitis, diarrhoea, dementia), Sore mouth and tongue	Urinary N-methyl-nicotinamide
Vitamin B_5 (Pantothenic acid)	5-10 mg	Weakness, Fatigue, Parasthesias,Tenderness of heels and feet	Urinary pantothenic acid
Vitamin B_6 (Pyridoxine)	12 mg	Cheilosis, Glossitis, Seborrheic dermatitis, Peripheral neuropathy, Convulsions, Hypochromic anaemia,	Plasma pyridoxalphosphate
Vitamin B_7 (Biotin)	100-200 µg	Alopecia, Seborrheic dermatitis, Myalgia, Seizures, Hyperesthesia	Plasma biotin
Vitamin B_9 (Folic acid)	400 µg	Megaloblastic anaemia, Glossitis,Diarrhoea, Increased homocysteine	Serum folic acid RBC folic acid
Vitamin B_{12} (Cobalamin)	5 µg	Megaloblastic anaemia, Decreased Vibratory and position sense, Ataxia, Paraesthesias, Dementia, Diarrhoea	Serum cobalamin, Serum methylmalonic acid
Vitamin C(Ascorbic acid)	100 mg	Gingival inflammation and bleeding, Purpura, Petechiae, Ecchymosis, Scurvy, Weakness, Depression, Joint effusion, Poor wound healing	Plasma ascorbic acid Leukocyte ascorbic acid
Vitamin D (Ergocalciferol)	400 IU	Rickets-Skeletal deformity-Rachitic rosary, Bowed legs, Osteomalacia, Osteoporosis, Bone pain, Muscle weakness, Tetany	Serum 25 hydroxy-Vitamin D
Vitamin E (Alpha tocopherol)	10-15 IU	Neuropathy, Abnormal clotting, Retinopathy, Haemolysis, Spino-cerebellar ataxia	Serum tocopherol, Total lipid-TGL:TC
Vitamin K (Phyloquinone)	80 µg	Easy bruising / Bleeding	Prothrombin time
Chromium	30-200 µg	Glucose intolerance, Peripheral Neuropathy, Encephalopathy	Serum chromium
Zinc	15 mg	Impaired taste and smell, Alopecia, Dermatitis (Acro-orificial lesion) Hypogonadism, Delayed sexual maturation, Growth retardation, Dementia	Plasma zinc
Copper	2 mg	Anaemia, Neutropenia, Osteoporosis, Defective keratinization and pigmentation of hair	Serum copper Plasma ceruloplasmin
Manganese	1.5 mg	Dementia, Dermatitis, Hypercholesterolemia, Impaired growth and skeletal development	Serum manganese
Selenium	100-200 µg	Cardiomyopathy, Muscle weakness	Serum selenium, Blood glutathione – Peroxidase activity
Iodine	150 µg	Hypothyroidism, Goiter	TSH, Urine iodine
Iron	10-15 mg	Hypochromic microcytic anaemia,Impaired congenital development,Pre-mature labor, Increased peri-natal and maternal mortality	Serum Iron,Total iron binding capacity, Serum ferritin
Molybdenum		Severe neurological abnormalities	

The state of nutrition can be assessed in the following ways:

1. Ideal body weight (IBW): IBW = 22.5 × (height in metres)^2

    Overweight   - More than 10% of IBW
    Underweight   - Less than 20% of IBW
    Obesity   - More than 20% of IBW

2. *Body mass index: BMI = Weight in kg / (height in metres)^2*

    BMI   - In Males 20 to 25
                      In Females - 18 to 23
    Overweight   - BMI is between 25 to 30
    Underweight   - For Males BMI below 18
                      For Females - BMI below 16
    Obesity   - BMI is more than 30
    Grading of obesity:
        Grade I: BMI - 25 to 30 (over weight)
        Grade II: BMI - 30 to 40 (obese)
        Grade III: BMI - more than 40 (gross obesity)

3. *Skin-fold thickness:*

    It can be estimated by using special pair of calipers over the triceps, biceps, subscapular and suprailiac region.

    Normal triceps skin-fold thickness:
        Adult males - 12.5 mm
        Adult females - 16.5 mm

4. *Rough calculation of body weight in an adult (Broca's index):*

    Height in inches = weight in kg
    Height in cm - 100 = desired body weight in kg.

5. *Waist-hip ratio:*

    Waist - hip ratio is useful to assess the prognosis in a case of obesity.

    Waist-measurement of narrowest segment between ribcage and iliac crest

Hip-maximal measurement of the hip over the buttocks:

Waist-hip ratio	Type of obesity	Prognosis
0.8 or less	Pear shaped obesity	Good
0.9 or more	Apple shaped obesity	Increased morbidity.

    Apple shaped obesity is nothing but abdominal obesity, which is associated with hyperlipidemia, insulin resistance, diabetes mellitus and coronary artery disease.

6. *Waist circumference*

Waist circumference alone is enough to assess the prognosis in obesity.

Waist Circumference—Morbidity Risk

Sex	Moderate	High
Male	more than 94 cm (37")	more than 102 cm (40")
Female	more than 80 cm (32")	more than 88 cm (35")

Type of Obesity

1. Generalised obesity—Uniform deposition of excess fat throughout the body
2. Android obesity—Excess deposition of fat over the waist.
3. Gynoid obesity—Excess deposition of fat over the hips and thighs.
4. Superior or central type of obesity—Excess deposition of fat over the face, neck, and upper part of the trunk and the limbs are thin—Cushing's syndrome.

Aetiology

1. *Excess energy intake*
   With excess feeding, excess calories are stored in adipose tissue.
2. *Decreased energy expenditure*
   Physical activity is less in the obese than in the lean.
3. *Behavioural changes*
   High fat intake results in obesity.
   High fat diets do not switch off appetite.
   Little is used for energy expenditure and is mostly stored.
   - Frequent snacks in between standard meals.
   - Consumption of energy dense foods—sweets, ice-cream, soft-drinks
   - Alcohol—It provides energy and stimulates appetite.
   - Smoking—Energy expenditure is more in smokers and their appetite is lost. Most of the smokers are lean. Giving up smoking induces fall in expenditure and increases food intake.
4. *Age*
   Physical activity is decreased with aging.
5. *Familial and genetic factors*
   They play a major role.
   More than 20 genes and 12 chromosomes have been implicated in obesity.
   A. Lipoprotein lipase—This enzyme is synthesized in adipocytes. It induces obesity by causing deposition of fat calories in adipose tissue.
   B. Leptin—This hormone is produced by adipose tissue. It acts at the level of hypothalamus to suppress appetite. Elevated levels of leptin are seen in obesity similar to elevated insulin levels

Causes of Sinus Tachycardia

Physiological   Infants
                          Children
                          Emotion
                          Exertion.

Pathological
    Tachyarrhythmias: supraventricular, ventricular.
    High output states: anaemia, pyrexia, beriberi, thyro-toxicosis, pheochromocytoma, arteriovenous fistula.
    Acute anterior wall myocardial infarction.
    Cardiac failure, cardiogenic shock.
    Hypovolemia, hypotension.
    Drugs (atropine, nifedipine, beta agonists—salbutamol, thyroxine, catecholamines, nicotine, caffeine). ↓ vagal effect

Pulse Deficit (Apex-Pulse Deficit)

It is the difference between the heart rate and the pulse rate, when counted simultaneously for one full minute.

Causes

Atrial fibrillation
Ventricular premature beats.

Differentiating Features between VPC and AF

Features	Ventricular Premature Beats (VPCs)	Atrial Fibrillation (AF)
Pulse deficit	Less than 10 per min.	More than 10 per min.
'a' wave in JVP	Present	Absent
On exertion	Decreases or disappears	Persists or increases
Rhythm	Short pause (between normal beat and VPC) followed by a long pause (following VPC)	Pauses are variable and chaotic

Rhythm

Rhythm is assessed by palpating the radial artery. In certain conditions rhythm may be irregular.

Regularly Irregular Rhythm

Seen in
   (i) Atrial tachyarrhythmias (PAT and atrial flutter) with fixed AV block
   (ii) Ventricular bigemini, trigemini.

Irregularly Irregular Rhythm

Seen in
   (i) Atrial or ventricular ectopics

   (ii) Atrial fibrillation
   (iii) Atrial tachyarrhythmias (PAT and atrial flutter) with varying AV blocks.

Pulse Volume

Pulse volume is best assessed by palpating the carotid artery. However, the pulse pressure (the difference between systolic and diastolic BP), gives an accurate measure of pulse volume.

When pulse pressure is between 30 and 60 mm Hg, pulse volume is normal.

When pulse pressure is less than 30 mm Hg, it is a small volume pulse.

When pulse pressure is greater than 60 mm Hg, it is a large volume pulse.

Pulse volume depends on stroke volume and arterial compliance.

Pulse Character

Pulse character is best assessed in the carotid arteries (Figs 3.2 and 3.3).

Hypokinetic Pulse (Fig. 3.4)

Small weak pulse (small volume and narrow pulse pressure).

Causes

Cardiac failure
Shock
Mitral stenosis
Aortic stenosis.

Anacrotic Pulse (Parvus et Tardus) (Fig. 3.5)

A low amplitude pulse (parvus) with a slow rising and late peak (tardus). It is seen in severe valvular aortic stenosis.

Hyperkinetic Pulse (Fig. 3.6)

A high amplitude pulse with a rapid rise (large volume and wide pulse pressure).

Causes

High output states—Anaemia, pyrexia, beriberi
Mitral regurgitation
Ventricular septal defect.

Collapsing Pulse (Water-Hammer Pulse, Corrigans Pulse) (Figs 3.7 and 3.8)

It is a large volume pulse with a rapid upstroke (systolic pressure is high) and a rapid downstroke (diastolic pressure is low).

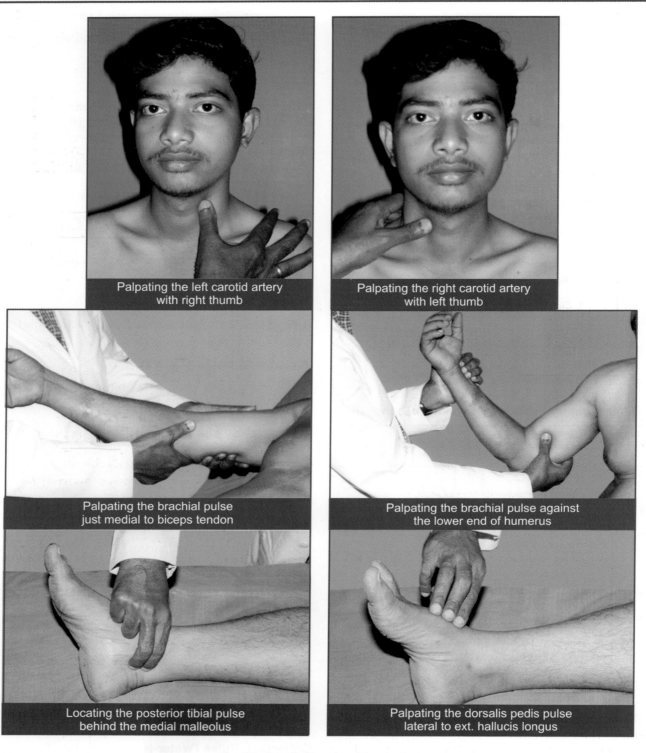

Palpating the left carotid artery
with right thumb

Palpating the right carotid artery
with left thumb

Palpating the brachial pulse
just medial to biceps tendon

Palpating the brachial pulse against
the lower end of humerus

Locating the posterior tibial pulse
behind the medial malleolus

Palpating the dorsalis pedis pulse
lateral to ext. hallucis longus

Fig. 3.2: Examination of peripheral pulses

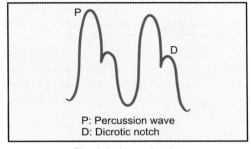

P: Percussion wave
D: Dicrotic notch

Fig. 3.3: Normal pulse

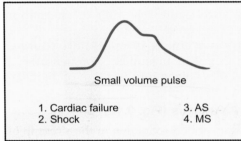

Small volume pulse

1. Cardiac failure   3. AS
2. Shock   4. MS

Fig. 3.4: Hypokinetic pulse

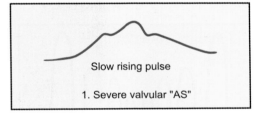

Slow rising pulse

1. Severe valvular "AS"

Fig. 3.5: Pulsus parvus et Tardus

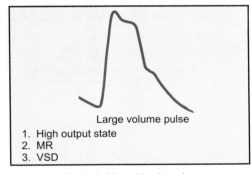

Large volume pulse
1. High output state
2. MR
3. VSD

Fig. 3.6: Hyperkinetic pulse

The rapid upstroke is because of an increased stroke volume. The rapid downstroke is because of diastolic run off into the left ventricle, and decreased peripheral resistance and rapid run off to the periphery.

Causes

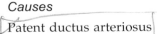
Patent ductus arteriosus

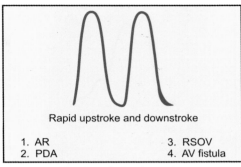

Rapid upstroke and downstroke

1. AR   3. RSOV
2. PDA   4. AV fistula

Fig. 3.7: Collapsing pulse

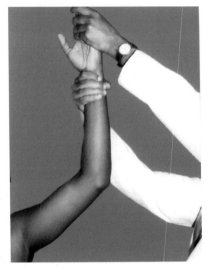

Fig. 3.8: Raise the arm to feel for the collapsing pulse

Aortic regurgitation
Arteriovenous fistula
Rupture of sinus of Valsalva.

Thready pulse is seen in shock.

Jerky pulse is seen in HOCM.

Pulsus Bisferiens (Fig. 3.9)

Pulsus bisferiens is a single pulse wave with two peaks in systole.

Causes   mainly AR

Aortic stenosis and aortic regurgitation
Severe aortic regurgitation
Hypertrophic obstructive cardiomyopathy (HOCM).

Pulsus Dicroticus (Fig. 3.10)

It is a single pulse wave with one peak in systole and one peak in diastole due to a very low stroke volume with decreased peripheral resistance.

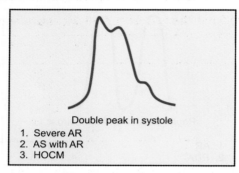

Double peak in systole
1. Severe AR
2. AS with AR
3. HOCM

Fig. 3.9: Bisferiens pulse

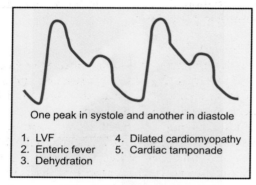

One peak in systole and another in diastole

1. LVF   4. Dilated cardiomyopathy
2. Enteric fever   5. Cardiac tamponade
3. Dehydration

Fig. 3.10: Dicrotic pulse

Causes

Left ventricular failure
Typhoid fever
Dehydration
Dilated cardiomyopathy
Cardiac tamponade.

Pulsus Alternans (Fig. 3.11)

Alternating small and large volume pulse in regular rhythm. It is best appreciated by palpating radial or femoral pulses, rather than the carotids.

Causes

a. It is a sign of severe left ventricular dysfunction

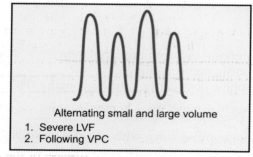

Alternating small and large volume
1. Severe LVF
2. Following VPC

Fig. 3.11: Pulsus alternans

b. It may occur following paroxysmal tachycardia
c. It may occur for several beats, following a premature beat, in an otherwise normal heart.

Coupled ventricular premature beats may also mimic pulsus alternans, but however the rhythm is irregular.

Pulsus alternans may be associated with S$_3$ and electrical alternans—alternate small and large ECG complexes (in 10% of cases).

Pulsus Bigeminus

A pulse wave with a normal beat followed by a premature beat and a compensatory pause, occurring in rapid succession, resulting in alternation of the strength of the pulse.

In pulsus alternans, compensatory pause is absent, whereas in pulsus bigeminus, compensatory pause is present. Pulsus bigeminus is a sign of digitalis toxicity.

Pulsus Paradoxus (Fig. 3.12)

It is an exaggerated reduction in the strength of arterial pulse during normal inspiration or an exaggerated inspiratory fall in systolic pressure of more than 10 mm Hg during quiet breathing.

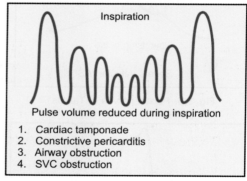

Inspiration

Pulse volume reduced during inspiration
1. Cardiac tamponade
2. Constrictive pericarditis
3. Airway obstruction
4. SVC obstruction

Fig. 3.12: Pulsus paradoxus

Causes

Cardiac tamponade
Constrictive pericarditis
Airway obstruction—acute severe asthma
SVC obstruction.

Reverse pulsus paradoxus is an inspiratory rise in arterial pressure.

Causes

Hypertrophic obstructive cardiomyopathy
Intermittent positive pressure ventilation
Atrioventricular dissociation.

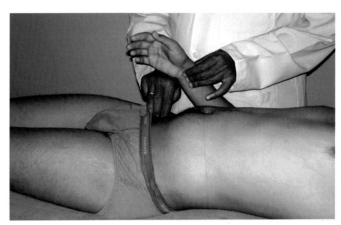
Fig. 3.13: Method of examination for radio-femoral delay

Radio-femoral Delay (Fig. 3.13)

Delay of the femoral compared with the right radial pulse is found in coarctation of the aorta.

Blood Pressure

The lateral force exerted by the blood column per unit area of the vascular wall that is expressed in mm of Hg.

Korotkoff Sounds

Korotkoff sounds should be examined preferably with bell of the stethoscope. There are five phases of korotkoff sounds, i.e., the sounds produced by the flow of blood as the constricting BP cuff is gradually released.

Phase I — First appearance of clear, tapping sound. It represents the systolic blood pressure
Phase II — Tapping sounds are replaced by soft murmurs
Phase III — Murmurs become louder
Phase IV — Muffling of sounds
Phase V — Disappearance of sounds.

Diastolic pressure closely corresponds to phase V. However, in aortic regurgitation, the disappearance point is extremely low, sometimes 0 mm Hg and so phase IV is taken as diastolic BP in adults as well as children.

When Korotkoff sounds are not heard while recording BP, ask the patient to raise the cuffed upper limb and ask him to open and close the fist of that hand repeatedly and then record the BP.

The length of the bladder is approximately twice that of the width. The average length of the rubber bag is 25 cm.

The air bag within the cuff should extend for at least 2/3rd of the arm length and circumference.

Various Cuff Sizes for BP Measurement

Age in Years	Width of the bladder of the cuff
< 1 yr	2.5 cm
1–5 yrs	5 cm
6–10 yrs	10 cm
Normal adult	12.5 cm
Obese adult	14 cm
Thigh	20–25 cm

The midportion of the rubber bag within the cuff should lie over the brachial artery.

After inflation, the cuff should be deflated at a rate of 2–3 mm Hg per second.

Auscultatory Gap

Occasionally, after the initial appearance of the Korotkoff sounds, indicating the systolic pressure, the sounds disappear for sometime, to reappear again and finally disappear at the diastolic pressure.

This phenomenon of a silent gap is found in certain patients with hypertension. It overestimates the diastolic pressure and underestimates the systolic pressure thereby necessitating the palpatory method of BP recording to always precede the auscultatory method.

Auscultatory gap occurs when there is venous distension or reduced velocity of arterial flow in the arm.

Blood Pressure in the Basal Condition

In order to determine BP in basal condition the patient should have rested in a quiet room for 15 minutes. He should not have consumed coffee or tea for the preceding one hour or smoked for the preceding 15 minutes. He should not be on adrenergic stimulants and there should be no bladder distension.

It is desirable to record the BP in both the arms as the differences in systolic pressure exceeding 10 mm Hg between the two arms when measured simultaneously or in rapid sequence suggest obstructive lesions of aorta, innominate or subclavian arteries.

In vertebrobasilar insufficiency, a difference in pressure between the arms may signify that a subclavian steal is responsible for cerebrovascular symptoms.

Normally systolic pressure in the legs is up to 20 mm Hg higher than in the arms, but diastolic BP is the same.

When systolic pressure in the popliteal artery exceeds that in brachial artery by > 20 mm Hg (Hill's sign), AR is usually present.

Measuring lower limb BP is useful in detecting coarctation of aorta or obstructive disease of the aorta or its immediate branches.

Postural or Orthostatic Hypotension

BP must be recorded in lying, sitting and standing positions especially when postural hypotension is suspected.

When there is a fall in systolic pressure of > 20 mm Hg after standing for 3 minutes, from the lying posture, the patient is said to have postural hypotension.

Causes

1. Hypovolaemia (blood or fluid loss)
2. Autonomic neuropathy (diabetes mellitus, old age)
3. Drugs (ganglion blocking agents, centrally acting anti-hypertensives)
4. Myocardial pump failure
5. Secondary hypertension* (pheochromocytoma).

In atrial fibrillation, an average of three BP recordings in the same limb must be taken.

Normal Blood Pressure

Systolic 100-140 mm Hg.
Diastolic 60-90 mm Hg.

Pulse pressure is the difference between systolic and diastolic blood pressure.

Normal pulse pressure is 30–60 mm Hg.

Mean arterial pressure is the product of cardiac output and total peripheral resistance. It is the tissue perfusion pressure.

Mean arterial pressure = Diastolic blood pressure + 1/3 of pulse pressure.

Normal mean arterial pressure is approximately 100 mm Hg.

To confirm the presence of hypertension, multiple BP recordings should be taken with a mercurial manometer on several occasions. Home monitoring and ambulatory monitoring are preferable as they eliminate anxiety.

JNC 7 Classification of Hypertension

(The seventh report of the joint national committee on prevention, detection, evaluation and treatment of high blood pressure)

Category	Systolic pressure (mm Hg)	Diastolic pressure (mm Hg)
Normal	< 120	< 80
Pre-hypertension	120-139	80-89
Hypertension		
Stage 1	140-159	90-99
Stage 2	>160	>100

*When there is a rise in diastolic BP in the standing posture, it is more in favour of essential hypertension.

When the diastolic pressure is below 90 mm Hg, a systolic pressure

below 140 mm Hg indicates normal blood pressure.

between 140-149 mm Hg indicates borderline isolated systolic hypertension

140 mm Hg or higher indicates isolated systolic hypertension.

When there is an elevation of systolic pressure of > 30 mm Hg and a diastolic pressure of > 20 mm Hg from the basal original level, it indicates presence of hypertension.

Common Causes of Hypertension

1. Essential or primary hypertension (94%)
2. Secondary hypertension (6%)
   a. Renal (4%)
   b. Endocrine (1%)
   c. Miscellaneous (1%).

Isolated Systolic Hypertension

This is said to be present when systolic blood pressure is > 140 mm Hg and diastolic blood pressure is < 90 mm Hg. It is commonly seen in old age (above 65 years).

Accelerated Hypertension

A significant recent increase in blood pressure over previous hypertensive levels, associated with evidence of vascular damage on fundoscopic examination, but without papilledema.

Malignant Hypertension

A triad of blood pressure of > 200/140 mm Hg, grade IV retinopathy (papilledema) and renal dysfunction.

Hypertensive Urgency

This is a situation in which the BP is markedly elevated, but without any evidence of end organ damage. In this condition the control of the elevated BP can be done gradually.

Hypertensive Emergency

This is a situation in which the BP is markedly elevated, but with evidence of some end organ damage. In this condition, the control of the elevated BP has to be done immediately in order to prevent further end organ damage.

White Coat Hypertension

A transient increase in blood pressure in normal individuals, when BP is recorded in a physician's consulting room, or in a hospital.

Pseudohypertension

A false increase in blood pressure recording due to stiff and noncompliant vessels (Osler's sign), occurring in old age. In these individuals, actual intra-arterial BP is lower than the BP measured by a sphygmomanometer.

Transient Hypertension

This may be seen in
   Acute cerebrovascular accidents
   Acute myocardial infarction
   Acute glomerulonephritis
   Pregnancy
   Acute intermittent porphyria.

It is systemic hypertension seen for a transient phase of time when the patient is under stress or when he is having a disorder with a transient hypertensive phase, as may occur in the above-mentioned conditions.

Episodic or Paroxysmal Hypertension

This is seen in pheochromocytoma. However, a patient with pheochromocytoma may be normotensive, hypotensive or hypertensive.

Labile Hypertension

Patients who sometimes, but not always have arterial pressure within the hypertensive range, are classified as having labile hypertension.

Paradoxical Hypertension

In this form of hypertension, patients paradoxically show an increase in BP, even when on antihypertensive drugs.

Examples

1. Patients with DM and HTN, on β blockers, on developing hypoglycaemia show a paradoxical rise over previously well-controlled BP. This is because the excess adrenaline released secondary to hypoglycaemia, acts unopposed on the α_1 receptors and thereby raises the BP.
2. With high doses of clonidine, the peripheral α_1 receptors are stimulated, apart from its central action, thereby raising the BP.
3. In patients with bilateral renal artery stenosis, administration of ACE inhibitors, results in a paradoxical rise in BP.
4. Administration of β blockers in patients with pheochromocytoma leads to uninhibited α receptor stimulation by epinephrine leading to paradoxical rise in BP.

Hypertensive States

These are situations in which there is a marked increase in both systolic and diastolic BP, occurring in normal individuals, as during sexual intercourse or on diving into cold water.

Measurement of BP may be useful in detecting
1. Pulsus paradoxus
2. Pulsus alternans.

Pulsus Paradoxus

Inflate the BP cuff to suprasystolic level and deflate slowly at a rate of 2 mm Hg per heart beat. The peak systolic pressure during expiration is noted. The cuff is then deflated even more slowly, and the pressure is again noted when Korotkoff sound becomes audible throughout the respiratory cycle. Normally the difference between the two pressures should not exceed 10 mm Hg during quiet respiration. If it is more than 10 mm Hg, pulsus paradoxus is said to be present.

Paradox: Heart sounds are still heard over the precordium at a time when no pulse is palpable at the radial artery.

Pulsus Alternans

Inflate the BP cuff to suprasystolic level and deflate slowly. Pulsus alternans is present if there is an alteration in the intensity of Korotkoff sound.

Examination of Neck Veins

Examination of the neck veins has a two-fold purpose.
1. To assess approximately the mean right atrial pressure.
2. To study the waveforms.

Jugular Venous Pressure

Jugular venous pressure is expressed as the vertical height from the sternal angle to the zone of transition of distended and collapsed internal jugular veins. When measured with the patient reclining at 45° is normally about 4-5 cm.

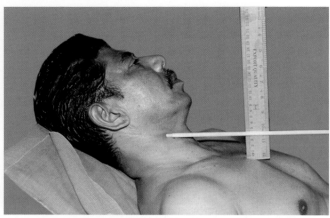

Fig. 3.14: Measurement of jugular venous pressure

The right internal jugular vein is selected because it is larger, straighter and has no valves. It is situated between two heads of sternomastoid.

Patient Position in Examination of JVP

Since right atrial pressure is often very low, optimal positioning of the patient to visualize the column of venous blood above the level of the clavicle is critical. The examiner must position the patient's upper thorax so that the column of blood in the internal jugular vein is visible in the neck. In general, in positioning the patient, the lower the pressure in the venous system, the more supine the patient's position should be; the higher the pressure, the more upright the patient's position should be (Fig. 3.14).

JVP as Indicator of Mean Right Atrial Pressure

The overall height of the pulsating column is an indicator of mean right atrial pressure, which can be estimated based on a simple anatomic fact, that in most individuals, the centre of the right atrium is approximately 5 cm from the sternal angle of Louis. This relation is maintained in every position between supine and upright posture. Thus, the vertical height of the column of blood in the neck can be estimated from the sternal angle, to which 5 cm is added to obtain an estimate of mean right atrial pressure in centimeters of blood. This amount can be converted to millimeters of mercury by multiplying by 0.736. Normal values are less than 8 cm of blood or less than 6 mm Hg. This estimation may be erroneous in patients with deformed chest walls or malpositioning of the heart (Fig. 3.15).

Causes of Elevated JVP

1. Unilateral nonpulsatile	Innominate vein thrombosis
2. Bilateral nonpulsatile	SVC obstruction
	Massive right sided pleural effusion
3. Bilateral pulsatile	
a. Cardiac	Cardiac failure
	Tricuspid stenosis
	Tricuspid regurgitation
	Constrictive pericarditis
	Cardiac tamponade
b. Pulmonary	COPD/cor pulmonale
c. Abdominal	Ascites
	Pregnancy
d. Iatrogenic	Excess IV fluids

Most common cause of raised JVP is CCF.

Causes of Fall in JVP

Hypovolaemia
Shock
Addison's disease.

Jugular Venous Pulse (JVP)

JVP is the reflection of phasic pressure changes in the right atrium and consists of three positive waves (a, c, v) and two negative troughs (x, y) (Fig. 3.16).

Abnormalities of JVP

'a' wave
Absent
    Atrial fibrillation
Present
    Prominent 'a' waves
    a. Pulmonary stenosis
    b. Pulmonary hypertension
    c. Tricuspid atresia or stenosis.

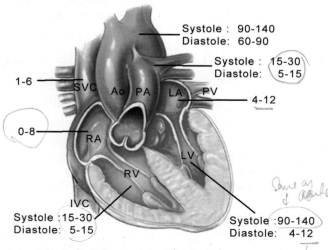

Systole : 90-140
Diastole: 60-90

Systole : 15-30
Diastole: 5-15

1-6

SVC   Ao   PA   LA   PV

4-12

0-8

RA

LV

RV

IVC

Systole :15-30
Diastole: 5-15

Systole :90-140
Diastole: 4-12

Fig. 3.15: Pressure in heart chambers (in mm Hg)

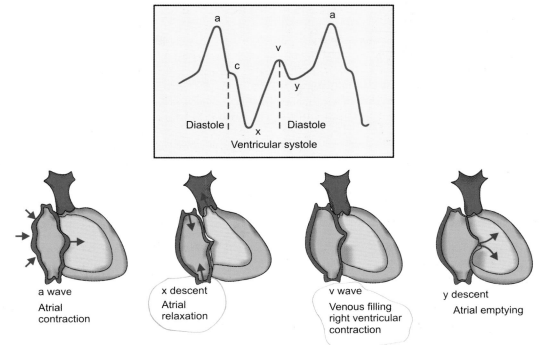

Fig. 3.16: Jugular venous pulse

Differentiating Features Between Carotid Artery Pulse and JVP

Carotid artery pulse	Jugular venous pulse
Seen internal to the sternomastoid	Seen in the triangle formed by the two heads of the sternomastoid and the clavicle
Better palpable	Better visible
Predominant outward movement	Predominant inward movement
One peak per heart beat	Two peaks per heart beat
No variation with posture or respiration	Variation with posture, respiration, abdominal compression.
Not obliterable	Obliterable

Waves in JVP	Cardiac event
'a' wave (atrial wave)	Right atrial contraction
'c' wave (closure wave)	Carotid artery impact Tricuspid valve ascends
'x' wave	Right atrial relaxation
'x'-wave	Tricuspid valve descends
'v' wave (ventricular wave)	Venous filling into atrium
'y' wave	Tricuspid valve opens
'a' wave precedes Sl	'x' wave precedes S2
'c' wave succeeds S1	'y' wave succeeds S2

Cannon waves (Giant 'a' waves seen in arrhythmias)

Regular	Junctional rhythm
Irregular	Multiple ectopics
	Complete heart block

Independent 'a' waves		Complete heart block
'v' wave	Prominent	Tricuspid regurgitation
'x' descent	Prominent	Constrictive pericarditis
'y' descent	Slow	Tricuspid stenosis
	Fast	Tricuspid regurgitation
	Absent	Cardiac tamponade.

Kussmaul's sign is an inspiratory increase in JVP.

Friedreich's sign is the rapid fall (steep 'y' descent) and rise of JVP seen in constrictive pericarditis and tricuspid regurgitation.

Causes of Kussmaul's sign

Constrictive pericarditis
Restrictive cardiomyopathy
Right ventricle infarct
Right ventricle failure.

Abdominal Jugular Reflux

Firm compression is given in the periumbilical area for 30 seconds. In normal individuals the JVP rises transiently by less than 3 cm and falls down even when pressure is continued, whereas in patients with right or left heart failure, the JVP remains elevated.

Abdominal jugular reflux is positive in right or left heart failure and/or tricuspid regurgitation. In the absence of these conditions, a positive abdominal jugular reflux suggests an elevated pulmonary artery wedge or central venous pressure. It is negative in Budd-Chiari syndrome.

General Examination

External Features of Cardiac Disease

a. In congenital heart disease look for:
   Cyanosis
   Clubbing
   Polycythaemia
   Hypertelorism
   Low set ears
   High arched palate
   Webbed neck
   Syndactyly, Polydactyly, Arachnodactyly
   Cubitus valgus, Absent radius
   Pectus excavatum, carinatum
   Kyphoscoliosis, Shield chest
   Abdominal hernia, Cryptorchidism
   Upper segment/Lower segment inequality
   Dwarfism
   Gigantism
b. In acquired heart disease look for:
   1. *Markers of Rheumatic Fever*
      Joint swelling (Migrating polyarthritis involving major joints, leaving no residual deformities)
      Erythema marginatum
      Subcutaneous nodules.
   2. *Markers of Infective Endocarditis*
      Anaemia, jaundice
      Clubbing, splinter haemorrhages
      Osler's nodes
      Janeway lesions
      Arthritis.
   3. *Markers of Coronary Heart Disease*
      Arcus senilis
      Xanthelasma, xanthomas
      Earlobe creases
      Nicotine stains on fingers and teeth
      Obesity.

Fundus in Cardiology

A. *Infective endocarditis*—Roth's spot
B. *Hypertensive retinopathy* (Fig. 3.17)

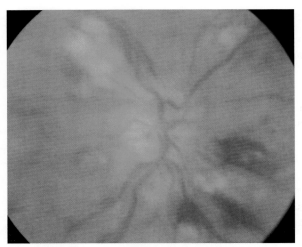

Fig. 3.17: Malignant hypertension—grade IV retinopathy

Keith-Wagner-Barker Grading of Hypertensive Retinopathy

Degree	AV Ratio (Ratio of Arterial to Venous Diameter)	Haemor-rhages	Exudates	Papill-oedema
Normal	3 : 4	0	0	0
Grade I (focal spasm)	1 : 2	0	0	0
Grade II (AV nipping)	1 : 3	0	0	0
Grade III	1 : 4	+	+	0
Grade IV	fine, fibrous cords	+	+	+

C. *Arteriosclerotic retinopathy*

Grades	Vessels
Normal	Fine yellow lines
I	Broad yellow lines
II	Copper wire appearance
III	Silver wire appearance
IV	Fibrous cords

D. *Cor pulmonale*—Papilloedema.

Inspection

Precordium is the anterior aspect of chest overlying the heart.

Precordial bulge indicates the presence of right ventricular hypertrophy presenting since early childhood.

Visible Pulsations

Carotid artery pulsation

Hyperdynamic states
Aortic regurgitation

	Coarctation of aorta Systemic hypertension
Aortic pulsation	Dilatation of ascending aorta Aortic aneurysm Aortic regurgitation
Pulmonary artery pulsation	Pulmonary artery dilatation High output states Pulmonary hypertension Pulmonary hypercirculation (ASD)
Suprasternal pulsation	Aortic regurgitation Aortic arch aneurysm Thyrotoxicosis Coarctation of aorta
Supraclavicular pulsation	Aortic regurgitation Subclavian artery aneurysm
Sternoclavicular pulsation	Aortic regurgitation Aortic dissection Aortic aneurysm Right sided aortic arch (TOF)
Left parasternal pulsation	Right ventricular hypertrophy Mitral regurgitation
Apical pulsation	May be due to left ventricular or right ventricular enlargement
Ectopic pulsation	Ischaemic heart disease Left ventricular dysfunction or aneurysm Cardiomyopathies
Inter and infra scapular pulsations	Coarctation of aorta (Suzman's sign)
Epigastric pulsation	Aortic aneurysm (expansile pulsation) Tumour or nodes over the aorta (transmitted pulsation) Aortic regurgitation Right ventricular hypertrophy Hepatic pulsation (left lobe of liver)
Hepatic pulsation	Tricuspid stenosis Tricuspid regurgitation Aortic regurgitation
Chest wall defects Sternum	Pectus excavatum, Pectus carinatum
Costal cartilages	Costochondritis
Spine	Kyphosis, scoliosis Ankylosing spondylitis Straight back syndrome.

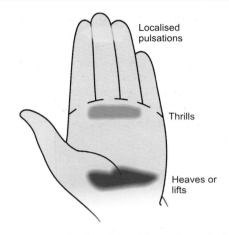

Fig. 3.18: Application of hand in cardiac palpation

Palpation

General rule (Fig. 3.18): The fingertips are used to feel pulsations, the base of fingers for thrills and hand base for heaves. Ideal position is supine or upper trunk elevated to 30°.

Apical Impulse

Apical impulse is the lower most and outer most point of definite cardiac impulse with a maximum perpendicular thrust to the palpating finger.

Normal apical impulse is produced by left ventricle and the left ventricular portion of the interventricular septum.

Normal site of the apical impulse is about
  1 cm medial to midclavicular line or 10 cm lateral to midsternal line at the left 5th intercostal space in adults.
  Normal displacement is 1 cm laterally in left lateral decubitus position.
  Normal apical impulse is confined to one intercostal space and has an area of 2.5 cm².
  Normal duration of thrust of apical impulse is less than 1/3 of systole.

Golden Rules

Before commenting on the position and character of apical impulse, look for the presence of chest wall or spinal deformities, and the tracheal position.

When the apical impulse is not localisable on the left side, palpate the right hemithorax for its presence (dextrocardia or pseudo-dextrocardia) (Figs 3.19 to 3.21).

Abnormalities of Apical Impulse

1. Absent apical impulse	Behind the rib or sternum Dextrocardia

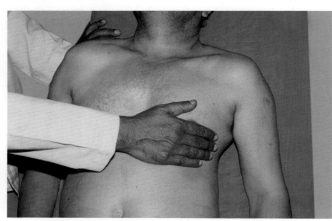

Fig. 3.19: Palpating the apical impulse with hand

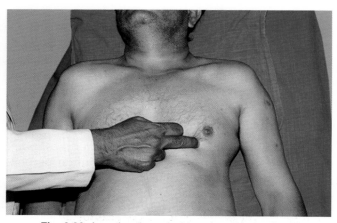

Fig. 3.20: Locating the apical impulse with the finger

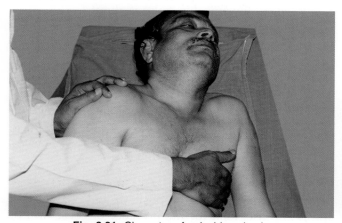

Fig. 3.21: Character of apical impulse is best studied in left lateral position

2. Tapping apical   Palpable S$_1$ (closing snap),
   impulse   e.g. Mitral stenosis
3. Hypodynamic apical   Obesity
   impulse (felt with   Acute myocardial infarction
   decreased thrust)   Pleural effusion

Pericardial effusion
Constrictive pericarditis
COPD

4. Hyperdynamic apical impulse is one in which there is an increase in amplitude without an increase in duration.

5. Heaving apical impulse is one in which there is increase in both amplitude and duration.

Differentiating Features between Heaving and Hyperdynamic Apical Impulse

Features	Heaving	Hyperdynamic
Time	Increased	Normal
Amplitude	Increased	Increased
Duration	> 2/3 of systole	> 1/3 to < 2/3 of systole
Location	Occupies one intercostal space	Occupies more than one intercostal space
Causes	LV pressure overload, e.g. AS, HTN, Coarctation of aorta	LV volume overload, e.g. AR, MR, VSD, PDA, High output states

6. Diffuse apical   Left ventricular aneurysm
   impulse   Left ventricular dysfunction
7. Double apical   HOCM
   impulse   Left ventricular aneurysm
                         AS with AR
                         Left bundle branch block
8. Triple or quadruple   HOCM
   apical impulse
9. Retractile apical   Constrictive pericarditis
   impulse   Severe TR.

Parasternal Impulse

Parasternal impulse is the anterior movement of lower left parasternal area (Fig. 3.22).

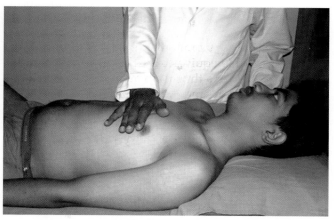

Fig. 3.22: Method of palpation for parasternal heave. Place the base of hand over the left parasternal area

Grading of parasternal impulse (AIIMS grading)
Grade I   Visible but not palpable
Grade II   Visible and palpable but obliterable
Grade III Visible and palpable but not obliterable.

Parasternal impulse can be seen in
Right ventricular enlargement or
Left atrial enlargement

Causes of Right Ventricular Enlargement

Volume overload: Fast, ill-sustained parasternal impulse—
Left to right shunts, e.g. ASD, VSD.

Pressure overload: Slow, sustained parasternal impulse,
e.g. PS.

Left Atrial Enlargement

Left atrial enlargement is seen in mitral stenosis and
mitral regurgitation. Aneurysmal dilatation of left
atrium (giant left atrium) is seen in severe mitral
regurgitation.

Shocks

Shocks are palpable equivalents of heart sounds.

Site	Shock	Cause
Aortic area	A₂	Systemic hypertension
	Aortic ejection click	Congenital valvular aortic stenosis
		Aortic root dilatation
Pulmonary area	P₂	Pulmonary hypertension
	Pulmonary ejection click	Pulmonary valvular stenosis
		Pulmonary artery dilatation
Apical	S₁	Mitral stenosis
	Opening snap	Mitral stenosis
	S₃	DCM
	S₄	HOCM

Thrills

Thrills are palpable vibrations in time with cardiac cycle.
They are palpable equivalents of heart murmurs.
The presence of a thrill indicates that the murmur is
most of the time organic. As a general rule apical thrills
are diastolic and basal thrills systolic. However, apical
thrill may be systolic (as in severe MR) and basal thrills
may be diastolic (as in acute severe AR).

Carotid Thrill (Carotid Shudder)

In aortic stenosis, systolic thrill (Carotid shudder) is
palpated over the carotids.

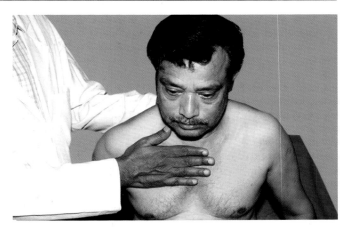

Fig. 3.23: Palpating base. Aortic thrills are better felt in leaning
forward position

Aortic Thrills (Fig. 3.23)

Systolic thrill	Aortic stenosis
Diastolic thrill	a. Acute severe aortic regurgitation due to eversion, infection or perforation of the valve
	b. Syphilitic aortic regurgitation.

Pulmonary Thrills

Systolic thrill	Pulmonary stenosis
	Atrial septal defect (30%)
	Ventricular septal defect
	Patent ductus arteriosus
Continuous thrill	Patent ductus arteriosus
	Rupture of sinus of Valsalva.

Left Lower Parasternal Thrills

Systolic thrill	Ventricular septal defect

Apical Thrills

Diastolic thrill	Mitral stenosis
Systolic thrill	Mitral regurgitation
	Aortic stenosis (as sometimes, aortic events are best appreciated in the mitral area).

*Carey Coombs' murmur and Austin Flint murmur are not
associated with a thrill.*

Percussion

Percussion may be useful in the following conditions
only. It is useful in detecting aortic dilatation as in
aneurysm of aorta and pulmonary artery dilatation as
in pulmonary hypertension or idiopathic pulmonary
artery dilatation.

It is also helpful for finding out the position and enlargement of heart as in

a. *Dextrocardia with or without situs inversus
b. Pericardial effusion
c. Dilated cardiomyopathy.

Auscultation

Ideal Stethoscope should have well fitting earpieces and a thick long tube of 25 cm length and diameter of 0.325 cm, a diaphragm of 4 cm diameter and a bell of 2.5 cm diameter.

Bell of Stethoscope is Used to Auscultate (Fig. 3.24)

Low pitched sounds and murmurs
    Third heart sound
    Fourth heart sound
    Mid diastolic murmurs.

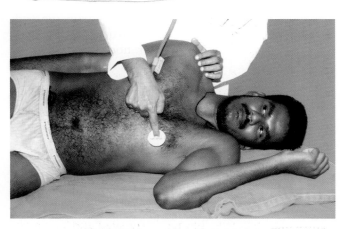

Fig. 3.24: Auscultate with bell in left lateral position (for mitral stenosis)

Diaphragm of Stethoscope is Used to Auscultate (Fig. 3.25)

High pitched sounds and murmurs
    First heart sound
    Second heart sound
    Clicks
    Opening snaps
    Tumour plops
    Pericardial rubs, knocks
    Systolic murmurs
    Early diastolic murmurs.

---

*Congenital heart disease is commonly associated with isolated dextrocardia rather than when dextrocardia is associated with situs inversus.

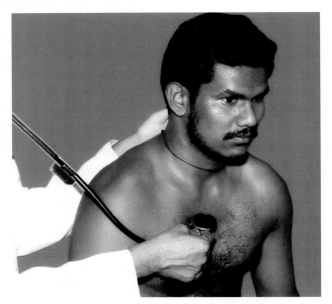

Fig. 3.25: Auscultate with the diaphragm in leaning forward position (for aortic murmurs)

Auscultatory Areas (Fig. 3.26)

Areas of Auscultation over Precordium

• Mitral area corresponds to cardiac apex.
• Tricuspid area corresponds to the lower left para-sternal area.
• Aortic area corresponds to the 2nd right intercostal space close to the sternum.
• Pulmonary area corresponds to the 2nd left intercostal space close to the sternum.
• Erb's area (second aortic area) corresponds to 3rd left intercostal space close to the sternum.
• Gibson's area corresponds to left first intercostal space close to sternum. PDA murmur is best heard here (Gibson's murmur).

Other Areas of Auscultation

Carotids
Inter and infrascapular areas
Axilla
Supra- and infraclavicular areas.

The heart is auscultated for
1. Heart sounds
2. Presence of murmurs
3. Presence of added sounds (S_3, S_4, OS, pericardial rub, diastolic knock, tumour plop, prosthetic valve sounds).

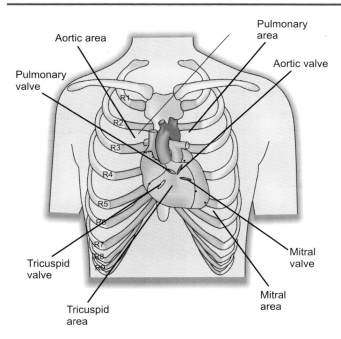

Fig. 3.26: Cardiac valves and auscultatory areas

Heart Sounds

Hearts sounds are defined as relative, brief, auditory vibrations of variable intensity, frequency and quality.

First Heart Sound (S_1)

First heart sound is produced primarily by closure of atrioventricular valves, Mitral (M_1) and Tricuspid (T_1). Associated vibrations of heart muscles, vessels and adnexal structures are also responsible for production of S_1 on phonocardiogram.

Abnormalities of S_1

S_1 may be soft, loud or variable in intensity.

Soft S_1

Mitral regurgitation
Tricuspid regurgitation
Right or left ventricular dysfunction
Tricuspid stenosis (valve calcification)
Mitral stenosis (valve calcification)
Obesity
Aortic regurgitation—acute
Prolonged PR interval.

Loud S_1

Mitral stenosis
    Mitral valve leaflets are kept widely open till the end of diastole as there is a wide pressure gradient across the mitral valve. During ventricular systole, there is a wide excursion and forceful closure (because of a normal LV contraction) of thickened mitral valve leaflets, producing a loud S_1. Loud S_1 is also due to the summation effect of M_1 and T_1, as M_1 is delayed.

Tricuspid stenosis
High output states
Short PR interval
Atrial myxoma (rarely).

Prolonged PR interval produces soft S_1 except in Ebsteins anomaly. Short PR interval produces loud S_1 except in Wolff-Parkinson-White syndrome.

Variable S_1

Atrial fibrillation
Extrasystoles
Complete heart block.

Cannon sound
Complete heart block.

Splitting of S_1

Normally the two major components of S_1 audible are the louder M_1, heard best at the apex, followed by T_1, heard best at the left sternal border. They are separated by only 20–30 msec and are usually heard only as a single sound in the normal subject.

When apparent splitting of S_1 is audible at the apex, it is usually caused by a combination of mitral valve closure with a preceding atrial sound or subsequent ejection sound.

In right bundle branch block, the onset of right ventricular systole is frequently delayed and T_1 may be heard sufficiently late to be easily recognized as a sound separated from M_1. The two components are more readily heard if RBBB is present in pulmonary hypertension.

Causes of splitting of S_1

1. RBBB with pulmonary hypertension
2. Left ventricular pacing
3. Ectopic beats and idioventricular rhythms from LV
4. Ebstein's anomaly.

Causes of reverse splitting of S_1

1. Right ventricular pacing
2. Ectopic beats and idioventricular rhythms from RV.

Second Heart Sound (S_2)

Second heart sound is produced by closure of the Aortic (A_2) and pulmonary (P_2) Valves.

It is useful to memorize the paired leads which are perpendicular to each other (Lead I to aVF, lead II to aVL, lead III to aVR). Similar method can be adopted for determining the 'P' wave and 'T' wave axis.

Simple Methods (Not accurate)

- Lead I and II show predominantly positive QRS complex – Normal axis
- QRS complex predominantly positive in lead I and negative in lead III – Left axis
- QRS complex predominantly positive in lead III and negative in lead I – Right axis
- Left axis deviation is more negative than -30°
- Right axis deviation is more positive than +90°

Left Atrial Enlargement (Fig. 3.40B)

P mitrale—P-wave is broad and bifid occupying > 0.11 sec in Lead II or biphasic P-wave in V_1.

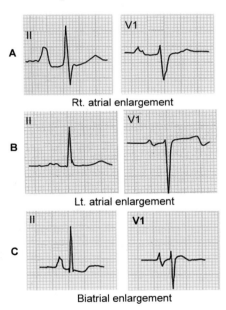

Fig. 3.40: Atrial enlargement

Right Atrial Enlargement (Fig. 3.40A)

Tall P-waves of amplitude > 2.5 mm in Lead II (P-pulmonale).

Left Ventricular Hypertrophy (Fig. 3.42)

a. Sum of the S-wave in lead V_1 and R-wave in lead V_6 should not exceed 35 mm normally. If it does, it constitutes presumptive evidence of LVH.
b. S-wave in V_1 is 20 mm or more in depth.
c. R-wave in LI is 20 mm or more in height, or in V_6 > 25 mm.

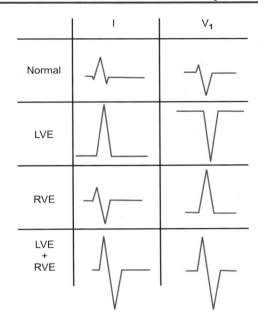

Fig. 3.41: QRS complexes in ventricular enlargement

d. R-wave in V_6 equals or exceeds the R-wave in V_5.
e. Total QRS voltage in all 12 leads is less than 175 mm in normal. Values greater than 175 mm constitute a good criterion of LVH (Fig. 3.41).
f. R-wave in aVL > 13 mm.
g. Any R + any S > 45 mm.

In LVH due to systolic overload, there is attenuation or disappearance of small initial q-wave in left oriented leads (LI, aVL, V_5, V_6). There may be ST depression and T-wave inversion.

In LVH due to diastolic overload, there are deep narrow q-waves in left oriented leads. There may be tall and symmetrical T-waves in left precordial leads.

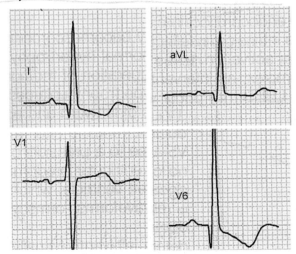

Fig. 3.42: Left ventricular hypertrophy

Right Ventricular Hypertrophy (Fig. 3.43)

a. Right axis deviation
b. Dominant R-waves in right oriented leads. This is often expressed as R : S ratio. If this ratio exceeds 1, RVH is diagnosed
c. R-wave is > 5 mm in amplitude in V_1
d. Dominance of S-wave in left precordial leads
e. Sum of R-wave in V_1 and S-wave in V_6 is more than 10
f. Terminal S-waves in all standard leads—SI, SII, SIII syndrome.

Tall 'R'-wave in V_1
(a) RVH
(b) RBBB
(c) WPW (Type A)
(d) Dextrocardia
(e) Posterior wall MI
(f) HOCM.

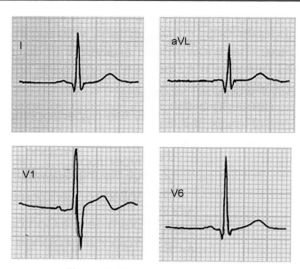
Fig. 3.44: Biventricular enlargement

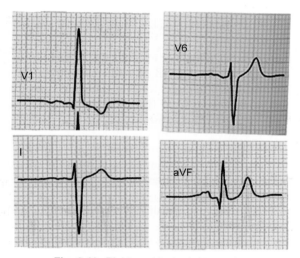
Fig. 3.43: Right ventricular hypertrophy

Biventricular Hypertrophy (Fig. 3.44)

a. ECG evidence of LVH + Right axis deviation
b. ECG evidence of LVH + clockwise electrical rotation
c. ECG evidence of LVH + R : S ratio > 1 in V_1
d. Large equiphasic QRS in midprecordial leads (Katz-Wachtel phenomenon)
e. LAE + R : S ratio in V_5 and $V_6 \leq 1$ or S-wave in V_5 and $V_6 \geq 7$ mm or right axis deviation.

Right Bundle Branch Block (RBBB)
Complete RBBB (Fig. 3.45)

a. Wide S-wave in LI, V_5 and V_6
b. In V_1, tall, wide notched R deflection

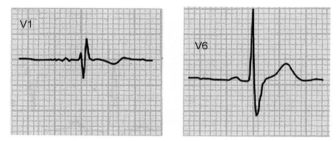
Fig. 3.45: Right bundle branch block

c. QRS duration ≥ 0.12 sec in V_1, V_2
d. Secondary S-T, T changes.

Incomplete RBBB

a. Diminution of S in V_2 (earliest sign of RBBB)
b. QRS duration < 0. 12 sec.

Significance

RBBB may be physiological.
It may also occur with
    Coronary artery disease
    ASD
    Atypical Ebstein's anomaly
    Cardiomyopathy
    Massive pulmonary embolism.

Left Bundle Branch Block (LBBB) (Fig. 3.46)
Complete LBBB

a. Prolonged QRS duration > 0. 12 sec; may be as long as 0.20 sec.

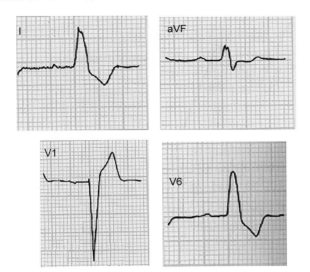

Fig. 3.46: Left bundle branch block

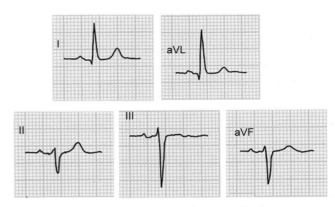

Fig. 3.47: Left anterior fascicular block

b. RsR complex or a wide, unnotched complex in aVL
c. LI, V_5, V_6 show RR or M-shaped complexes
d. Secondary S-T, T changes opposite in direction to terminal QRS deflection.

Incomplete LBBB

a. Initial 'q' in V_5 and V_6 disappears and it results in single tall R-wave
b. Small initial 'r'-wave of rS complex in V_1 disappears and it results in a QS complex.

Significance

LBBB indicates organic heart disease. It is commonly seen in IHD or hypertensive heart disease.

Hemiblocks (Fascicular Blocks)

Left Anterior Hemiblock (LAHB)

Causes

Coronary artery disease
Cardiomyopathy
Longstanding systemic hypertension
Longstanding CCF
May be due to MI (divisional peri-infarction block).

ECG Features (Fig. 3.47)

1. Left axis deviation
2. rS complex in lead II; No terminal r or R-wave as in inferior wall MI
3. Lead I and aVL may reflect a prominent initial 'q'-wave followed by a tall ensuing R-wave
4. Lead aVR may reflect a late, slurred terminal r-wave

5. Lead V_5 and V_6 show no initial 'q'-waves which are normally seen. There is attenuation of R-waves and prominence of S-waves in these leads
6. T-waves are in opposite direction to the main QRS deflection.

   LAHB when occurs in association with RBBB, it usually indicates a poor prognosis and may lead to complete AV block. When it occurs with LBBB, prognosis is worse.

Left Posterior Hemiblock (LPHB)

Occurrence of LPHB is very rare.

ECG Features (Fig. 3.48)

1. Right axis deviation
2. Prominent small initial q-waves in lead II, III and aVF; and a small initial r-wave in standard lead I
3. The distal limb of the tall R-wave in lead III is notched or slurred
4. Low to inverted T-waves in leads II, III and aVF and upright T-waves in lead I.

   LPHB with sinus tachycardia may denote pulmonary embolism.

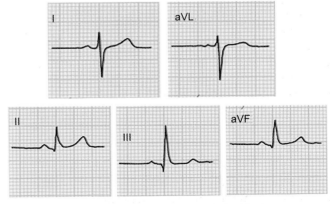

Fig. 3.48: Left posterior fascicular block

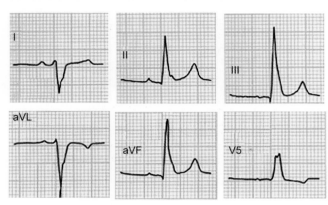

Fig. 3.49: Bifascicular block (RBBB + LPHB)

Bifascicular Block (Fig. 3.49)

It is the combination of RBBB and left bundle hemiblock (manifest as an axis deviation, e.g. LAD in left anterior hemiblock).

Trifascicular Block (Fig. 3.50)

It is the combination of bifascicular block and first degree heart block.

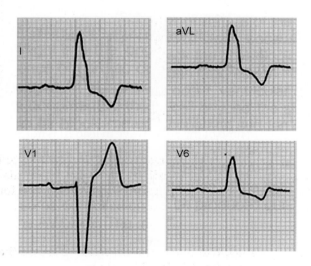

Fig. 3.50: Trifascicular block (first degree heart block + LBBB)

Causes of ST Segment Elevation

1. Coronary vasospasm (Prinzmetal's angina)
2. Organic stenosis of coronary arteries (MI)
3. LV aneurysm
4. Pericarditis (elevated concave upwards S-T segment associated with tall, peaked T-waves and no reciprocal changes in the opposite leads)
5. Early repolarization.

Causes of S-T Segment Depression

1. In coronary insufficiency
   a. Horizontal S-T Segment (earliest sign)
   b. Upward sloping S-T segment depression (It may be a physiological change also. A hypothetical parabola joining the distal limb of the P-wave, the P-R segment, the S-T segment and the proximal limb of the T-wave will be smooth and unbroken in physiological junctional S-T segment depression, whereas the parabola is broken in abnormal junctional S-T segment depression)
   c. Plane S-T segment depression
   d. Downward sloping S-T segment depression (This reflects a severe form of impaired coronary blood flow).
2. Hypokalaemia
3. Hypothermia
4. Tachycardia
5. Hyperventilation
6. Anxiety
7. Post prandial, cold drinks
8. MVP
9. CVA
10. Smoking
11. Pheochromocytoma
12. Digoxin therapy
13. RBBB and LBBB.

ECG in Coronary Artery Disease (Fig. 3.51)

Myocardial Necrosis

This is by the appearance of pathological Q-waves (depth of the Q-wave is more than 25% of the height of succeeding R-wave and its width is more than 0.04 sec.) This may also manifest as QS complexes.

Myocardial Injury

This is characterised by S-T segment elevation on the ECG. An elevation of > 1 mm is significant.

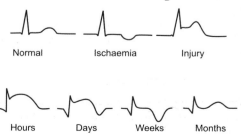

Fig. 3.51: ECG changes in coronary artery disease

Myocardial Ischaemia

This is characterised by inverted, symmetrical, pointed and sometimes deep T-waves.

Localisation of MI

Left Ventricular Infarct

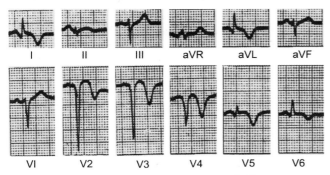

Fig. 3.52: Extensive anterior wall MI

a. Extensive anterior wall MI (Fig. 3.52)—LI, aVL and precordial leads.
b. Anteroseptal wall MI—V_1 to V_4
c. Anterolateral wall MI—LI, aVL, V_4, V_5, V_6
d. Apical wall MI—V_5, V_6
e. Inferior wall MI (Fig. 3.53)—LII, LIII and aVF
f. Inferolateral wall MI—LII, LIII, aVF, V_5 and V_6.

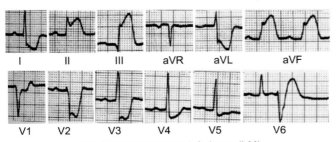

Fig. 3.53: Hyperacute inferior wall MI

Right Ventricular Infarct (Fig. 3.54)

a. This is suspected in the setting of acute inferior wall infarction. There is an elevated S-T segment (of 1 mm) in extreme right oriented leads V_1 and V_4R (to V_6R).
b. There is failure of reciprocal S-T segment depression in the right precordial leads in cases of inferior wall MI.

True Posterior Wall Infarct (Fig. 3.55)

Right precordial leads V_1 to V_3, especially lead V_2, reflect the inverse change or mirror image of a classic anterior wall MI, i.e.,

1. Mirror image of QS complex is reflected by a tall and slightly widened 'R'-wave.

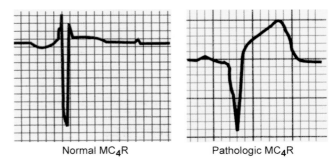

Normal MC₄R   Pathologic MC₄R

Fig. 3.54: Right ventricular MI

2. Mirror image of the coved and elevated S-T segment is reflected by a depressed, concave upward S-T segment. Usually, this change is not seen.
3. Mirror image of inverted, symmetrical T-wave is reflected by an upright, widened and usually tall T-wave. Diagnosis of true posterior wall MI should not be entertained without this change.

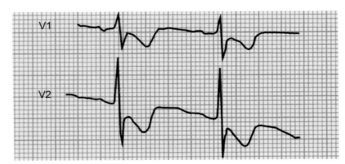

Fig. 3.55: Posterior wall MI

Subendocardial Infarct

ECG presents with ST depression and deeply inverted T-waves in the midprecordial and lateral precordial leads as well as in LI and LII. These changes persist for several days (mirror image of epicardial infarction).

MI with LBBB

It is very difficult to detect the presence of MI in the presence of associated LBBB (Fig. 3.56).

The various ECG signs that are proposed for diagnosis of acute MI in the presence of LBBB are:

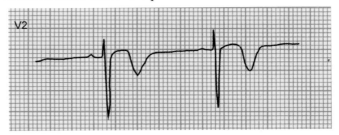

Fig. 3.56: Non-Q wave MI (non-ST elevation MI)

1. ST segment elevation ≥ 1 mm and concordant with QRS complex
2. ST segment depression ≥ 1 mm in leads V_1V_2 (or) V_3
3. ST segment elevation ≥ 5 mm and discordant with QRS complex
4. Presence of Q-waves in two contiguous precordial leads or in two limb leads
5. Left axis deviation > −30°
6. R-wave regression from V_1–V_4
7. QS pattern from V_1–V_4
8. Terminal S-wave in V_5 or V_6
9. Positive T-waves in V_5 or V_6
10. Notching ≥ 0.05 sec. in the ascending limb of S-wave in V_3 or V_4 (*Cabrera's sign*)
11. Notching ≥ 0.05 sec in the ascending limb of R-wave in Ll, aVL, V_5 (or) V_6 (*Chapman's sign*).

* Infarct pattern is not masked in LII, LIII, aVF and premature beats.

MI with RBBB

The presence of RBBB does not interfere with the diagnosis of associated MI.

Acute Pericarditis (Fig. 3.57)

ECG shows
Sinus tachycardia
An elevated, concave upwards S-T segment
Upright, tall, peaked T-waves (earliest change)
No reciprocal changes in the opposite leads.

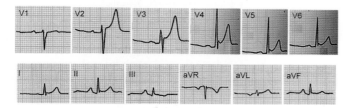

Fig. 3.57: Pericarditis

Pericardial Effusion (Fig. 3.58)

ECG shows
Low to inverted 'T'-waves in most leads
Low voltage complexes (Voltage of QRS is < 5 mm in limb leads and < 10 mm in chest leads)
Potential electrical alternans.

Causes of Low Voltage Complexes

Obesity
Thick chest wall
Global ischaemia
Cardiomyopathy

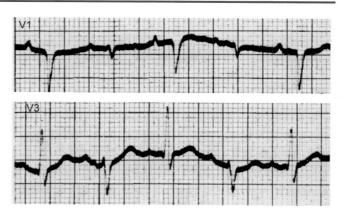

Fig. 3.58: Pericardial effusion

Hypothyroidism
Hypopituitarism
Hypothermia
Emphysema.
Amyloid heart disease
Pericardial effusion
Incorrect standardization

Electrical Alternans

Electrical alternans is an ECG manifestation in which there is alternation in the amplitude of QRS complexes and/or the T-waves. It often accompanies fast rates. When found with slow rates, it indicates left ventricular failure. This is occasionally seen in pericardial effusion.

When pulsus alternans is also present in addition to electrical alternans, it is said to be complete. When electrical alternans is in isolation, it is said to be incomplete.

ECG in Electrolyte Imbalance

Hyperkalaemia

1. Absent 'P'-wave
2. Widening of QRS complex
3. A bizarre, intraventricular conduction disturbance

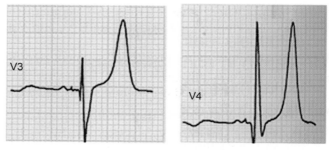

Fig. 3.59: Hyperkalaemia (peaked 'T' waves)

4. Tall, peaked 'T'-waves (Fig. 3.59)
5. Disappearance of the ST segment.

Hypokalaemia (Fig. 3.60)

1. Disappearance of 'T'-wave
2. Progressive increase in the amplitude of 'U'-wave
3. First and second degree AV block
4. ST segment depression.

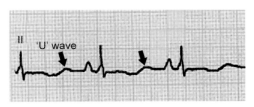

Fig. 3.60: Hypokalaemia

Hypermagnesemia

ECG findings are similar to hyperkalaemia.

Hypomagnesemia

ECG findings are similar to hypokalaemia.

Hypocalcaemia (Fig. 3.61)

Prolonged QT interval (due to an increase in duration of ST segment). QT prolongation is inversely proportional to serum calcium level. T-waves are normal.

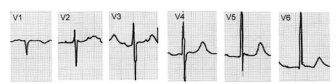

Fig. 3.61: Hypocalcaemia (prolonged QT interval 0.43S)

Hypercalcaemia

Shortening of QT interval (due to shortening of ST segment). 'T'-waves may also become flattened or inverted.

Uraemia

ECG findings are similar to hypocalcaemia and hyperkalaemia (prolonged QT interval + tall, peaked T-waves).

Causes of Tall Symmetrical T-waves

1. Acute subendocardial ischaemia, injury or infarct
2. Recovering inferior wall MI
3. Hyperacute anterior wall MI

4. Prinzmetal angina
5. True posterior wall MI
6. Hyperkalaemia.

Absent P-waves

1. Atrial fibrillation
2. Sinoatrial arrest or block
3. Nodal rhythm
4. Hyperkalaemia.

Inverted 'P' in LI

1. Nodal rhythm
2. Dextrocardia
3. Reversed limb leads.

ECG Changes with Drug Intoxication

Digoxin Effect (Fig. 3.62)

1. ST depression and T-wave inversion in V_5, V_6 (inverted check mark sign)
2. Short Q-T_c interval
3. Bradycardia, PAT, PAT with block, ventricular extrasystoles, bigeminy, ventricular tachycardia, ventricular fibrillation, 1st, 2nd (Wenkebach type) and 3rd degree heart blocks.

Bundle branch blocks and Mobitz type II second degree AV block are never a complication of digoxin toxicity (Fig. 3.62).

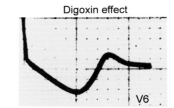

" T" wave rises above the baseline

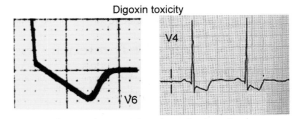

"T" wave does not rise above the baseline

Fig. 3.62: Digoxin effect and toxicity

Quinidine Effect (Fig. 3.63)

1. Prolongation of the Q-T interval and PR interval
2. Prolongation of the QRS complex (LBBB or RBBB may be associated)

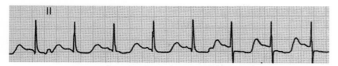

Fig. 3.63: Quinidine effect (Prolonged QT interval)

3. Occasional ST segment depression
4. Torsades de pointes.

Causes of Prolonged Q-T$_c$ Interval (Normally, QT interval is less than 50% of RR interval)

1. During sleep
2. Hypocalcaemia
3. Acute myocarditis
4. Acute MI
5. Quinidine effect
6. Procainamide effect
7. Tricyclic and tetracyclic antidepressant drugs, phenothiazines
8. Cerebral injury
9. Hypothermia
10. HOCM
11. Advanced or complete block, with torsades de pointes
12. The Jervell-Lange-Nielsen syndrome (congenital deafness, syncopal attacks and sudden death)
13. The Romano-Ward syndrome (no deafness)
14. Hypothyroidism
15. MVP
16. Pulmonary embolism
17. Increased ICT.

The prolonged Q-T syndromes are characterised by a prolonged Q-T interval on the ECG, ventricular arrhythmias, and sudden death especially in the familial long Q-T syndromes.

The Q-T$_c$ interval in familial long Q-T syndromes ranges from 0.40–0.60 sec., whereas it is 0.38–0.47 sec. in the non-familial conditions.

Causes of Shortened Q-T$_c$ Interval

1. Digitalis effect
2. Hypercalcaemia
3. Hyperthermia
4. Vagal stimulation.

ECG in Acute Pulmonary Embolism (Fig. 3.64)

In addition to sinus tachycardia
1. Low voltage deflections
2. S$_1$ Q$_3$ T$_3$ pattern (Prominent S in lead I, Q in lead III and inverted T in lead III)

3. Right axis deviation
4. RBBB
5. ST segment depression or a staircase ascent in lead I and II
6. ST segment elevation or depression in left precordial leads
7. Prominent S in V$_6$
8. T inversion in right precordial leads
9. P-pulmonale
10. Sinus tachycardia alone.

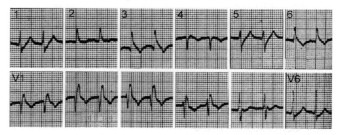

Fig. 3.64: Acute pulmonary embolism

ECG Features of COPD (Fig. 3.65)

1. Low voltage complexes
2. RVH (Right axis deviation, RBBB and prominent S in V$_5$, V$_6$)
3. P-pulmonale
4. Prominent terminal S-waves in leads I, II and III (SI, SII, SIII syndrome)
5. Non-progression of R-waves in precordial leads.

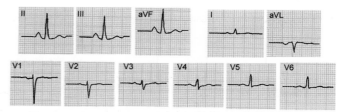

Fig. 3.65: COPD 'P' pulmonale, poor 'R' wave progression

ECG Features of Hypothermia (Fig. 3.66)

It is characterised by J-wave or junctional wave, a hump like deflection which occurs at the junction of the distal limb of QRS complex with the S-T segment. There is a delay in the inscription of the intrinsicoid deflection (> 0.06 sec), that might be an early sign of impending VF.

Sinus bradycardia and prolonged Q-T interval may also occur.

J-wave is also known as 'Osborne' wave.

Causes of Pathological Q-wave

1. Transmural MI

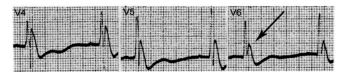

Fig. 3.66: Hypothermia (Osborn waves)

2. HOCM
3. WPW syndrome
4. Cardiac contusion and myocarditis
5. Amyloid heart
6. Anomalous origin of coronary arteries
7. Racial.

ECG in Various Arrhythmias

I. Tachyarrhythmias

Tachyarrhythmias are defined as heart rhythms with a rate in excess of 100 beats per minute. These arrhythmias can further be classified into supraventricular tachycardia (origin above the bifurcation of bundle of His) and ventricular tachycardia (Fig. 3.67).

When the origin of impulse is not traced these arrhythmias can be classified morphologically into narrow complex tachycardia (duration of QRS < 120 msec, i.e. 3 small squares) and wide complex tachycardia (duration of QRS > 120 msec).

Analysis of ECG

• Frequency, morphology and regularity of 'P' waves

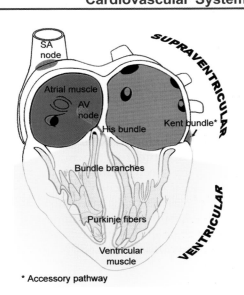

* Accessory pathway

Fig. 3.67: Classification of arrhythmias (based on origin)

• Look for sinus 'P' wave/Ectopic P'2 deflection/ Flutter wave/Fibrillation wave
• Relationship between atrial and ventricular activity
• QRS morphology during sinus rhythm/tachyarrhythmia
• Response to carotid sinus massage/vagal manoeuvres.

Rule of Hundreds for Tachycardias

The rule refers to atrial rate.
Atrial tachycardia – 200 ± 50

Narrow Complex Tachycardia (SVT)

	P-wave			QRS- Complex		
	Rate	Contour	Rhythm	Rate	Rhythm	Contour
Sinus tachycardia	100-180	Normal /Peaked	Regular	100-180	Regular	Normal
Atrial flutter	250-350	Saw -toothed	Regular	75-175	Regular except drugs/disease	Normal
Atria fibrillation	400-600	Absent 'P' with 'f' waves	Irregular	100-160	Irregularly irregular	Normal
Atrial tachycardia with block	150-250	Abnormal 'P' waves	Regular or may be irregular	75-200	Regular except drugs/disease	Normal
AVNRT	150-250	Retrograde 'P'/merged	Regular except onset/termination	150-250	Regular except onset/end	Normal
AVRT	150-250	Retrograde 'P'/merged	Regular except Onset/termination	150-250	Regular except Onset/end	Normal
Non-paroxysmal AV junctional tachycardia	60-100	Normal	Regular	70-130	Regular	Normal

Atrial flutter — 300 ± 50

Atrial fibrillation – 400 ± 50

Ventricular tachycardia has the same range as atrial tachycardia – 200 ± 50, but usually has a rate on the slower side.

A. Paroxysmal Supraventricular Tachycardia

Electrophysiological studies have demonstrated that reentry is responsible for the majority of SVT. Anatomical site has been localized to the sinus node, atrium, AV node or a macroentry circuit involving AV node and AV bypass tract. The mechanism of PSVT can be traced on the basis of R-P interval, the time interval between the peak of an R wave and the subsequent P wave during tachycardia (Fig. 3.68).

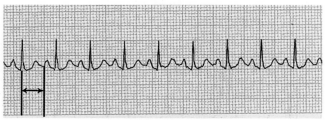

Long R-P tachycardia

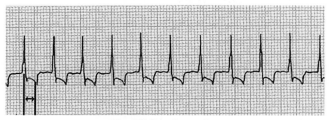

Short R-P tachycardia

Fig. 3.68: R-P interval

1. Short R-P tachycardia

They have an R-P interval that is less than 50% of the R-R interval. These include:

a. *'Typical' AV nodal re-entrant tachycardia (AVNRT):*
   It occurs in patients who have functional dissociation of the AV node into 'slow' and 'fast' pathways. Conduction proceeds antegradely down the slow pathway and retrograde conduction up the fast pathway resulting in atrial and ventricular excitation concurrently. P waves are hidden within the QRS complexes and can be distinguished only by the comparison of QRS morphologies in tachycardia and in sinus rhythm.

b. *Orthodromic AV re-entrant tachycardia (O-AVRT):*
   It is an accessory pathway mediated re-entrant rhythm. (Anterograde conduction to the ventricle through the AV node and retrograde conduction to

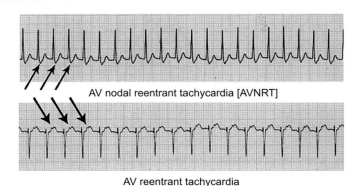

AV nodal reentrant tachycardia [AVNRT]

AV reentrant tachycardia
[AVRT-orthodromic conduction)

Accessory pathway

A   AVNRT

B   AVRT
Orthodromic cond.

C   AVRT
Antidromic cond.

Fig. 3.69: Mechanisms in PSVT

the atrium through the accessory pathway. P waves are seen shortly after QRS complexes (Fig. 3.69).

c. *Sinus tachycardia or ectopic atrial tachycardia with first degree AV block*

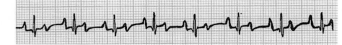

Fig. 3.70: Paroxysmal atrial tachycardia with 2:1 AV block

d. *Junctional tachycardia:*
   It is a narrow-complex tachycardia arising from the AV junction. The impulse is conducted to the atrium and ventricle simultaneously and the P wave is not easily discernible. It is seen in acute MI, mitral/aortic valve surgery or digitalis toxicity.

2. Long R-P Tachycardia

They have an R-P interval that is greater than 50% of the R-R interval.

a. *Sinus tachycardia or ectopic atrial tachycardia with normal PR intervals.*

b. *'Atypical' AVNRT:*
   Anterograde conduction proceeds over the fast AV nodal pathway and the retrograde conduction over the slow AV nodal pathway in patients with dual AV nodal physiology. Because of the slow retrograde conduction P wave is well seen after the QRS complex (Fig. 3.70).

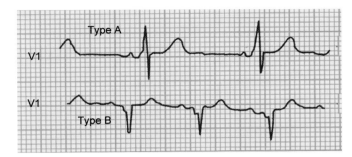

Fig. 3.71: Wolf-Parkinson-White syndrome

c. *O-AVRT mediated by an accessory bypass tract with slow or decremental conduction properties.*

3. WPW Syndrome

Preexcitation is as a result of anterograde activation of the ventricle via an accessory pathway as well as the AV node, resulting in a short PR interval with a delta wave slurring the upstroke of the QRS complex (Fig. 3.71). The presence of accessory pathway predisposes the individuals for SVT (narrow complex orthodromic AVRT).

a. *Antidromic AVRT:(5% of patients with WPW)*
   The conduction to the ventricle proceeds down the accessory pathway and the retrograde conduction through the His-Purkinje system and the AV node to the atria.

b. *Atrial fibrillation:*
   Atrial fibrillation in patients with WPW syndrome may facilitate rapid ventricular response since the accessory pathway has no decremental properties and ultimately VF.

4. Multifocal Atrial Tachycardia (Fig. 3.72)

Multifocal atrial tachycardia is revealed by 3 or more varying 'P' wave morphologies with irregular QRS complexes. This tachycardia is commonly seen in COPD patients especially when on theophylline therapy.

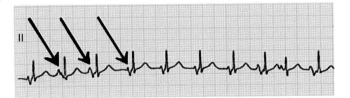

Fig. 3.72: Multifocal atrial tachycardia

5. Atrial Tachycardia with Complete Heart Block

This is often a manifestation of digoxin toxicity unless proved otherwise.

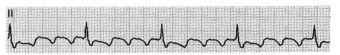

Fig. 3.73: Atrial flutter

B. Atrial Flutter (Fig. 3.73)

It is as a result of single re-entrant circuit around functional or structural (scar due to prior cardiac surgery) conduction barriers within the atria. Flutter waves are negative in inferior leads (II, III and aVF) and positive in V_1 with 'sawtooth' appearance. Atrial rate is usually 300 beats / minute with 2:1 or varying conduction to the ventricle.

C. Atrial Fibrillation (Fig. 3.74)

It is the most common sustained tachyarrhythmia seen in many patients.

Common Causes

- 10% of elderly > 75 years
- Lone AF - < 65 years (normotensive with normal heart)
- Valvular heart disease
- Hypertensive heart disease
- Coronary artery disease
- Myocarditis and cardiomyopathy
- Cardiac surgery
- Hypothyroidism
- Hyperthyroidism
- Pheochromocytoma
- Pericarditis

Atrial rate is 400-600/minute with an irregularly irregular rapid ventricular response (> 100 beats/minute).

The ECG is characterized by irregular baseline with no discernible P waves. The AF waves may be either fine (AF of recent onset) or coarse (AF of long standing duration) The R-R interval is irregularly irregular. The R-R interval may be deceptively regular and slow in

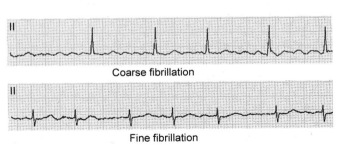

Coarse fibrillation

Fine fibrillation

Fig. 3.74: Atrial fibrillation

patients with complete heart block, either due to conduction system disease or digoxin toxicity.

Symptoms of AF (Due to rapid ventricular rate):

*   Acute pulmonary oedema
*   Syncope
*   Angina
*   Palpitations
*   Thromboembolic (cerebral, peripheral, renal, coronary).

Prolonged episodes of rapid ventricular rate may cause a tachycardia mediated cardiomyopathy.

Management of Narrow Complex Tachycardia (SVT)

Initial therapy of acute episodes of narrow complex tachycardia includes hospitalization, administration of oxygen, establish IV line, vagal manoeuvres such as Valsalva manoeuvre, carotid massage with caution (avoid in the presence of carotid bruit, acute ischaemia and digoxin toxicity) and if it fails, administer IV bolus either one of the short acting drugs that slow or block AV nodal conduction.

*   Adenosine (Drug of choice) 6 mg IV and repeat if necessary every 2 minutes using 12 mg or
*   Metoprolol 5 mg IV every 5 minutes
*   Verapamil 5 mg IV (over 3 minutes) and repeat after 15-30 minutes
*   Diltiazem 0.25 mg/kg over 3 minutes and repeat the bolus after 30 minutes
*   Esmolol 40 mg IV over one minute followed by IV infusion 4 mg /minute and titrated upto 12 mg / minute
*   Digoxin maximum IV dose 0.5 mg over 3 minutes and repeat if needed once.
*   Amiodarone IV infusion 300 mg over one hour
*   Over-drive pacing.

Use the above drugs in the absence of following adverse signs:

*   Hypotension – BP < 90 mm Hg
*   Acute severe chest pain
*   Heart failure
*   Altered conscious level
*   Heart rate > 200 bpm

In the presence of above adverse signs- give sedation and synchronized cardioversion.

Synchronized Cardioversion

*   100 J – 200 J – 300 J
    (If refractory or to maintain sinus rhythm use)
*   Amiodarone 150 mg IV over 10 minutes and then 300 mg over one hour

Chronic therapy of SVT: (use either one of the drugs)

*   Diltiazem sustained release 120-360 mg PO qd
*   Verapamil sustained release 120-480 mg PO qd
*   Metoprolol 25-100 mg PO bid
*   Atenolol 25-100 mg PO qd
*   Digoxin 0.25-0.5 mg PO qd.

Radiofrequency Ablation

It offers definitive cure for different type of SVTs:
*   AVNRT / AVRT
*   Accessory pathway mediated tachycardias
*   Focal atrial tachycardia
*   Atrial flutter.

Complications of radiofrequency ablation (Less than 1%)

*   Groin haematomas
*   Bleeding
*   Cardiac perforation
*   Cardiac tamponade
*   Complete heart block
*   Stroke

With the advent of successful radiofrequency ablation, antiarrhythmic agents are rarely indicated for the management of SVT.

Specific Management

Sinus tachycardia: The cause has to be identified and treated accordingly.

Atrial tachycardia: It is rare and usually due to digoxin toxicity. Stop digoxin and maintain potassium level at 4-5 mmol/L. Digoxin-specific Fab antibody fragments should be used.

Multifocal tachycardia: It is most commonly seen in COPD. After correcting hypoxia and hypercapnia, if the heart rate remains > 110 b/minute verapamil should be used.

Junctional tachycardia: If vagal manoeuvres fail adenosine can be used. If it recurs beta-blocker and amiodarone should be used. Radio-frequency ablation is most ideal in the management.

Atrial fibrillation: Management protocol consists drugs to reduce rate, rhythm correction and to prevent thrombo-embolism by using anticoaglants.

Acute AF (< 72 hours) – Treat the associated acute illness such as MI /Pneumonia.
*   Control ventricular rate with digoxin
*   For persistent fast ventricular rate add either verapamil or beta-blocker.

- Drug – Cardioversion can be tried with either amiodarone or flecainide.

Amiodarone: 5 mg/kg over one hour – then 100 mg over two hours with central line – maximum of 1-2 grams in 24 hours or PO 200 mg tid in the firstweek – 200 mg bid second week – 100-200 mg od for maintenance.

Flecainide: 2 mg/kg IV over 30 minutes (maximum of 150 mg) or

PO 50-200 mg q 12th hourly.

Ibutilide: 1mg IV over 10 minutes – Repeat 1 mg if required.

Dofetilide: PO 125-500 mcg q 12 h

- DC – Cardioversion is indicated electively following the first attack of AF with an identifiable cause and as an emergency if the patient is compromised (200 J – 360 J – 360 J).

Anticoagulation with warfarin is essential for 3 weeks before and 4 weeks after cardioversion to prevent thrombo-embolic episodes.

Paroxysmal AF: Sotalol 80-320 mg q 12 h PO or amiodarone

Chronic AF: Digoxin is the ideal drug to control the ventricular rate. Amiodarone is the most effective antiarrhythmic agent for the maintenance of sinus rhythm.

Anticoagulation: Anticoagulation is not required if AF is of recent onset with structurally normal heart on echo, but aspirin may be given. In all other cases of AF, anticoagulation with warfarin should be given. It is further categorized as AF with high and moderate risk factors.

AF with high risk factors:
- Age greater than 75 years
- Previous stroke or TIA
- Systemic embolus
- Valvular heart disease
- Poor LV systolic function.

AF with moderate risk factors:
- Age between 65-75 years
- Diabetes mellitus
- Hypertension
- CAD with normal LV function.

Use warfarin to keep the INR 2-3 in patients with one high risk factor or more than 2 moderate risk factors. Warfarin is not indicated for patients without risk factors and in them, use aspirin 325 mg od.

Atrial flutter: Management is similar to AF including anticoagulation. If drugs fail, consider 'cavotricuspid isthmus' ablation. This flutter isthmus is low in the right atrium.

Atrial Extrasystoles (Fig. 3.75)

This is characterised by the presence of a bizarre P-wave, which may be pointed, notched, biphasic, or inverted and which occurs earlier than the next anticipated sinus P-wave. The width of the QRS complex is normal. The compensatory pause is relative.

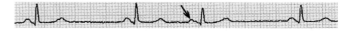

Fig. 3.75: Atrial extrasystole

AV Node
AV Nodal Extrasystole (Fig. 3.76)

This is similar in appearance to atrial extrasystole on the ECG. P-waves may either precede, merge with, or follow the QRS complex depending on whether the ectopics arise from the upper, mid or lower part of the AV node respectively.

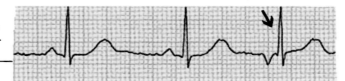

Fig. 3.76: AV nodal extrasystole

Paroxysmal AV Nodal Tachycardia

This may be defined as a succession of three or more AV nodal extrasystoles and has similar characteristics as that of atrial tachycardia.

Ventricular
Ventricular Extrasystole

This is characterised by the appearance of a premature and bizarre (widened and slurred or notched) QRS complex, with associated secondary ST-T changes (when the QRS complex is dominantly upright, the ST segment is depressed and T-wave is inverted. When the QRS complex is dominantly downwards, the ST segment is elevated and T-wave is upright). The ventricular extrasystole is followed by an absolute compensatory pause.

Ventricular ectopics may be benign, due to excessive ingestion of coffee, tea, alcohol, cold water, smoking, or emotional stress.

T-wave inversion if present in normal complex immediately following the ventricular ectopic indicates the presence of underlying ischaemia (*Poor man's stress test*).

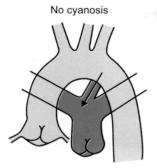

No cyanosis

Left to right shunt

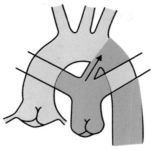

Bilateral lower limb cyanosis

Right to left shunt

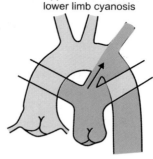

Left upper limb and bilateral lower limb cyanosis

Right to left shunt ductal

Fig. 3.99: Patent ductus arteriosus

2. Trisomy 18.
3. Fetal hydantoin syndrome (Hypertelorism, growth and mental retardation, short phalanges, bowed upper lip).
4. Incontinentia pigmenti (patchy alopecia, irregular pigmented skin lesions, hypodontia).
5. Crouzon syndrome (ptosis with shallow orbit, craniosynostosis, maxillary hypoplasia).
6. Rubinstein-Taybi syndrome (broad thumbs and toes, maxillary hypoplasia, slanted palpebral fissure).
7. Conradi-Hunermann syndrome.

Clinical Features

Grade IV continuous murmur heard best over the left second intercostal space at midclavicular line.

Differential Diagnosis of Continuous Murmurs

Location	Underlying Disease Entity
Left upper sternal border and below left clavicle	PDA
Second to fourth intercostal spaces	Aortopulmonary septal defect
Along the lower left sternal border	Rupture of sinus of Valsalva aneurysm
Over lower or mid-sternal border or entire precordium	Coronary arteriovenous fistulae
May be audible anywhere over the chest	Pulmonary arteriovenous fistulae

ECG

Left atrial enlargement is commonly seen.

Left ventricular enlargement may be seen (volume overload). Right ventricular enlargement may be seen (pressure overload).

Chest X-ray

The lung fields are plethoric (Fig. 3.100).

The angle between the main pulmonary artery and aortic knuckle can be obliterated by presence of a patent ductus.

Calcification at the site of ductus indicates a fibrosed or a calcified ductus.

PDA can close spontaneously after early infancy.

Ductal endarteritis is common either near the ductal orifice in the pulmonary artery or in the pulmonary end of the ductus.

Aneurysms or rupture (secondary to development of aneurysm or calcification) of the PDA can occur.

Congestive cardiac failure is the commonest cause of death.

Treatment

Medical: Administration of indomethacin within the first two to seven days of life.

Note: Indomethacin favours ductal closure by reducing prostaglandin levels especially PG-E.

Surgical: Ligation and excision of patent ductus. Ideal age for surgery is below two years.

Transcatheter closure of patent ductus using a variety of approaches using coils, buttons, plugs and umbrellas can be done (Fig. 3.101).

Conditions where PDA is Essential for Survival
1. Pulmonary atresia
2. Hypoplastic left heart syndrome
3. Preductal coarctation of aorta
4. Complete TGV without septal defects.

Eisenmenger Syndrome

It is the condition in which left to right shunt gets reversed (right to left) with the development of severe pulmonary hypertension, resulting in central cyanosis (Fig. 3.99), clubbing, and secondary polycythaemia (Fig. 3.101).

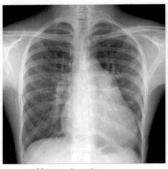
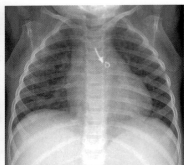
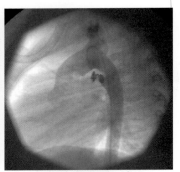

X-ray showing   PDA-Coil occlusion   Angiogram showing
pulmonary plethora   coil occlusion of PDA

Fig. 3.100: Patent ductus arteriosus

Its incidence is equal in both males and females.

Since this syndrome is uncommon below two years of age, surgical closure of left to right shunt lesions is advocated below two years of age.

Haemoptysis is uncommon, but when it occurs, prognosis is bad, as it is caused by rupture of thin-walled, fragile pulmonary arteries or their small aneurysms.

Conditions that cause systemic vasodilatation (exercise, fever, hot bath, hot weather) may exaggerate the shunt from right to left resulting in systemic desaturation and poor tolerance.

Clinical Features

- Generalised cyanosis occurs in presence of VSD and ASD.
- Differential cyanosis involving the lower limbs occurs in the presence of PDA (Fig. 3.99).

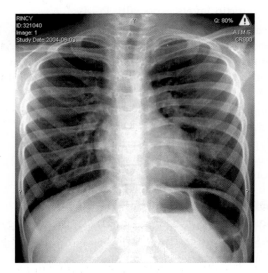

Fig. 3.101: VSD with Eisenmenger's syndrome

- P_2 is loud and palpable.
- There is a prominent parasternal heave.

Eisenmenger syndrome occurs earlier in life in VSD, a little later in PDA, and very late in adult life in ASD.

In ASD with reversal   Narrowly fixed split of S_2
In VSD with reversal   Single S_2 and decreased
(Eisenmenger complex)   intensity of murmur
In PDA with reversal   Closely split S_2 which varies
                          normally with respiration.

Surgery is not contraindicated in the early phase of Eisenmenger's syndrome, developing as the result of volume overload without evidence of increased pulmonary vascular resistance (normal pulmonary wedge pressure).

Death is caused by
1. CCF
2. Pulmonary infection
3. Pulmonary thrombosis (pulmonary infarction)
4. Brain abscess
5. Infective endocarditis
6. Severe haemoptysis
7. Ventricular arrhythmias.

Pregnancy must be avoided or terminated with development of Eisenmenger's syndrome.

The only curative treatment of Eisenmenger's syndrome is heart-lung transplantation.

Differential Diagnosis

1. Primary pulmonary hypertension
2. Recurrent pulmonary embolism
3. Idiopathic dilatation of pulmonary artery.

Tetralogy of Fallot (TOF) (Fig. 3.102)

It is the most common cyanotic congenital heart disease in patients who survive infancy.

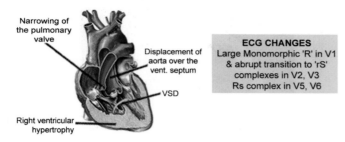

ECG CHANGES
Large Monomorphic 'R' in V1 & abrupt transition to 'rS' complexes in V2, V3 Rs complex in V5, V6

Fig. 3.102: Tetralogy of Fallot

It is composed of 4 distinct anatomic abnormalities
1. Large non-restrictive VSD
2. Right ventricular outflow tract obstruction* (infundibular pulmonary stenosis)
3. Overriding of the aorta
4. Right ventricular hypertrophy.

Embryology

TOF occurs as the result of anterocephalad malalignment of the infundibular septum, resulting in a ventricular septal defect, right ventricular outflow tract obstruction (subpulmonic obstruction) and overriding of the aorta.

Cyanotic Fallot

When the resistance to pulmonary outflow is greater than the systemic resistance, right to left shunting of blood across the VSD occurs, resulting in central cyanosis.

Acyanotic Fallot

When the resistance to the pulmonary outflow is lower than the systemic resistance, then a predominant left to right shunt occurs across the VSD and cyanosis is absent.

Initially, in TOF, cyanosis is episodic, occurring during feeding, crying, fever, exercise, etc., when systemic vasodilatation occurs causing an increased right to left shunting across the VSD.

A baby born cyanotic is unlikely to have TOF.

Cyanosis becomes more prominent after about 5-6 months of life due to the following reasons:
a. HbF is the predominant Hb present in the first few years of life. It binds less avidly to O_2 and releases it easily at times of need. Hence when an infant with TOF, in the first 5 to 6 months of life develops cyanotic spells, O_2 is easily released from HbF and hence cyanosis is minimal.

After 5-6 months of age, HbF is replaced by HbA_2. HbA_2 binds O_2 more avidly and releases it less readily at times of need and so the child becomes cyanotic.
b. With the growth of the child, the O_2 demand for growth increases and cyanosis becomes more prominent.

TOF may be associated with other cardiac anomalies like:
1. Patent foramen ovale
2. ASD
3. AR
4. Right sided aortic arch (It is the most common anomaly, seen in 25 to 30% of cases, its likelihood increasing with increasing severity of RVOT obstruction and particularly in pulmonary atresia)
5. PDA
6. Anomalous origin of the coronary arteries
7. Absence of left pulmonary artery.

Pentology of Fallot

Presence of ASD along with TOF is called pentology of Fallot.

Triology of Fallot

Right ventricular outflow tract obstruction with RV hypertrophy and right to left shunt across interatrial septum in the absence of VSD is called triology of Fallot (PS, RVH, and ASD).

TOF Associated Syndromes

1. TAR (thrombocytopenia and absent radius)
2. Down syndrome (hypotonia, mental retardation, mongoloid facies, hyperextensible joints)
3. Di-George syndrome (Thymic hypoplasia, parathyroid hypoplasia, ear anomalies)
4. CHARGE association (coloboma, choanal atresia, mental and growth retardation, genital and ear anomalies)
5. Velocardiofacial.

Clinical Features

A silent precordium is often characteristic.

On auscultation, a loud, single S_2 (representing aortic valve closure) and an ESM is best heard over the 3rd and 4th left intercostal spaces.

The intensity and duration of the murmur is inversely proportional to the severity of RVOT obstruction.

---

*Rarely valvular PS or a combination of infundibular and valvular PS may be present.

Because of a large ventricular septal defect, VSD murmur is inconspicuous.

ECG

ECG shows right axis deviation. A large monophasic R-wave is present in V_1, with abrupt transition to a rS complex in V_2, V_3 and Rs complexes in V_5, V_6.

X-ray Chest

This shows a normal sized heart with a characteristic appearance termed as 'Coeur en Sabot' or 'boot shaped heart' (tilted apex). There is pulmonary oligemia. Boot shaped heart (Fig. 3.103) is due to the prominence of RV and concavity in the region is due to underdeveloped RVOT and main pulmonary artery.

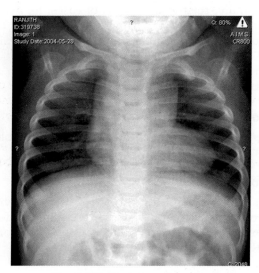

Fig. 3.103: Boot shaped heart

Complications

1. Marked secondary polycythaemia may result in intravascular thrombosis leading to cerebrovascular accidents and paradoxical emboli.
2. Cerebral abscess (common causative organism being Streptococcus) (Fig. 3.104).
3. Incidence of pulmonary tuberculosis and tuberculoma is high.
4. Infective endocarditis (common causative organism being Streptococcus).
5. CCF is a rare complication and if present, may be secondary to
   a. Infective endocarditis
   b. Pregnancy
   c. Anaemia
   d. Systemic hypertension
   e. Aortic regurgitation

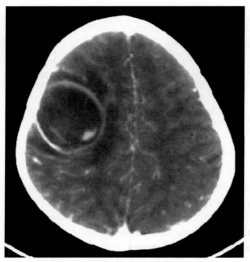

Fig. 3.104: Brain abscess in a TOF patient

f. Acquired calcific stenosis of the bicuspid aortic valve
g. Pulmonary atresia with large systemic arterial collaterals –RV failure
h. Accessory tricuspid leaflet occluding the VSD – RV failure.

Treatment

Medical

Treatment of cyanotic spells by
a. squatting or knee chest position
b. nasal O_2
c. morphine
d. β-blockers (propranolol).

Morphine and β-blockers (propranolol) help to relieve infundibular spasm.

Propranolol initially at the dose of 0.01 mg/kg IV followed by oral dose of 3-5 mg/kg/day is advocated. Morphine sulphate is given at the dose of 0.1mg/kg IV.

e. Correct metabolic acidosis with sodium bicarbonate—1 mEq/kg IV.

Surgical

Total correction is advocated and is the definitive treatment.

If pulmonary arteries are excessively small, then early definitive correction of TOF is not possible and a palliative procedure (Blalock-Taussig shunt) is done till the time when the pulmonary arteries have enlarged sufficiently.

Blalock-Taussig Procedure: In left sided aortic arch— Left subclavian to left pulmonary artery. In right sided aortic arch—Right subclavian to right pulmonary artery.

This procedure results in absent radial pulse on the side of anastomosis and a continuous murmur at the site of anastomosis.

Waterston procedure: Ascending aorta to right pulmonary artery.

Pott's procedure: Descending aorta to left pulmonary artery.

Pulmonary Stenosis (PS)

Pulmonary stenosis may occur as an isolated defect or may accompany other anomalies, notably ventricular septal defect. It may occur at various levels (Fig. 3.105)
a. Supravalvular
b. Valvular
c. Infundibular
d. Subinfundibular.

Congenital stenosis of the valve presents as a dome-shaped diaphragm, consisting of fused cusps, with small central aperture, and bulging into the pulmonary artery.

In infundibular stenosis, the infundibular impedance may consist of localized fibrous stricture or diffuse obstructive infundibular hypertrophy.

Supravalvular pulmonary stenosis occurs at the level of the pulmonary trunk, pulmonary arteries, or its peripheral branches. This is often a manifestation of the congenital rubella syndrome.

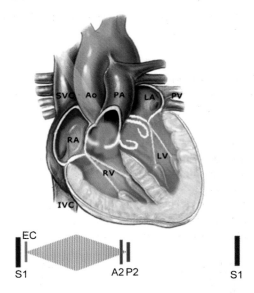

Fig. 3.105: Pulmonary stenosis

Concentric hypertrophy of the right ventricle occurs.

Reduced right ventricular compliance may raise right atrial pressure, enough to force open the foramen ovale, with resultant right-to-left shunt.

Marked pulmonary stenosis causes dyspnoea and fatigue, and central cyanosis may develop (secondary to right-to-left shunt across foramen ovale).

PS Associated Syndromes

1. Maternal rubella

Assessment of Severity of Pulmonary Stenosis

	Features	Mild	Moderate	Severe
1.	Symptoms	Absent	Absent or minimal	Dyspnoea and fatigue
2.	Central cyanosis	Absent	Absent	Present
3.	Pulse	Normal volume	Normal volume	Small volume
4.	JVP	Normal	'a'-wave prominent	Giant 'a'-wave seen
5.	Parasternal heave	Grade I	Grade II	Grade III
6.	Systolic thrill over pulmonary area	No thrill	Thrill may or may not be palpable	Thrill palpable
7.	P_2	Heard	Faint and delayed	Absent
8.	Pulmonary ejection click	Prominent	Less prominent and occurs earlier (close to S_1)	Very faint or absent
9.	Duration and contour of ejection systolic murmur	Short duration of murmur with intensity peaking in early systole	Medium duration murmur with intensity peaking in mid-systole	Long duration of murmur with intensity peaking in late systole
10.	Area of pulmonary valve orifice (normal area is 3–4 cm²)	> 1 cm²	0.8–1 cm²	< 0.8 cm²
11.	Right ventricular systolic pressure (normal pressure is 25 mm Hg.)	30–50 mm Hg.	50–80 mm Hg.	> 80 mm Hg.
12.	Treatment	Medical	Medical or surgical	Surgical

2. Noonan syndrome (webbed neck, pectus excavatum, cryptorchidism).
3. Williams syndrome (Elfin facies, mental retardation, loquacious personality, coarse voice).
4. Foetal hydantoin syndrome.
5. Cutis laxa (generalised disruption of elastic fibres, diminished skin resilience, hernias)
6. Alagille syndrome (biliary hypoplasia, vertebral anomalies, prominent forehead, deep set ears)
7. LEOPARD syndrome (broad facies, basal cell naevi, rib anomalies and deafness).

Clinical Features

- A raised JVP, with prominent 'a'-wave.
- Lower left parasternal heave.
- Systolic thrill felt over pulmonary area.
- S_2 is widely split (mild PS).
- P_2 is soft and delayed, in valvular PS (in other types, P_2 is normal).
- Pulmonary ejection click may be heard, in valvular PS (other types not heard).
- Harsh, loud ejection systolic murmur heard over the pulmonary area, increasing in intensity with inspiration.

ECG

ECG shows right ventricular hypertrophy. RBBB may be seen.

X-Ray Chest

Right atrial and right ventricular enlargement. Prominence of the main pulmonary artery (poststenotic dilatation).

Complications

i. Right ventricular failure
ii. Infective endocarditis
iii. Sudden death.

Treatment

Patients with mild stenosis do well with medical management, consisting of antibiotic coverage of bacteremic events, and with periodic examination.

Patients with severe stenosis warrant corrective surgery. Pulmonary balloon valvuloplasty is preferred. Other corrective surgeries are:
1. Pulmonary valvotomy
2. Pulmonary valve repair
3. Pulmonary valve replacement.

Differentiating Severity of Pulmonary Stenosis in Isolated Pulmonary Stenosis and Tetralogy of Fallot

In isolated pulmonary stenosis, the intensity of the murmur (ESM) across the stenosed pulmonary valve is directly proportional to the severity of stenosis. Hence, the more severe the stenosis, the louder the murmur and later is the peaking of its intensity.

In TOF, the intensity of the murmur (ESM), across the infundibular stenosis, is inversely proportional to the severity of stenosis. This occurs because as the infundibular stenosis becomes more severe, the blood is directed to the overriding aorta, thereby reducing the pulmonary blood flow and therefore also the intensity of the murmur.

Congenital Aortic Stenosis

It is one of the most common congenital defects in both children and adults.

Types

1. Supravalvular
2. Valvular
3. Subvalvular.

Both valvular and subvalvular aortic stenosis may be associated with:
a. PDA
b. VSD
c. Coarctation of the aorta.

Supravalvular Aortic Stenosis (Williams Syndrome)

Features
a. Supravalvular aortic stenosis (localised constriction immediately above the sinuses of Valsalva or a diffuse narrowing of the ascending aorta)
b. Elfin facies (prominent forehead, widely spaced eyes, blunt upturned nose, underdeveloped mandible, dental hypoplasia and malocclusion, large mouth and patulous lips)
c. Mental retardation
d. Hypercalcaemia (due to vitamin D excess or intolerance).

Valvular Aortic Stenosis EC + ESM

This usually consists of a dome-shaped diaphragm with an eccentric aperture and fused commissures.

Poststenotic dilatation of the ascending aorta is common.

In supravalular harsh murmur (R) lt 1C usually w/AR, ↑BP by 30 mm Hg

Subvalvular Aortic Stenosis

This consists of a fibrous or fibromuscular shelf encircling the outflow tract beneath the valve.

w/AR & ESM in mid/lower (L) sternal on (L) side

Congenital AS Associated Syndromes

Williams syndrome and fetal hydantoin syndrome.

Clinical Features

Congenital valvular stenosis causes physical findings similar to those of acquired valvular stenosis. The congenital valve remains flexible in contrast to the thick, calcified stenotic valve of acquired aortic stenosis. Hence, aortic ejection sounds and normal aortic closure sounds (A_2) are usually heard in congenital valvular stenosis. The harsh aortic ejection systolic murmur is heard.

Congenital subvalvular aortic stenosis causes clinical findings similar to those of valvular stenosis. Aortic regurgitation is more common and ejection sounds are not heard. The ejection systolic murmur is sometimes maximal along the mid or lower left sternal edge.

Congenital supravalvular aortic stenosis causes a harsh aortic ejection systolic murmur that occasionally is maximal in the first right interspace. Ejection sounds are not heard. Aortic regurgitation may be present. Systolic blood pressure is usually higher in the right arm than in the left arm, by approximately 30 mm Hg.

ECG

ECG shows left ventricular hypertrophy; occasionally congenital valvular stenosis is associated with partial or complete atrioventricular block.

X-ray Chest

CXR shows left ventricular enlargement. Poststenotic dilatation of the ascending aorta may be seen in valvular stenosis.

Treatment

Treatment is surgical repair of the stenotic lesion obstructing the left ventricular outflow tract.

In case of infravalvular stenosis, the defect must be corrected immediately after its detection, as it may lead to progressive obstruction, valvular deformity and development of AR if uncorrected. AR may also develop as a result of infective endocarditis.

In supravalvular AS, surgery is recommended when aortic arch hypoplasia is less and when the obstruction is discrete and significant (gradient > 50 mm Hg).

In case of valvular aortic stenosis, corrective surgery may be performed only after the patient becomes symptomatic (develops angina, syncope or left ventricular failure) or when the patient develops left ventricular dysfunction, as evidenced by echo, whichever may be earlier. Surgery is in the form of valve replacement and this procedure is delayed as complications developing with a prosthetic valve (infective endocarditis) is more than with the native valve.

Coarctation of the Aorta (Figs 3.106 and 3.107)

In adults, coarctation of the aorta typically consists of a discrete, diaphragm-like ridge that extends into the aortic lumen in the region of the ligamentum arteriosum.

Postductal coarctation: Narrowing of the thoracic aorta immediately distal to the origin of the ductus and left subclavian artery.

Preductal coarctation: Diffuse coarctation of the ascending aorta and transverse aortic arch, often in association with a hypoplastic left ventricle, aortic valve or mitral valve.

In this condition upper half of the body is perfused via the systemic circulation, whereas flow to the lower half of the body comes from the pulmonary artery through a patent ductus arteriosus. This results in "differential cyanosis", where the lower extremities are cyanotic.

Pseudocoarctation: Anatomically there is buckling or kinking of the aorta in the vicinity of ligamentum arteriosum but there is no gradient or development of systemic hypertension or collaterals.

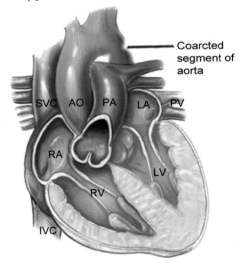

Fig. 3.106: Coarctation of aorta

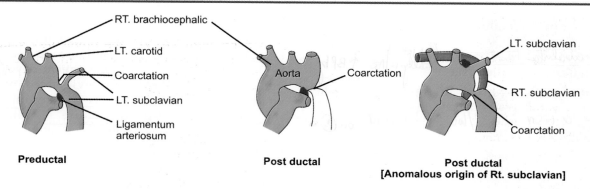

Fig. 3.107: Coarctation of aorta

Associated Cardiac Abnormalities

1. PDA
2. Bicuspid aortic valve
3. VSD.
   85% of patients with COA have bicuspid aortic valve
   15% of patients with bicuspid aortic valve have COA

Coarctation of Aorta Syndromes

Turner syndrome, foetal hydantoin syndrome, Crouzon syndrome.

Clinical Features

- Systolic arterial pressure is higher in the arms than in the legs, but the diastolic pressures are usually similar.
- In comparison to the radial or brachial pulses, the femoral pulses are weak and delayed.
- Systolic thrill may be palpable in the suprasternal notch and left ventricular enlargement may be present.
- A systolic ejection click often is audible (from a bicuspid aortic valve).
- A characteristic rough ejection systolic murmur may be audible along the left sternal border and in the back.
- A continuous murmur may be heard over the interscapular or infrascapular areas, indicating blood flow through collateral channels.
- Coarctation of the abdominal aorta may be associated with renal artery stenosis.

ECG

Evidence of left ventricular hypertrophy is seen.

X-ray Chest

Left ventricular enlargement is seen.

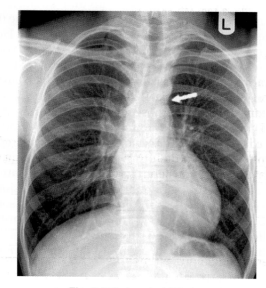

Fig. 3.108: Inverted 'E' sign

Notching of the ribs, due to increased collateral flow through the intercostal arteries, develops along the inferior and posterior aspect of 3rd to 8th ribs, bilaterally.

"Reversed E sign" (due to pre and poststenotic aortic dilatation and dilatation of the subclavian artery) (Fig. 3.108).

Fundus—Cork-screw appearance of retinal arteries.

Complications

1. Bacterial endocarditis (at the site of the coarctation, bicuspid aortic valve or associated collateral channels) (Fig. 3.109).
2. Aortic dissection and rupture of the proximal ascending aorta may occur, sometimes during pregnancy.
3. Leak or rupture of a berry aneurysm (these patients have increased incidence of berry aneurysms of the circle of Willis).

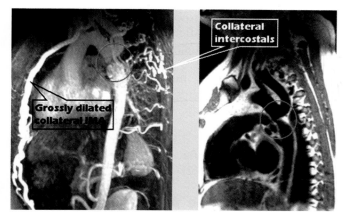

Fig. 3.109: MR angiography showing coarcted segment and collaterals

Treatment

Medical treatment consists of control of hypertension. Surgical treatment consists of resection of the coarctation and reanastomosis or by aortoplasty. Elective surgery should be preferably performed at 4 to 5 years of age, since earlier surgical therapy is likely to result in restenosis of the aortic lumen and later repair may be associated with persistent hypertension.

Anomalous Pulmonary Venous Connection

The term anomalous pulmonary venous connection is used when any (in partial anomalous connection PAPVC) or all (in total anomalous connection— TAPVC) of the pulmonary veins drain into a site other than the left atrium.

TAPVC

In patients with TAPVC, the pulmonary veins may connect to a systemic vein within the thorax (supra-diaphragmatic) or portal vein in abdomen (subdia-phragmatic) (Fig. 3.110).

Associated Cardiac Malformations

1. Common atrium
2. Single ventricle
3. PDA
4. Pulmonary valve stenosis
5. Truncus arteriosus.

Clinical Features

- Almost all patients are cyanotic.
- Some patients may have a continuous murmur along the left sternal border due to flow through the anomalous pulmonary venous channels.
- Pulmonic component of S_2 is accentuated with development of PHT and the murmur becomes less marked or is even absent.
- Patients with TAPVC, with large left to right shunt, without pulmonary hypertension or pulmonary venous obstruction, show clinical findings resembling that of an uncomplicated ostium secundum ASD (except for the presence of cyanosis).

X-ray Chest

Snow man or figure of eight appearance (Fig. 3.111).

PAPVC

This implies that one or more (but not all) of the pulmonary veins are connected to the right atrium or its venous tributaries.

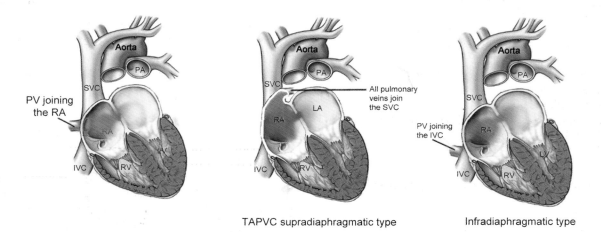

TAPVC supradiaphragmatic type   Infradiaphragmatic type

Fig. 3.110: Types of total anamolous pulmonary venous connection (TAPVC)

- Calcification of annulus or leaflets
- Signs of pulmonary venous hypertension and pulmonary oedema.

Echocardiogram

Dilated LA (giant or aneurysmal left atrium) and LV; Dynamic LV (unless LVF predominates) Regurgitation detectable.

Cardiac Catheterisation

Dilated LA, LV; mitral regurgitation demonstrated; pulmonary hypertension may be present.

Management
Medical

Same as for MS.

ACE inhibitors are useful in the treatment of chronic MR. Intravenous nitroprusside or nitroglycerine reduce the afterload and thereby the volume of regurgitant flow and thus useful in stabilizing patients with acute and or severe MR.

Surgical

- *Indication for surgery* – LV end-systolic dimension of < 45 mm or LVEF < 60 % or both in echocardiogram

Surgery is indicated when there is progressive deterioration in LV function despite antifailure measures.
- Plastic reparative procedure of mitral valve (in young patients).
- Valve replacement in older patients.

Causes of Acute MR

1. Infective endocarditis
2. Trauma
3. Acute rheumatic fever
4. Myocardial infarction (rupture of papillary muscle especially in inferior wall MI)
5. Myocardial abscess
6. Prosthetic valve endocarditis
7. Left atrial myxoma
8. Connective tissue disorders
9. Myxomatous degeneration of the valve.

Surgery for Acute MR

- Failure of medical therapy to stabilize the patient in acute MR
- Stable MR in infective endocarditis surgery is delayed till the completion of antibiotic therapy (If unstable immediate surgery under antibiotic coverage).

Difference between Acute MR and Chronic MR

Features	Acute MR	Chronic MR
Symptoms	Sudden onset of dyspnoea, PND, orthopnoea	Gradual onset of symptoms
Signs:		
Apex beat	Unremarkable	Displaced and dynamic
First heart sound	Soft	Normal/Soft
Murmur	Early/Holosystolic	Holosystolic

Fourth heart sound is heard mainly in the MR of recent onset.

ECG	Normal except in acute myocardial ischaemia	Left atrial enlargement (P-mitrale), Atrial fibrillation, LVH
Radiology and Fluoroscopy	Heart size—Normal	Cardiomegaly (LVH); left atrial enlargement; on fluoroscopy, calcium on valve leaflets
ECHO	Cause of acute MR may be demonstrated (Flail leaflet, ruptured chordae or vegetations)	Cause of chronic MR may be defined

Mitral Valve Prolapse Syndrome (MVPS) (Fig. 3.124)

MVPS is also known as systolic click—murmur syndrome, Barlow syndrome, floppy valve syndrome.

There is excessive or redundant mitral leaflet tissue, with myxomatous degeneration and increased concentrations of acid mucopolysaccharide.

Posterior leaflet is commonly involved. Involvement of anterior leaflet alone is very rare.

Conditions Causing or Associated with MVP

- Idiopathic/Unknown (in majority)
- Genetically determined collagen tissue disorder
- Marfan's syndrome
- Acute rheumatic fever
- Chronic rheumatic heart disease
- Following mitral valvulotomy
- Ischaemic heart disease
- Cardiomyopathies
- Ostium secundum ASD
- Trauma
- LV aneurysm
- Connective tissue disorders.

MVP is more common in females; MVP may present with only a systolic click and murmur with a mild prolapse of the posterior leaflet or with severe MR.

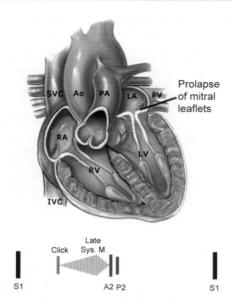

Fig. 3.124: Mitral valve prolapse

MVP is the most common cause of isolated severe MR.

Symptoms

a. Palpitations (due to tachyarrhythmias)
b. Chest pain.

Signs

A mid or late systolic click (about 0.14 sec after S_1) due to sudden tensing of slack, elongated chordae tendineae or by prolapsing mitral valve which reaches its maximum excursion. Clicks may be multiple due to scalloping of the redundant mitral valve.

A high pitched late systolic crescendo-decrescendo murmur (whooping or honking) heard best at the apex.

Click and murmur occur earlier with standing (decreased LV volume); squatting and isometric exercise (increased LV end diastolic volume) delay the click and murmur and may even make them disappear.

Complications

a. Transient cerebral ischaemic attacks (due to emboli from mitral valve)
b. Infective endocarditis when MVP is associated with MR.

ECG

Biphasic or inverted 'T'-waves in leads II, III and aVF and occasional supraventricular or ventricular extrasystole.

Echocardiogram

Useful in identifying the abnormal position and prolapse of the mitral valve leaflets. Mitral valve prolapse is diagnosed when systolic displacement of mitral leaflets >2 mm into the left atrium with coaptation superior to the plane of mitral annulus (Fig. 3.125).

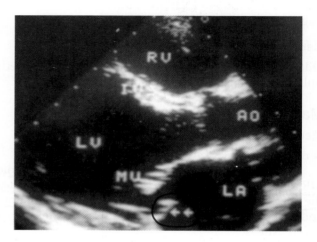

Fig. 3.125: Mitral valve prolapse—flail posterior mitral leaflet pointing towards left atrium

Management

Medical

*   Reassurance
*   Prevention of infective endocarditis, when there is MR
*   Beta blockers for chest pain and tachyarrhythmias
*   Antiarrhythmic agents for VPC's and tachyarrhythmias
*   Aspirin for TIA.

Surgical

When MR becomes severe, either reconstruction or valve replacement may be done.

Most common cause of combined mitral stenosis and mitral regurgitation is rheumatic heart disease.

Aortic Stenosis (AS) (Fig. 3.126)

Common Causes

*   Congenital aortic stenosis (supravalvular AS, valvular AS, subvalvular AS)
*   Rheumatic aortic stenosis
*   Degenerative (senile) calcific aortic stenosis
*   Atherosclerotic aortic stenosis (common after 65 years).

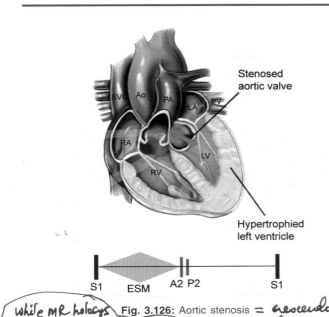

Stenosed
aortic valve

Hypertrophied
left ventricle

S1	ESM	A2 P2	S1

while MR holocys =

Fig. 3.126: Aortic stenosis = crescendo decrescendo ESM

Patients with rheumatic aortic stenosis almost always have concomitant mitral valve involvement.

Symptoms

Angina, dyspnoea, syncope, dizziness, sudden death (may be as a result of intolerance to complete heart block or atrial tachyarrhythmia).

Pure aortic valve disease may remain asymptomatic for 10–15 years.

Signs

- Slow rising, small volume pulse } same as MS°
- Heaving apex beat   } MR = hyperdynamic apex
- S_4 may be heard
- Ejection click (indicates valvular AS and excludes supra and subvalvular AS; disappears on calcification of aortic valve)
- Carotid thrill (shudder) is felt
- A rough, ejection systolic murmur loudest in the aortic area radiating to the carotids and the apex.

Severity

1. *According to S_2*
   Mild stenosis A_2 followed by P_2
   Moderate stenosis A_2 is delayed giving rise to single S_2
   Severe stenosis   Reverse splitting of S_2 (P_2-A_2).

2. *According to valve area*
   Normal aortic valve area is 3 cm^2–4 cm^2
   In severe aortic stenosis, valve area is < 0.75 cm^2/m^2 body surface area.

In critical aortic stenosis, valve area is < 0.5 cm^2/m^2 body surface area.

3. *Long murmur and late peaking of murmur indicate severe AS.*

4. *According to the gradient across aortic valve*
   Normal gradient   0 mm Hg
   Stenotic gradient
     Mild AS   < 30 mm Hg
     Moderate AS   30–50 mm Hg
     Severe AS   > 50 mm Hg

   compare. 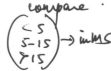 → in MS

5. *Presence of S_4 and absent A_2 indicate severe AS.*

6. *Presence of S_3 in AS means severe systolic dysfunction and elevated filling pressure.*

Silent AS

Severe AS with CCF (low cardiac output).

In this situation, AS murmur is not heard. But murmur reappears on treating failure.

When MS is associated with AS, usually MS masks the signs of AS.

Complications

Left ventricular failure
Arrhythmias including sudden death
Complete heart block
Infective endocarditis.

Investigations

ECG

- LVH with strain pattern
- LBBB, complete heart block if calcification of valve extends into the conducting system.

X-ray Chest

Post stenotic dilatation of ascending aorta in valvular AS; Calcification of aortic valve on fluoroscopy or lateral view.

Echocardiogram

Calcified valve, hypertrophied LV, Doppler estimate of gradient.

Cardiac Catheterisation

Systolic gradient between LV and aorta; post stenotic dilatation of aorta; regurgitation of aortic valve may be present.

Coronary Angiogram

To rule out coronary artery disease only in patients with AS developing symptoms of angina.

Prognosis

Patients developing angina have a life expectancy of about 4 years. Patients developing syncope have a life expectancy of about 3 years. Patients developing LVF have a life expectancy of about 2 years.

Management

Medical

Treatment of cardiac failure
Rheumatic fever prophylaxis
Infective endocarditis prophylaxis.

Use diuretics with caution to avoid volume depletion in the management of cardiac failure. Similarly digitalis and vasodilators – ACE inhibitors should be avoided in moderate or severe aortic stenosis. Nitroglycerine is useful for the relief of angina. Statins are useful in the management of degenerative calcific aortic stenosis.

Surgical

- Patients are prone for Stokes-Adams attacks and sudden death and so valve replacement is normally needed.
- *Valve replacement* when systolic gradient across the valve is > 50 mm Hg and when there is progressive LV dysfunction.
- If patient is unfit for surgery, *percutaneous, transluminal aortic valvuloplasty* can be tried. It is also useful in children and young adults with congenital AS, and also as a bridge to surgery in patients with severe LV dysfunction.
- *Simple commissural incision* under direct vision is done in children and adolescents with non-calcific congenital AS; it is indicated in symptomatic patients and also for asymptomatic patients with pressure gradient above 50 mm Hg, i.e., aortic valve orifice is < 0.75 cm².

Aortic Regurgitation (AR) (Fig. 3.127)

Causes

Aortic Valve Involvement

Rheumatic heart disease
Infective endocarditis
Congenital bicuspid aortic valve.

Aortic Wall Involvement

Syphilis
Rheumatoid arthritis
Ankylosing spondylitis
Marfan's syndrome

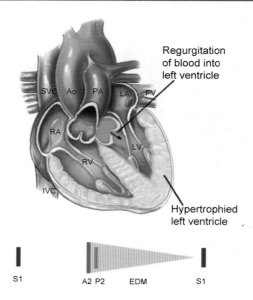

Fig. 3.127: Aortic regurgitation

Ehlers-Danlos syndrome
Takayasu's arteritis – *due TB antigens*
Aortic dissection
Systemic hypertension.

Symptoms

Dyspnoea, palpitation, angina (in severe AR).

Signs of Wide Pulse Pressure

1. *Light house sign* (alternate flushing and blanching of forehead).
2. *Landolfi's sign* (Change in pupillary size in accordance with cardiac cycle and not related to light).
3. Retinal artery pulsations (*Becker's sign*).
4. *de Musset's sign* (head bobbing with each heart beat).
5. *Muller's sign*—Systolic pulsations of uvula.
6. *Quincke's sign* (capillary pulsations) can be detected by pressing a glass slide on patients lip or nail bed.
7. Dancing carotids (*Corrigan's sign*).
8. Locomotor brachii.
9. Collapsing or water-hammer pulse (↑ systolic pressure and ↓ diastolic pressure); usually pulse pressure is more than the diastolic pressure.
10. Bisferiens pulse.
11. Pistol shot femorals (*Traube's sign*).
12. *Duroziez's sign*—systolic murmur heard over femoral artery when it is compressed proximally and a diastolic murmur when it is compressed distally using the 'bell' of the stethoscope.

Duroziez murmur—diastolic murmur heard with the diaphragm of the stethoscope when distal pressure is applied.

13. *Hill's sign*—popliteal cuff systolic pressure exceeds brachial cuff pressure by > 20 mm Hg.

Mild AR	20–40 mm Hg
Moderate AR	40–60 mm Hg
Severe AR	> 60 mm Hg.

14. *Rosenbach's sign*—pulsations of liver.
15. *Gerhardt's sign*—pulsations over enlarged spleen.

Other Signs

- Apical impulse is displaced downwards and outwards and hyperdynamic in nature.
- Soft S_1 (only in acute AR)
- S_3 may be heard
  A high frequency decresendo early diastolic murmur immediately after A_2, best heard in left 3rd or 4th spaces with the diaphragm of the stethoscope with the patient leaning forwards, in expiration.
- Flow ESM across aortic valve heard at heart base, conducted to carotids.
- Flow MDM across mitral valve (*Austin-Flint murmur*). In MS, there is loud S_1 and there is opening snap.

Severity

The presence of the following indicate severe AR:

a. Duration of murmur (> 2/3 of diastole) is directly proportional to the severity. In moderate to severe AR, murmur becomes holodiastolic and may have a rough quality.
b. Bisferiens pulse
c. Hill's sign > 60 mm Hg.
d. Apical impulse (down and out)
e. Austin-Flint murmur
f. Marked peripheral signs.

In the presence of heart failure, due to peripheral vaso-constriction, there may be a rise in arterial diastolic pressure. This may cause an erroneous judgement as to the severity of AR. Proper assessment can be done, only after correcting the failure.

ECG

LV enlargement (volume overload) – 'q'-waves in V_5, V_6.

X-ray Chest

- Gross cardiomegaly (Cor Bovinum)
- In syphilitic AR, there may be calcification of ascending aorta

- In bicuspid aortic valve or rheumatic AR, there may be calcification of the aortic valve.

Echocardiogram

Dilated LV, hyperdynamic ventricle, fluttering anterior mitral leaflet; Doppler detects reflux (Fig. 3.128).

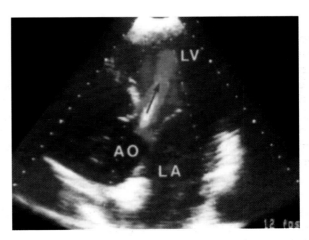

Fig. 3.128: Colour Doppler flow imaging aortic regurgitation

Cardiac Catheterisation

Dilated LV, aortic regurgitation
Dilated aortic root.

Management

Medical

Antifailure measures
Rheumatic fever prophylaxis
Infective endocarditis prophylaxis.
Vasodilators like ACE inhibitors are very useful in the management of AR.

Surgical

Early left ventricular systolic dysfunction even in the absence of symptoms is an indication for surgery

a. Valve replacement
b. Surgical repair in case of perforation of a leaflet by infective endocarditis or in case of a torn leaflet.
c. Narrowing of annulus or excising a portion of the aortic root without replacing the valve.
d. Echocardiogram must be performed every year and aortic valve replacement is indicated in patients with end-systolic dimension >55 mm or end-systolic volume >55 ml/m² or ejection fraction <55% (Rule of 55) or end-diastolic dimension >75 mm.

than 125 mEq/L to prevent arrhythmias and neurologic abnormalities. Water intake may be ad libitum in all but the most severe forms of CCF.

Dialysis and Ultrafiltration

This procedure is indicated in severe HF with renal dysfunction. Therapeutic paracentesis, phlebotomy, rotating tourniquet are other mechanical methods of fluid removal which are useful in the management of refractory failure.

B. Pharmacologic Therapy

1. Diuretics

a. *High potency loop diuretics (Furosemide, Bumetanide, Ethacrynic acid):* These drugs are most useful in severe heart failure and also in the presence of impaired renal function. Furosemide causes direct venodilatation and reduces preload. It also prevents reabsorption of Na^+ and Cl^- from thick ascending limb of loop of Henle and also from proximal tubule. In severe failure, IV route is preferable since the GIT mucosal congestion may interfere with absorption of orally administered drug.

Dose
Furosemide—40 to 200 mg/day
Bumetanide—0.5 to 2 mg—maximum 10 mg/day
Ethacrynic acid—25 to 100 mg/day
Torsemide – 5 mg IV / 10 mg od or bid.

Adverse effects: Hypokalaemia, hypomagnesemia, hypocalcemia, hyperglycemia, hyperuricemia, ototoxicity, rash, vasculitis and postural hypotension. Allergic reactions are less with ethacrynic acid than with other loop diuretics and thiazides due to absence of sulfhydryl moiety.

b. *Medium potency thiazide diuretics:* They are useful in mild cardiac failure and in the presence of normal renal function. They act in the distal tubule except metolazone which acts in the proximal and distal tubule. Indapamide is a long acting drug and it has fewer side effects on serum lipids.

Dose:
Chlorothiazides—250 to 500 mg/day
Hydrochlorothiazide—25 to 100 mg/day
Chlorthalidone—25 to 100 mg/day
Metolazone—2.5 to 20 mg/day
Indapamide—5 to 10 mg/day.

Adverse effects: Hypokalaemia, hyponatraemia, hypomagnesemia, hyperglycaemia, hypercalcaemia, hyperuricaemia, hyperlipidaemia, alkalosis, pancreatitis, vasculitis, rash.

c. *Low potency potassium sparing diuretics:* They are weak diuretics and they act in the distal tubule and collecting duct. They are contraindicated in the presence of renal failure. Concomitant use of ACE inhibitors, NSAIDs, and presence of DM increase the risk of hyperkalaemia.

Dose
Spironolactone—50 to 200 mg/day
Triamterene—100 to 200 mg/day
Amiloride—5 to 10 mg/day.

Adverse effects: Hyperkalaemia, acidosis, and in addition, for spironolactone, gynaecomastia and for triamterene, renal stone and ARF when used with indomethacin.

2. Vasodilator Therapy

Vasodilators are used to minimize the workload to the heart. Arterial dilators reduce the afterload and the venodilators reduce the preload to the heart. In the presence of volume depletion with hypotension, vasodilators should be used with caution. Vasodilators are not beneficial in HF with outflow tract obstruction and predominant diastolic dysfunction (Restrictive or hypertrophic cardiomyopathy or tamponade).

a. *Oral Vasodilators*

i. *ACE inhibitors:* They inhibit the formation of angiotensin II (powerful vasoconstrictor) by blocking angiotensin converting enzyme and this blockade results in reduction of preload and afterload.

Dose
Captopril—6.5 to 25 mg tid
Enalapril—2.5 to 20 mg bid
Lisinopril—2.5 to 10 mg od
Quinapril—10 to 40 mg od
Ramipril—1.25 to 5 mg bid
Fosinopril—5 to 10 mg od can be used bid
Benazepril—5 to 10 mg od can be used bid
Moexipril—5 to 7.5 mg od can be used bid
Trandolapril—1 to 2 mg od
Spirapril—12.5 to 50 mg bid
Cilazapril—2.5 to 5 mg bid
Perindopril—1 to 16 mg bid

Adverse effects: First dose hypotension, (withhold the diuretics for 24 hours before starting ACE inhibitors), dry cough, altered taste, skin rash, hyperkalaemia. They should not be given when the serum creatinine is more than 3 mg% and in bilateral renal artery stenosis. Agranulocytosis and angioedema are common with captopril because of the presence of sulfhydryl moiety.

Verapamil } DHP ℗
diltiazem } (ditropdisopyrnidine)

ACE inhibitor is very useful in postinfarction failure with reduced ejection fraction below 40%. The reduction in workload allows the ventricle to remodel and reduce the incidence of development of severe cardiac failure.

In ACE inhibitors intolerant patients angiotensin receptor blockers can be used with equal efficacy.

ii. *Nitrates:* They are predominantly venodilators and are useful in CHD with HF. It relieves venous and pulmonary congestion.

Dose
Isosorbide dinitrate—5 to 20 mg qid
Isosorbide mononitrate—10 to 20 mg tid
Nitroglycerin sustained release—2.5 to 9 mg bid
Transdermal nitroglycerin patches—5 to 15 mg bid.
 Headache is the main adverse effect and that might subside with sustained therapy; nitrate tolerance can be prevented by nitrate free interval of at least 10 to 12 hours/day.

iii. *Hydralazine:* It is an arterial dilator and it reduces the afterload. It is useful in the presence of valvular regurgitant lesions with volume overload. By combining it with nitrate a balanced preload and afterload reduction can be achieved.

Dose: Hydralazine—25 to 100 mg tid.

Adverse effects: Reflex tachycardia (use with caution in IHD), headache, flushing, nausea, vomiting, fluid retention and SLE like syndrome.

iv. *Adrenergic blockers*

a. *Alpha-Blockers:* They are powerful vasodilators and they reduce the systemic vascular resistance and thereby reduce the afterload. However, the adverse effects like orthostatic hypotension and reflex tachycardia limit their role in the management of heart failure.

b. *Beta-Blockers:* The adverse effects of endogenous catecholamines on the failing heart can be antagonised by beta-blockers. Beta-blockers with ISA activity like pindolol, xamoterol have been tried. A minimum of two months therapy is required to demonstrate improvement in ejection fraction and exercise tolerance. Caution must be exercised in advocating beta-blockers in HF with low ejection fraction. They are useful in hypertrophic cardiomyopathy, dynamic outflow tract obstruction and those with diastolic dysfunction.

The drugs approved for use in cardiac failure are carvedilol, metoprolol and bisoprolol.

v. *Calcium Channel Blockers:* Even though they dilate the vascular smooth muscle, their negative inotropic

effect limit the usage in HF. Amlodipine and felodipine are preferable than verapamil and diltiazem in the management of heart failure especially in the presence of diastolic dysfunction. They enhance the diastolic relaxation of the ventricle (lusitropic effect). They are absolutely contraindicated in cardiac failure with low ejection fraction (below 40%).

b. *Parenteral Vasodilators*

They are useful in severe HF. Central haemodynamic monitoring and optimal titration of dosage are essential.

Nitroglycerin: It is a potent venodilator and it relieves systemic and pulmonary venous congestion. This drug is useful in myocardial infarction with HF and also in unstable angina. The dose is 10 to 200 μg/minute. The adverse effects are hypotension and nitrate tolerance.

Sodium nitroprusside: It is a potent arterial dilator and it is very useful in severe hypertensive heart failure and in valvular regurgitant lesions with volume overload.

Dose: 10 to 300 μg/minute
In IHD it can cause coronary steal. Serum thiocyanate level should be monitored. Levels above 10 mg/dl is manifested as abdominal pain, nausea, seizure, change in the conscious level and metabolic acidosis especially in the presence of renal failure.

Enalaprilat: It can be used in the dose of 1.25 to 5 mg IV six hourly. The indications and adverse effects are similar to oral form of enalapril.

Recombinant BNP-Nesiritide: It can be used as a parenteral vasodilator in a dose of 2μg/kg IV bolus followed by continuous IV infusion of 0.01 – 0.03 μg/kg/minute. Hypotension is the most common side effect of nesiritide. Avoid using it in cardiogenic shock and in patients with systolic blood pressure < 90 mm of Hg. Episodes of hypotension can be treated with volume expansion vasopressor drugs.

3. Digitalis

Digoxin is the most effective drug in the management of heart failure especially in the presence of:
a. Supraventricular tachycardia
b. Dilated left ventricle (increased TCD, 3rd heart sound)
c. Impaired systolic function (low ejection fraction).
It causes reversible inhibition of sarcolemmal sodium-potassium adenosine triphosphatase. This enhances the myocardial contractility (positive inotropic effect). It slows conduction and prolongs refractory

NB

↑ contractility (+ve inotropic)
↓ conduction (-ve chronotropic)

period in AV node, and purkinje fibres (negative chronotropic effect) and thus reduces the ventricular rate. However, it shortens the refractory period and enhances the excitability in the atria, ventricles and accessory conduction pathways (atrial and ventricular tachyarrhythmias as in toxic doses).

Conduction velocity and effective refractory period are increased in atrium and ventricle. It improves cardiac output and augments ejection fraction. It has little value in hypertrophic cardiomyopathy, myocarditis, constrictive pericarditis, mitral stenosis in sinus rhythm without right ventricular involvement and chronic cor pulmonale. It has no effect in HF with diastolic dysfunction with preserved systolic function and good ejection fraction. The toxic therapeutic ratio is narrow. Hypokalaemia, hypoxaemia, hypomagnesemia and hypercalcaemia potentiates digitoxicity. Digoxin should be administered with caution in elderly patients with hypothyroidism and in renal failure.

Dose

Digitalising dose: Adult—1 to 1.5 mg. Initiate with 0.5 mg and follow it with 0.25 mg qid. This schedule is implemented in patients who have not received digitalis therapy earlier.

Maintenance dose: Digoxin—0.25 mg od or bid. Maintain serum level of digoxin between 1 to 2 ng/ml.

Drug interactions: Antacids, cholestyramine, kaolin-pectin, bran, neomycin, sulfasalazine and PAS can impair the absorption of digoxin. Digoxin levels are increased by oral erythromycin and tetracycline, quinidine, verapamil, flecainide and amiodarone.

Adverse effects

GIT symptoms: Anorexia, nausea, vomiting, diarrhoea are signs of digitoxicity (if the above symptoms occur only after the initiation of digitalis therapy and not present earlier due to GIT mucosal congestion).

Neurological symptoms: Headache, fatigue, malaise, disorientation, delirium, confusion, convulsions, visual symptoms like scotomas, flickering halos, altered colour vision.

Cardiac toxicities: Bradycardia, multiple VPCs, ventricular bigemini (hallmark of digitoxicity), PAT, VT, VF and any type of cardiac arrhythmias except sinus tachycardia, bundle branch block and Mobitz type II block.

Other manifestations: Gynaecomastia, skin rash and sexual dysfunction.

Management of digitoxicity: Stop digoxin and correct the electrolyte abnormalities, titrate the dose of diuretics. Correct the bradycardia with IV atropine 0.6 mg or temporary pacing. Treat the atrial or ventricular arrhythmias with phenytoin, beta-blockers or lidocaine (never treat with quinidine or verapamil). Cardioversion is usually contraindicated in digitalis induced arrhythmias. However, as a last resort it can be tried in low joules after discontinuing the digitalis, under cover of lidocaine infusion.

Digoxin specific Fab antibody fragment: Fab antibody fragments are considered when other modes of therapy fail. Each 40 mg vial (add 4 ml sterile water) is given in the form of infusion in 100 ml of normal saline in 30 minutes (80 drops/mt). It will neutralize 0.6 mg of digoxin. Dose can be calculated as follows:

Number of vials =   Serum level (ng/ml) × Weight in kg/100.

4. Sympathomimetic Amines

Norepinephrine, epinephrine, isoprenaline, dopamine and dobutamine. These drugs improve cardiac output and improve tissue perfusion at the expense of increased oxygen demand.

Dopamine: It increases renal blood flow, GFR and sodium excretion by stimulating specific dopaminergic receptors at doses of 1 to 3 µg/kg/minute. By stimulating beta$_1$ adrenoreceptors at doses of 3 to 5 µg/kg/minute, it increases the myocardial contractility (inotropic effect) and heart rate. At a higher doses of 5 to 10 µg/kg/minute it causes vasoconstriction by stimulating alpha-adreno-receptors resulting in elevation of blood pressure. Dopamine should be used primarily to stabilize the hypotensive patient. When large doses of dopamine are required for inotropic effect, nitroprusside or nitroglycerin can be infused simultaneously to counteract the vasoconstrictor action. It is widely used in the management of acute heart failure.

Dobutamine: It is a synthetic catecholamine with marked beta$_1$ and weak beta$_2$ and alpha receptor activity. In contrast to dopamine, dobutamine is not a renal vasodilator. A low dose infusion of dopamine may be added to dobutamine to obtain a balanced renal vasodilator and inotropic effect. The dose is 2.5 to 10 µg/kg/minute.

Adverse effects: Precipitation of myocardial ischaemia, ventricular arrhythmias; dopamine can cause severe peripheral vasoconstriction resulting in digital gangrene and local tissue necrosis at the site of extravasation. Inject at the site of extravasation 5 mg of phentolamine mixed with saline to prevent tissue necrosis.

Digitoxicity : Ventricular bigemini

5. Phosphodiesterase Inhibitors
Inamrinone

(Amrinone, Milrinone, Enoximone, Pimobendan)

They exert positive inotropic and vasodilator effect through the inhibition of phosphodiesterase III which is a membrane bound enzyme responsible for the breakdown of cyclic AMP. They are indicated for short term treatment of refractory heart failure. They reduce the pulmonary and systemic vascular resistance and have a favourable effect on myocardial oxygen consumption. Long-term administration increases the mortality in chronic failure.

Dose
Amrinone—750 μg/kg bolus followed by 2.5 to 10 μg/kg/minute.
Milrinone—50 μg/kg bolus followed by 0.5 to 0.75 μg/kg/minute.

Adverse effects: Cardiac arrhythmias and thrombocytopenia.

Mechanical Circulatory Support

This may be considered when medical measures fail either in transient myocardial dysfunction or when alternative procedures like CABG or cardiac transplantation are planned.
a. Intra-aortic balloon pump
b. Ventricular assist devices
c. Enhanced external counterpulsation
d. Resynchronization therapy/biventricular pacing.
   Cardiac resynchronization therapy or biventricular pacing in cases of refractory failure with conduction abnormalities like LBBB may be beneficial.

Management of cardiogenic pulmonary oedema:
1. Strict bed-rest to reduce cardiac workload.
2. Sitting position to improve pulmonary function by relieving pulmonary congestion.
3. Oxygen by nasal cannula or mask to raise PaO_2 more than 60 mm of Hg.
4. *Morphine sulphate* (2 to 5 mg IV) is used to relieve anxiety and it results in pulmonary and systemic venous dilatation.
5. *Furosemide*—A potent venodilator 40 to 80 mg IV relieves pulmonary congestion even before the commencement of diuresis.
6. *Nitroglycerin* (5 μg/minute) potentiates the effect of furosemide. Avoid hypotension and keep the systolic pressure above 90 mm of Hg.
7. *Nitroprusside* is more useful in pulmonary oedema resulting from valvular regurgitant lesions or systemic hypertension.
8. *Dobutamine-dopamine-phosphodiesterase inhibitors* are used in the presence of cardiogenic shock.
9. *Aminophylline*—250 to 500 mg slow IV is given in some cases to relieve bronchoconstriction and to augment myocardial contractility.
10. Mechanical aids: a) Rotating tourniquets b) Phlebotomy.
11. Treat the precipitating cause.

Systemic Hypertension (Fig. 3.132)

Seventh Report of the Joint National Committee: (JNC 7)

Category	Systolic pressure (mm Hg)	Diastolic pressure (mm Hg)
Normal	< 120	< 80
Pre-hypertension	120-139	80-89
Hypertension		
Stage 1	140-159	90-99
Stage 2	>160	>100
Isolated systolic Hypertension	>140	< 90

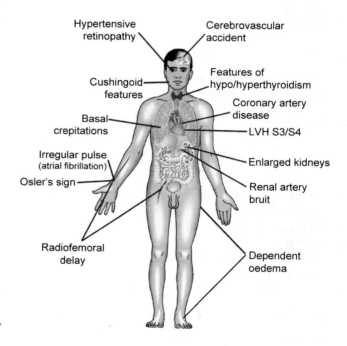

Fig. 3.132: Systemic hypertension

Primary (Essential)—94%

Secondary—6%

Renal (4%)
Vascular   Renal artery stenosis
Parenchymal   Glomerulonephritis (acute/chronic)

Chronic pyelonephritis
Polycystic kidneys
Amyloidosis
Diabetes.

Endocrine (1%)
Acromegaly
Hyperthyroidism
Hypothyroidism
Hyperparathyroidism
Cushing's syndrome
Conn's syndrome
Pheochromocytoma.

Miscellaneous (1%)
Drugs
1. Steroids
Anabolic steroids
Corticosteroids
Oral contraceptive pills
2. Cyclosporine
3. Beta receptor agonists
4. Sympathomimetics (Cold remedies/Nasal Drops)
5. NSAIDs.
Coarctation of aorta.

Causes of Isolated Systolic Hypertension

1. Atherosclerosis (old age)
2. Coarctation of aorta
3. Severe AR
4. Thyrotoxicosis.

Factors Influencing Prognosis

I. Used for Risk Stratification

a. Levels of systolic and diastolic BP (grade I-III)
b. Men > 55 years
c. Women > 65 years
d. Smoking
e. Total cholesterol 250 mg%
f. Diabetes mellitus
g. Family history of premature CVD

II. Other Factors Adversely Influencing Prognosis

a. Reduced HDL cholesterol
b. Raised LDL cholesterol
c. Microalbuminuria in diabetes/HT
d. Impaired glucose tolerance
e. Obesity
f. Sedentary lifestyle
g. Raised fibrinogen
h. High-risk socioeconomic group
i. High risk ethnic group
j. High risk geographic region

III. Target Organ Damage (TOD)

a. LVH
b. Proteinuria or slight elevation of plasma creatinine (1.2-2 mg%)
c. Radiological evidence of atherosclerotic plaque (carotid, femoral, iliac, aorta)
d. Generalised or focal narrowing of retinal arteriole

IV. Associated Clinical Conditions (ACC)

a. Cerebrovascular disease (infarcts, haemorrhages, TIA)
b. Heart disease (MI, angina, CCF, coronary revascularisation)
c. Renal disease (nephropathy, renal failure—P. creatinine > 2 mg%)
d. Vascular disease (dissecting aneurysm, symptomatic arterial disease)
e. Advanced hypertensive retinopathy (grade III and IV)

Risk stratification to quantify prognosis

Other risk factors and disease history	BLOOD PRESSURE (mmHg)		
	Grade I	Grade II	Grade III
I. No other risk factor	Low risk	Medium risk	High risk
II. 1 to 2 risk factors	Medium risk	High risk	Very high risk
III 3 or > risk factors or TOD or Diabetes	High risk	High risk	Very high risk
IV. ACC	Very high risk	Very high risk	Very high risk

Investigations

Investigation of Hypertension (All Patients)

- Urine analysis: protein, glucose, haematuria
- Plasma urea/creatinine
- Chest radiograph (cardiomegaly, heart failure, rib notching)
- ECG (left ventricular hypertrophy, ischaemia)
- Plasma electrolytes (hypokalaemic alkalosis in the absence of diuretic therapy may indicate primary or secondary hyperaldosteronism)
- Plasma cholesterol/triglycerides.

Investigation of Hypertension (Patients Suspected of having Secondary Hypertension)

- Intravenous urogram, ultrasound (if renal disease is suspected)

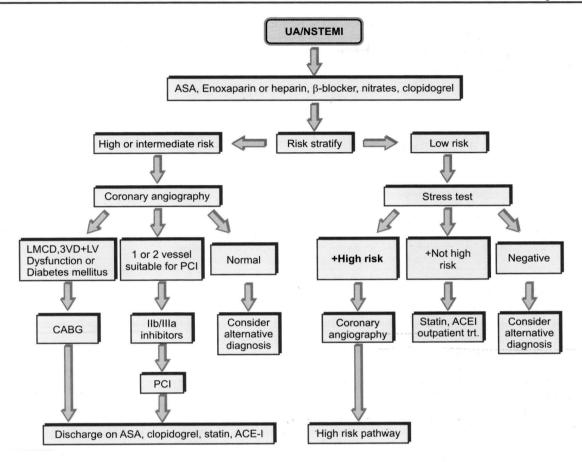

Fig. 3.134: Acute management of unstable angina or non-ST elevation myocardial infarction

is also distinguished from ST-elevation MI by the absence of persistent ST segment elevation.

Pathogenesis

1. Plaque rupture or erosion with superimposed non-occlusive thrombus (most common)
2. Progressive mechanical obstruction – either rapidly advancing coronary atherosclerosis or restenosis following percutaneous coronary intervention.
3. Increased discrepancy between myocardial oxygen demand and supply.

Management (Fig. 3.134)

Immediately assess the following:
- Clinical evaluation – history and physical examination
- 12 – lead ECG recording
- Measurement of cardiac specific markers – troponin and CK-MB.

All ACS patients should be placed on aspirin, β-blocker, nitrate and clopidogrel immediately.

Low risk patients – On observation if the patient remains pain-free with normal ECG and normal levels of cardiac markers, submit them for stress ECG. If the stress test is negative, consider alternative diagnosis. If the stress test is positive continue medication and invasive testing when required.

Intermediate and high risk patients – Patient has to be admitted in the intensive care unit and to be managed with anti-ischaemia, antiplatelet and anticoagulant group of drugs. In the meantime coronary angiography is planned.

Antiplatelet Therapy

A. Aspirin (75-150 mg/day after lunch or immediately on admission) reduces subsequent MI and cardiac death.

Risk Stratification of ACS

Features	High risk	Intermediate risk	Low risk
Clinical history	Accelerating tempo of ischaemic symptoms in preceding 48 hours	Prior MI, peripheral or cerebro-vascular disease, CABG orprior aspirin use	
Classical pain	Prolonged ongoing> 30 min rest pain	Prolonged > 20 min rest angina, now resolved, with high likelihood of CAD, rest angina < 20 min relieved with SL-TNG	New-onset or Progressive angina in the past 2 weeks with moderate or high likelihood of CAD
Clinical findings	Pulmonary oedema, Worsening MR, S_3, Hypotension, tachycardia, bradycardia, Age > 75 years	Age > 70 years	
ECG	Transient ST changes> 0.05 mV, new bundle branch block or VT	T wave inversions> 0.2 mV Pathological Q waves	Normal or unchanged ECG
Biochemical cardiac markers	Elevated troponin or CK-MB (TnT or TnI> 0.1ng/mL)	Borderline elevation (TnT >0.01 but <0.1 ng/mL)	Normal

CRP (c-reactive protein) levels > 3 mg/L represent a high risk group.
Thrombolytic therapy is not indicated in ACS.

B. Clopidogrel (loading dose 300 mg followed by 75 mg/day) in aspirin intolerant patients.
   Added benefit in reducing the motality is achieved by combining both aspirin and clopidogrel and can be used for a minimum of one month if PCI is planned or maximum of 9 months.

C. Glycoprotein (GP) IIb/IIIa antagonists – abciximab (ReoPRO) or eptifibatide(Integrilin) or tirofiban (Aggrastat) should be considered for high risk patients. They should be used in conjunction with heparin. If early invasive strategy is planned any one of the molecule can be used. If early invasive strategy is not planned, one of the small molecule either eptifibatide or tirofiban can be used.

Anticoagulant Therapy

Dalteparin – (Fragmin) 120 IU/kg SC 12 hr (Maximum 10,000 IU bid)

Enoxaparin – (Lovenox) 30 mg IV bolus followed by 1 mg/kg SC bid

Heparin (unfractionated -UFH) 60-70 U/kg (maximum 5000 U)IV followed by infusion 12-15 u/kg/hr
(Initial maximum 1000 U/hr) titrated to achieve a PTT 1.5-2.5 times control.

Compared with UFH, LMWH produces more predictable anticoagulant response because of the better bioavailability, longer half-life and dose independent clearance. Enoxaparin 1 mg/kg bid subcutaneously is the only LMWH found to confer greater cardiac benefit.

Coronary Angiography

Coronary angiography is performed for high/intermediate risk patients (Fig. 3.136).

CABG: Left main disease, triple vessel disease, LV dysfunction or diabetes mellitus

GP IIb/IIIa receptor inhibitors in ACS -IV

Feature	Abciximab	Eptifibatide	Tirofiban
Drug type	Monoclonal antibody	Cyclic heptapeptide	Nonpeptide
Dosage	0.25 mg IV bolus then 0.125 mg/kg/min (max 10 µg/min) × 12 hr-ACS planned for PCI	180 µg/kg bolus then 2 µg/kg/min × 24-48 hours	0.4 µg/kg/min for 30 min, then 0.1 µg/kg/min × 24-48 hrs
Metabolism	Cellular catabolism	Renal –modify dose in renal failure	Renal – modify dose in renal failure
Recovery of platelet inhibition	48-96 hrs	4-6 hrs	4-6 hrs
Reversibility	Platelet transfusion	None	None

PCI: 1or 2 vessel disease –GP IIb/IIIa inhibitors followed by PCI.

If coronary angiography is normal consider alternative diagnosis.

Myocardial Infarction (MI)

Irreversible necrosis of part of the heart muscle is almost always due to coronary atherosclerosis.

Incidence

5/1000 per year. Fifty per cent of deaths due to MI occur within 1-2 hrs after the onset of symptoms.

Risk Factors

Category I (For which interventions have been proved to lower CVD risks)

1. Raised LDL cholesterol
2. Reduced HDL cholesterol
3. Atherogenic diet
4. Cigarette smoking
5. Hypertension
6. LVH
7. Thrombogenic factors

Category II (For which interventions are likely to lower CVD risks)

1. Diabetes mellitus
2. Physical inactivity
3. Increased triglycerides
4. Small dense LDL
5. Obesity

Category III (Associated with increased CVD risk that, if modified, might lower risk)

1. Psychosocial factors
2. Increased Lipoprotein a (normal level—0-3 mg/dl)
3. Hyperhomocysteinemias
4. No alcohol consumption
5. Oxidative stress
6. Postmenopausal status

Category IV (associated with increased CVD risk which cannot be modified)

1. Age
2. Male gender
3. Low socioeconomic status
4. Family history of early onset CVD

Symptoms

Anginal pain is of greater severity and is associated with nausea, vomiting, sweating and extreme distress.

Painless infarcts are common in diabetics and in the elderly, due to autonomic neuropathy.

Signs

Tachycardia, bradycardia, VPCs, gallop
There may be hyper or hypotension
Cold and clammy extremities
Cyanosis may be present
Mild pyrexia (< 38.5°C)
Features of complications (LV failure, pulmonary oedema, arrhythmias).

Syndrome X

- Ischaemic chest pain in the presence of normal coronary arteries
- It is probably due to microvascular disease of the heart
- Prognosis is good when compared with classic CAD patients.

Investigations

ECG

- May be normal initially and hence serial ECGs must be taken.
- ST elevation and T-wave inversion with pathological Q-waves are typically seen in leads adjacent to the infarcted segment of myocardium.
- Reciprocal ST depression or T-wave inversion in opposite leads.
- A non Q-wave infarct may occur and has a high risk of mortality (as they are prone to develop dangerous arrhythmias and recurrent angina).

X-ray Chest

Signs of heart failure or pulmonary oedema.

Cardiac Enzymes

a. *CPK-MB:* This cardiac isoenzyme starts rising within 4–6 hrs after development of acute MI, peaks during the 2nd day (4 fold rise) and disappears in 2–3 days.
   Other causes of total CK elevation:
   1. Skeletal diseases – Polymyositis, Muscle dystrophy, Myopathies
   2. Electrical cardioversion
   3. Skeletal muscle damage – trauma, convulsions, immobilization
   4. Hypothyroidism
   5. Stroke
   6. Surgery
b. *AST:* Starts rising on the 1st day, peaks in 2–3 days (3 fold rise) and disappears by 3rd day.

c. *LDH₁*: Starts rising by second day, peaks around 3–4 days (3 fold rise) and disappears in 10 days.

d. *Troponin T:* Cardiac troponin T is a regulatory contractile protein not normally found in blood. Its detection in the circulation has been shown to be a sensitive and specific marker for myocardial cell damage.

Troponin T and I reach a reliable diagnostic level in plasma by 12-16 hrs, maximal activity by 24-32 hrs, returns to normal in 10-12 days.

Troponin I : 0-0.4 ng/ml
Troponin T: 0-0.1 ng/ml

Cardiac troponins are detected in the serum by using monoclonal antibodies. These antibodies have negligible cross reactivity to skeletal muscle. Cardiac troponins I and T start to rise within 3-4 hours after myocardial infarction and remain raised for 4-10 days (Fig. 3.135).

Other causes of elevated cardiac troponins:

Cardiac causes:
• Cardiac contusion/surgery
• Myocarditis
• Cardiomyopathy
• Heart failure
• Cardioversion
• Percutaneous coronary intervention
• Cardiac amyloidosis
• Radiofrequency ablation
• Supraventricular tachycardia
• Post-cardiac transplantation

Non-cardiac causes:
• Primary pulmonary hypertension
• Pulmonary embolism
• Cerebrovascular stroke
• High dose chemotherapy
• Sepsis and septic shock
• Renal failure
• Critically ill patients
• Scorpion envenomation
• Ultra-endurance exercise (marathon)

e. *Myoglobin*
It is increased within 2 hrs of onset of symptoms and remains increased for at least 7-12 hrs. Normal level is 20-100 μg/L.

Complications

Cardiogenic Shock

Cardiogenic shock occurs when > 40% of LV is infarcted and rendered non-functional. It carries a high mortality rate (80–90%). The criteria for diagnosing cardiogenic shock are:

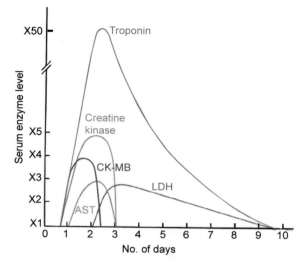

Fig. 3.135: Enzyme levels in acute MI

a. Signs of failure like thready pulse, cold and clammy extremities and pallor.
b. Systolic BP < 80 mm Hg
c. Cardiac index < 1.8 L/min/m²
d. Left ventricular filling pressure > 18 mm Hg
e. Urine output less than 20–30 ml/hr
f. Presence of tachycardia and S_3 and S_4 gallop rhythm
g. Features of pulmonary oedema.

Treatment of cardiogenic shock with drugs like dopamine, dobutamine, norepinephrine, amrinone or various combinations of these agents or with intra-aortic balloon (or external) counter-pulsation and use of anti-coagulants help to lower the mortality. Emergency PTCA or CABG can reduce the mortality by about half.

The prognosis, in the presence of cardiac failure, when untreated, is assessed by using the Killip classi-fication.

Killip Classification

Class	Features	Incidence	Mortality
I	No heart failure	40%	0.5%
II	Mild to moderate heart failure (S_3; rales no more than half way up the back)	40%	10–20%
III	Severe heart failure (pulmonary oedema)	10%	30–40%
IV	Cardiogenic shock	10%	80–90%

Arrhythmias

Nearly all patients with acute MI have arrhythmias. In many cases it is mild and of no haemodynamic significance.

Common arrhythmias seen in acute MI are:

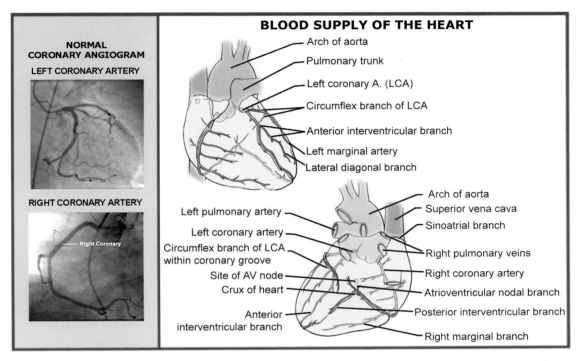

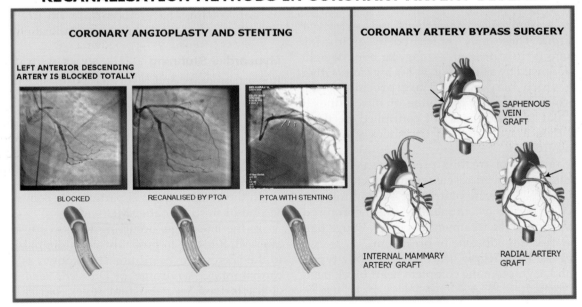

Fig. 3.136: Recanalisation methods in coronary artery disease

a. *Ventricular fibrillation:* This is a major cause of death within one hour of developing MI
b. Ventricular tachycardia
c. Accelerated idioventricular rhythm
d. Ventricular ectopics
e. *Atrial fibrillation:* Common and frequently transient.

May cause a rapid ventricular rate and hypotension
f. Atrial tachycardia
g. *Sinus bradycardia:* Should be treated if there is associated hypotension
h. *Heart block:* Following inferior wall MI is often temporary and may resolve without treatment, but

draining of the pericardial space if fluid reaccumulates. Surgical drainage through a limited thoracotomy may be required in recurrent tamponade or when tissue diagnosis is needed.

If pericardial drainage is delayed, IV saline is given to maintain adequate ventricular filling along with parenteral inotropic support to stabilize the patient. Do not use diuretics, nitrates or any other pre-load reducing agents.

Cardiac Arrest—Causes

Anatomical/Mechanical

Coronary artery disease   Atherosclerosis / Ischaemic heart disease

Anomalous left coronary artery from pulmonary artery (ALCAPA).

Kawasaki disease

Myocardial disorders   Primary
       Hypertrophic obstructive-cardiomyopathy
     Secondary
       Dilated cardiomyopathy
       Infiltrative cardiomyopathy
     Myocarditis

Valvular heart disease   Aortic stenosis, Pulmonary stenosis
     Mitral valve prolapse syndrome

Cardiac failure
Cardiac shock

Electrical

- Wolff-Parkinson-White syndrome
- Romano Ward syndrome (Long QT_c)
- Jervell-Lange-Nielsen syndrome (Long QT_c)
- Electric shock.

Physiological

Metabolic   Hypoxia
     Hypercapnia
     Hypocalcaemia
     Hypomagnesemia
     Hypokalemia
     Hyperkalaemia.

Toxins   Antiarrhythmics
     Digitalis
     Cocaine
     Adrenaline.

Cardiopulmonary Resuscitation (Basic Life Support)

Cardiopulmonary resuscitation (CPR) was developed to rescue patients with acute circulatory or respiratory failure or both.

The **ABCs** of basic life support are:

a. **A**irway
b. **B**reathing
c. **C**irculation.

and are essential for successful resuscitative efforts.

When one encounters an unconscious patient, the following procedures are recommended:

1. Determine responsiveness by gently shaking the patient. *Do not shake the head or neck unless trauma to this area has been excluded*
2. Position the patient on a firm, flat surface
3. Assess patency of airway and presence of respiration. Place the palm of one hand on the patient's forehead and apply firm pressure to tilt the head backward. At the same time, place the index and middle fingers of the other hand under the chin and displace the mandible anteriorly. This will raise the tongue away from the posterior pharynx. If a neck injury is suspected, the neck tilt should be avoided and the modified jaw thrust, by grasping the angles of the mandible with the fingers of both hands and moving the mandible anteriorly is done. With the airway thus made patent, the presence of spontaneous respiration is looked for.
4. *Assisted ventilation* is started when there is no spontaneous respiration. Gently pinch the nose closed with the index finger and thumb of the hand kept on the forehead. Make a tight seal over the patient's mouth and ventilate twice with slow, full breaths (1–1.5 seconds each). A two second pause should be interspersed between breaths. Alternatively, an Ambu bag may be used for ventilation. *Indicators of adequate ventilation* are the rise and fall of the chest and detection of escaping air during expiration.
5. *Palpate the carotid pulse* for at least 5 seconds. If a carotid pulse is palpable, assisted ventilation should be continued at a rate of 12 breaths per minute. If carotid pulse is not palpable, then cardiac resuscitation should be started.
6. *Cardiac resuscitation* is started by placing the patient on a firm surface. An initial blow to the chest over the sternum is delivered. Chest compressions are performed by placing the heel of one hand on the back of the other and placing it 1 inch above the

xiphoid process of the sternum, with the shoulders directly above the hands and the elbows in a locked position. With the heel of the hand, the sternum is compressed 3–5 cm., the thrust being applied straight down towards the spine.

Basic life support should be stopped for 5 seconds at the end of the first minute and every 2–3 minutes thereafter to determine whether the patient has resumed spontaneous breathing or circulation. The procedure should be continued till advanced cardiac life support is made available for revival.

CPR should be continued for a minimum period of 30 minutes. If, however, the pupils become dilated and fixed and the patient does not regain consciousness, CPR may be discontinued.

CPR need not be done in end organ failure or multisystem failure.

Cardioversion (DC Shock)

Cardioversion or DC shock is a safe means of terminating various tachyarrhythmias and restoring sinus rhythm.

Cardioversion is only effective for re-entrant arrhythmias, including atrial and ventricular fibrillation, but not for those caused by abnormal automaticity.

Indication for DC Shock

1. *Atrial fibrillation* is one of the most common indications for cardioversion. A minimum of 100 joules is required. Patients are unlikely to maintain sinus rhythm if atrial fibrillation is of longstanding duration or the echocardiographically determined left atrial dimension exceeds 4.5 cm. Cardioversion is more likely to be complicated by systemic emboli in patients with atrial fibrillation of more than 3 days' duration and hence anticoagulants should be administered for up to 3–6 weeks before the procedure, and for 1 week after the procedure.
2. *Atrial flutter* is one of the easiest rhythms to convert to sinus rhythm. Cardioversion frequently requires less than 50 joules.
3. *Re-entrant SVTs* require 25–100 joules for cardioversion.
4. *Ventricular tachycardia* requires synchronized cardioversion of 20–50 joules to be applied. If however the pulse and blood pressure are not recordable, 200 joules, followed by 360 joules (if no response) should be delivered.
5. *Ventricular fibrillation* requires repeated unsynchronized cardioversion, starting with 200 joules, followed by 3–4 applications of 360 joules.

If there is no response, then the following manoeuvres may be carried out:

CPR—Establish IV access—Epinephrine 1:10,000, 0.5-1 mg. IV stat—Intubation—DC shock of 360 joules—Lidocaine 1 mg/kg. IV stat—DC shock of 360 joules—Bretylium 5 mg/kg. IV stat—DC shock of 360 joules—Bretylium 10 mg/kg. IV stat—DC shock of 360 joules—Repeat Lidocaine and Bretylium—DC shock of 360 joules.

Sodium bicarbonate in a dose of 0.5 mEq/kg body weight may be administered intermittently every 10–15 minutes to counteract the developing acidosis.

Immediate Cardioversion is Mandatory if the Arrhythmia Causes Angina, Hypotension or Heart Failure.

Contraindications to Cardioversion

1. *Digitalis toxicity:* Elective cardioversion should not be performed in the presence of potentially toxic levels of digoxin. If cardioversion is necessary, then prophylactic lidocaine therapy should be given and cardioversion should begin at low energy levels.
2. Repetitive, short-lived tachycardias.
3. Multifocal atrial tachycardia or other automatic arrhythmias.
4. Patients with sick sinus syndrome, complete AV block or on β-blockers (as cardioversion may potentiate severe bradycardia).
5. Patients with supraventricular arrhythmias in hyperthyroidism should be made euthyroid before elective cardioversion.
6. Patients with AF secondary to mitral stenosis must have the underlying problem (MS) corrected before attempting to revert AF to sinus rhythm.
7. In patients with pacemaker (as pacemaker may be damaged).
8. Tachyarrhythmias developing immediately after cardiac surgery (as they cannot maintain sinus rhythm).
9. AF of long-standing duration (> 1 year duration).

Cardiac Transplantation

Cardiac transplantation is the therapy of choice for end stage heart disease, who are unlikely to survive for the next 6–12 months as evidenced by a decrease in ejection fraction of less than 20% or presence of serious ventricular arrhythmias.

Optimal candidates for transplantation are those who do not show evidence of end stage organ damage from cardiac failure and do not suffer from other systemic illnesses like collagen vascular disease or HIV. Long-standing pulmonary hypertension, recurrent pulmonary emboli or pulmonary infarction carries a high risk of intraoperative death.

Patients who are dopamine/dobutamine dependent to maintain an adequate cardiac output are those who get the highest priority for a donor heart.

A suitable donor is obtained by doing ABO matching and lymphocyte cross matching. He should also test negative for cytomegalovirus infection.

The donor heart is removed, except for posterior wall of RA, SVC and IVC. The LA along with the pulmonary veins are also left *in situ*. The donor heart is then sutured to the posterior wall of the two atria of the recipient's heart, the rest of the heart having been incised and removed.

Rejection of cardiac transplant is characterised by perivascular infiltration of killer T-lymphocytes, which may later migrate into the myocardium. This can be assessed by repeated percutaneous transvenous RV endomyocardial biopsies via the right internal jugular vein, every 3 months. Prolongation of isovolumetric relaxation time by echo may also provide an early clue to rejection.

Immunosuppressive therapy is given with cyclosporine, azathioprine and prednisolone. There is an increased risk of development of malignancy due to this.

The donor sinus node controls the rate of the transplanted heart. The controlling sinus node has no innervation by the autonomic nervous system and maintains a constant heart rate of 100–110 beats per minute.

The ECG taken after transplantation shows two P-waves (one from the recipient's SA node and the other from the donor's SA node). The P-wave from the recipient's SA node is dissociated from the QRS complexes as the impulse does not cross the suture line, whereas the P-wave arising from the donor SA node precedes the QRS complex.

Chronic rejection may occur in the form of accelerated atherosclerosis of the coronary arteries, affecting both the proximal and distal vessels and is the most important cause of death. Angina is rare, as the transplanted heart is devoid of autonomic innervation.

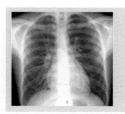

CHAPTER 4

Respiratory System

SYMPTOMS	SIGNS

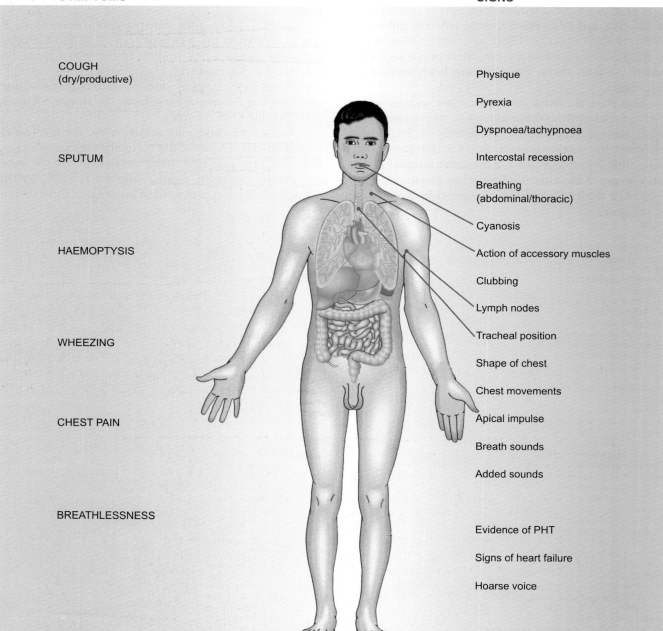

SYMPTOMS

COUGH
(dry/productive)

SPUTUM

HAEMOPTYSIS

WHEEZING

CHEST PAIN

BREATHLESSNESS

SIGNS

Physique

Pyrexia

Dyspnoea/tachypnoea

Intercostal recession

Breathing
(abdominal/thoracic)

Cyanosis

Action of accessory muscles

Clubbing

Lymph nodes

Tracheal position

Shape of chest

Chest movements

Apical impulse

Breath sounds

Added sounds

Evidence of PHT

Signs of heart failure

Hoarse voice

Anatomical Landmarks

The trachea bifurcates at the level of angle of Louis anteriorly and between the 4th and 5th thoracic spines posteriorly.

The second costal cartilage is connected to the angle of Louis. The ribs are counted downwards from the second rib.

Angle of Louis is the transverse bony ridge at the junction of the body of the sternum and the manubrium sterni.

Major interlobar fissure (Fig. 4.1) is marked by a line drawn from T_2 spine along the medial border of the scapula, with the arm kept hyperabducted, to the 6th rib at its costochondral junction, crossing the 5th rib at the mid axillary line. It corresponds to the upper border of the lower lobe.

Minor interlobar fissure (Fig. 4.1) is marked by a horizontal line drawn from the sternum at the level of 4th costal cartilage to meet the first line of the major interlobar fissure. It marks the boundary between the upper and middle lobes.

Bronchopulmonary Segments

Each main bronchus divides into three lobar bronchi. On the right side, one each to the upper lobe, middle lobe and lower lobe. On the left side, one each to upper lobe, lingular lobe and remainder of the lower lobe. Then these divide into segmental bronchi to individual segments.

The bronchopulmonary segments of the lungs on both the left and right side is given in the next column with their numbers.

Borders of the Lung

The apices of the upper lobes of both the lungs rise 2-3 cm. above the clavicles. From the apices of the upper lobe the inner margins of the lungs and their covering pleura start towards the sternum, meeting each other in the midline at the sternal angle. On the right, the margin of the lungs continue down the sternum as far as the 6th costal cartilage and then run outwards and downwards to meet the mid axillary line at the 8th rib, the scapular line at the 10th rib and the para vertebral line at the T_{10} vertebrae. The landmark of the left lung is the same except that the lung border turns away from the sternum at the 4th instead of 6th costal cartilage due to the position of the heart.

	Right side		*Left side*
Upper	Apical (1)	Upper	Apical (1)
	Posterior (2)		Posterior (2)
	Anterior (3)		Anterior (3)
Middle	Lateral (4)	Lingular	Superior (4)
	Medial (5)		Inferior (5)
Lower	Apical (6)	Lower	Apical (6)
	Medial basal (7)		Anterior basal (7)
	Anterior basal (8)		Lateral basal (8)
	Lateral basal (9)		Posterior basal (9)
	Posterior basal (10)		

Pleural Border

At the apices and along the inner margins of the lungs, the pleura lies close to the lungs to follow the same surface marking; but at the lower border of the lung the pleura extends 4–5 cm anteriorly and 9–10 cm posteriorly below the lung, lying at the level of eighth

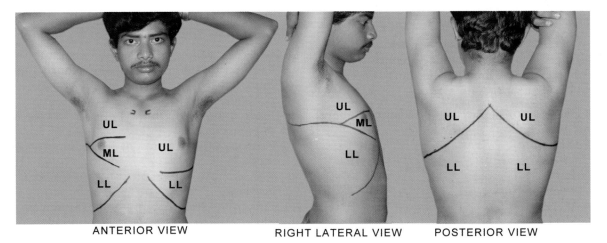

ANTERIOR VIEW   RIGHT LATERAL VIEW   POSTERIOR VIEW

Fig. 4.1: Surface marking of major (right and left) fissures and minor fissure (right)

rib in the mid clavicular line, tenth rib at the mid axillary line and twelfth rib at the scapular line.

Upper lobes of the lung are accessible from the front, lower lobes from the back and all the three lobes in the axilla.

Symptoms and Signs

Cough

It is the reflex act of forceful expiration against a closed glottis that helps in clearing the airways including foreign body.

Mechanism of Cough

It is brought about by contraction of respiratory muscles against the closed glottis with a resultant increase in intrathoracic pressure followed by opening of the glottis with forced expiration at very high air flow rate in the upper airways.

Types of Cough

1. *Dry cough:* Pleural disorders, interstitial lung disease, mediastinal lesions
2. *Productive cough:* Suppurative lung disease, chronic bronchitis, pulmonary TB
3. *Short cough:* It is seen in upper respiratory tract infections (common cold)
4. *Brassy cough:* Cough with metallic sound produced by compression of the trachea by intrathoracic space occupying lesions
5. *Bovine cough:* Cough with loss of its explosive nature, e.g. tumours pressing on recurrent laryngeal nerve
6. *Prolonged and paroxysmal cough:* It is present in chronic bronchitis and whooping cough
7. *Barking cough:* It is found in epiglottal involvement as well as in hysterical and nervous individuals.

Cough syncope (Post-tussive syncope): It is due to raised intrathoracic pressure, which reduces venous return to the heart, thereby diminishing cardiac output, resulting in cerebral hypoperfusion and syncope.

Nocturnal cough: It is present in the following conditions:
1. Chronic bronchitis
2. Left sided failure
3. Bronchial asthma
4. Aspiration
5. Tropical eosinophilia
6. Post-nasal drip.

Drug induced cough is present in drug therapy with ACE inhibitors.

Sputum

It is a mixture of tracheobronchial secretion, cellular debris, microorganisms and saliva. The character of sputum is determined by its amount, colour, chronology, consistency and smell.

Saliva contains squamous cells.

Sputum contains epithelial cells. If sputum contains epithelial cells and eosinophils then suspect.
a. Bronchial asthma
b. Allergic bronchopulmonary aspergillosis (ABPA).

Amount

Bronchorrhoea: When the quantity of sputum production is > 100 ml/day, it is termed as bronchorrhoea.

Copious sputum production is seen in conditions like:
1. Bronchiectasis
2. Lung abscess
3. Empyema rupturing into the bronchus
4. Necrotizing pneumonia
5. Alveolar cell carcinoma.

Copious sputum production upon changes in posture is seen in bronchiectasis and lung abscess. This postural relationship to cough is due to irritation of the healthy bronchial mucosa.

Large amount of colourless sputum is present in alveolar cell carcinoma.

Chronology

Chronic bronchitis: Sputum production is more in the early morning for many years.

Bronchial asthma: Sputum production is more either in the morning or at night. Recent onset of sputum production signifies severe infection.

Colour of the Sputum

a. Green or yellow coloured thick sputum indicates bacterial infections. The green colour to sputum is imparted by the enzyme myeloperoxidase (verdoperoxidase)
b. Black coloured sputum is present in coal worker's pneumoconiosis
c. Rusty sputum is present in pneumococcal pneumonia
d. Red currant jelly sputum is seen in *Klebsiella pneumonia*
e. Pink frothy sputum is present in pulmonary oedema
f. Blood stained sputum is present in tuberculosis
g. Anchovy sauce sputum is present in ruptured amoebic liver abscess.

Consistency

Serous: It is clear, watery and frothy. It is seen in broncho-alveolar carcinoma. It may be pink, as occurs in pulmonary oedema.

Mucoid: It is clear, greyish white or black in colour and frothy. It may be seen in conditions like chronic bronchitis and chronic asthma.

Mucopurulent or purulent: Yellowish or greenish brown in colour, seen in bacterial infection.

Bronchial asthma: Macroscopically the sputum is 'worm like', which are remnants of casts of bronchus. Microscopically the sputum consists of:

a. Eosinophils
b. Desquamated epithelium
c. Curschmann spirals (whorled mucous plugs)
d. Charcot-Leyden crystals (crystalloid debris of eosinophil membrane)
e. Creola bodies (exfoliated cells due to disruption of mucosal integrity).

Odour of Sputum

Offensive and foetid:

a. Lung abscess
b. Bronchiectasis
c. Anaerobic bacterial infection.

Haemoptysis

It is defined as expectoration of blood, or bloody sputum.

Types of Haemoptysis

Frank haemoptysis: It is the expectoration of blood only. Massive and fatal blood loss may occur. Frank haemoptysis daily suggests bronchogenic carcinoma.

Haemoptysis in suppurative lung disease: Large quantities of foul smelling sputum and blood suggests suppurative lung disease.

Spurious haemoptysis: Haemoptysis present secondary to upper respiratory tract infection, above the level of larynx.

Pseudohaemoptysis: It is due to pigment, prodigiosin produced by gram-negative organism, *Serratia marcescens.*

Endemic haemoptysis: Present in infection with *Paragonimus westermani* (lung fluke).

Severity of Haemoptysis

Mild	< 100 ml blood loss per day
Moderate	100–150 ml blood loss per day
Severe	Up to 200 ml blood loss per day
Massive	> 500 ml blood loss per day (or) rate of blood loss > 150 ml/hr (or) 100 ml blood loss per day for more than 3 days.

If there is > 500 ml blood loss per day, aggressive intervention (rigid bronchoscopy or surgery) is advocated. If the blood loss is submassive, after subsidence of haemoptysis, fibreoptic bronchoscopy is indicated.

Causes of Haemoptysis

Infection

a. Tuberculosis
b. Lung abscess
c. Bronchiectasis
d. Pneumonia
e. Fungal infection (aspergillosis, nocardiosis, blastomycosis).

Differences between Haemoptysis and Haematemesis

	Haemoptysis	*Haematemesis*
1.	Cough precedes haemoptysis	Nausea and vomiting precedes haematemesis
2.	Frothy due to admixture of air	Not frothy
3.	pH alkaline	pH acidic
4.	Mixed with macrophage and neutrophil	Mixed with food particles
5.	Malaena absent	Malaena present
6.	Bright red in colour	Dark brown in colour due to acid haematin
7.	Previous history of respiratory disease	Previous history of peptic ulcer disease
8.	Diagnosed by bronchoscopy	Diagnosed by gastroscopy

Neoplasm

a. Bronchogenic carcinoma
b. Bronchial adenoma
c. Metastatic tumour to lung.

Cardiovascular Disorders

a. Mitral stenosis
b. Pulmonary hypertension
c. Aortic aneurysm
d. Arteriovenous malformation
e. Pulmonary embolism.

Congenital

a. Bronchial cyst
b. Sequestration of lung
  (i) Intralobar
  (ii) Extralobar.

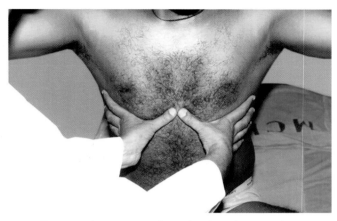

Fig. 4.16: Assessment of anterior thoracic expansion

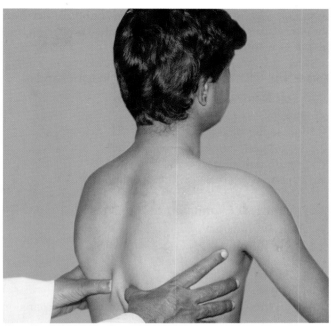

Fig. 4.18: Method 2 for assessing chest expansion

Tenderness over the Chest Wall

It may be due to:
1. Empyema
2. Local inflammation of parietal pleura, soft tissue and osteomyelitis
3. Infiltration with tumour
4. Non-respiratory cause (amoebic liver abscess).

Detection of Subcutaneous Emphysema

Spongy crepitant feeling on palpation suggests subcutaneous emphysema. It is present in:
1. Injury to chest wall and rib
2. Pneumothorax
3. Rupture of oesophagus.

Tactile Fremitus

These are palpable added sounds (rhonchi are better felt than crackles).

Friction Fremitus

It is a palpable pleural rub.

Vocal Fremitus

It is a vibration felt by the hand when the patient is asked to repeat ninety-nine or one-one-one, by putting the vocal cord into action. Identical areas of the chest are compared on both sides. It is felt with the flat of the

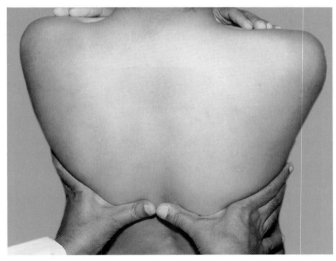

Fig. 4.17: Assessment of posterior thoracic movement

Assessment of Posterior Thoracic Movement

A similar procedure is carried out over the posterior aspect of the patient's chest (Fig. 4.17).

The difference in chest expansion can be assessed by holding a loose fold of skin in between the thumbs, approximated in the midline, whereby even a slight difference in chest expansion can be assessed easily. (The skin fold disappears on the side of good expansion) (Fig. 4.18).

Minimal difference in chest expansion of the two hemithoraces can be assessed in a cooperative patient, without dyspnoea in the following way. The patient is asked to expire fully thereby obtaining the residual lung volume, and then to inspire to his full capacity thereby attaining total lung capacity. The difference in expansion of each hemithorax can then be assessed.

hand or with the ulnar border of the hand for accurate localization. It is increased in consolidation. It is decreased in pleural effusion.

Special Clinical Features of Importance

General Restriction of Expansion

a. COPD
b. Extensive bilateral disease
c. Ankylosing spondylitis
d. Interstitial lung disease
e. Systemic sclerosis (hide bound chest).

Asymmetrical Expansion of the Chest

a. Pleural effusion
b. Pneumothorax
c. Extensive consolidation
d. Collapse
e. Fibrosis.

In all these above conditions, diminished expansion occurs on the affected side.

Percussion of the Lung Fields

General Principles

Position of the Patient

The sitting posture is the best position of choice for percussion. Supine posture is not desirable because of the alteration of the percussion note by the underlying structure on which the patient lies.

a. *Anterior percussion:* The patient sits erect with the hands by his side
b. *Posterior percussion:* The patient bends his head forwards and keeps his hands over the opposite shoulders. This position keeps the two scapulae further away so that more lung is available for percussion
c. *Lateral percussion:* The patient sits with his hands held over the head.

Objectives of Percussion

It is done to find out the degree of resonance over the symmetrical areas of the two sides of the chest and to map out areas in which percussion note is abnormal.

Cardinal Rules of Percussion

a. *The pleximeter:* The middle finger of the examiner's left hand should be opposed tightly over the chest wall, over the intercostal spaces. The other fingers should not touch the chest wall. Greater pressure

should be applied over a thick chest wall to remove air pockets
b. *The plexor:* The middle or the index finger of the examiner's right hand is used to hit the middle phalanx of the pleximeter
c. The percussion movement should be sudden, originating from the wrist. The finger should be removed immediately after striking to avoid damping
d. Proceed from the area of normal resonance to the area of impaired or dull note, as the difference is then easily appreciated
e. The long axis of the pleximeter is kept parallel to the border of the organ to be percussed.

Areas of Percussion (Fig. 4.20)

Anterior Chest Wall

a. *Clavicle:* Direct percussion is used and percussion is done within the medial 1/3rd of the clavicle (Fig. 4.19)

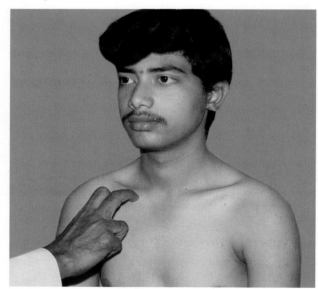

Fig. 4.19: Direct percussion—clavicle

b. *Supraclavicular region (Kronig's isthumus):* It is a band of resonance 5-7 cm size over the supraclavicular fossa. It is bounded medially by scalenus muscle of the neck, laterally by the acromion process of scapula, anteriorly by the clavicle and posteriorly by the trapezius. The percussion is done by standing behind the patient and the resonance of the lung apices is assessed by this method. Hyper resonance in this area indicates emphysema. Impaired resonance in this area indicates pulmonary TB or malignancy in the lung apex

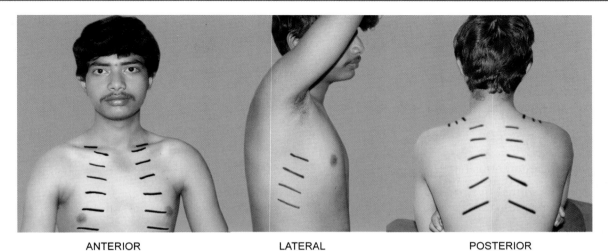

ANTERIOR   LATERAL   POSTERIOR

Fig. 4.20: Percussion areas

c. Infraclavicular
d. Second to sixth intercostal spaces. However the percussion note cannot be compared due to relative cardiac dullness on the left side.

Lateral Chest Wall

Fourth to seventh intercostal spaces.

Posterior Chest Wall

a. Suprascapular (above the spine of the scapula)
b. Interscapular region
c. Infrascapular region up to the eleventh rib.

	Types of percussion note	Lesions
1.	Tympanitic	Hollow viscus
2.	Subtympanitic (skodiac resonance or boxy quality)	Above the level of pleural effusion
3.	Hyper-resonant	Pneumothorax
4.	Resonant	Normal lung
5.	Impaired	Pulmonary fibrosis, cavity with surrounding fibrosis
6.	Dull *wooly*	Consolidation, collapse, Pleural thickening
7.	Stony dull	Pleural effusion, empyema, Parenchymal lung disorder with pleural thickening

Crack Pot Resonance

A type of tympanitic note which can be produced by clasping the moist hands loosely together and striking it against the knee. It may be elicited over a large cavity communicating with a bronchus.

Normal Percussion Note in Diseased Lung

1. Chronic bronchitis

2. Bronchial asthma
3. Interstitial lung disease
4. Diffuse emphysema.

Percussion on the Right Side

Liver dullness can be percussed from the right 5th intercostal space downwards in the midclavicular line up to the right costal margin.

Tidal Percussion

This is done to differentiate upward enlargement of liver or subdiaphragmatic abscess from right sided parenchymal or pleural disorder.

If on deep inspiration, the previous dull note in the fifth right intercostal space on the mid clavicular line becomes resonant, it indicates that the dullness was due to the liver, which had been pushed down by the right hemidiaphragm with deep inspiration. If the dullness persists on the other hand, it indicates underlying right sided parenchymal or pleural pathology, in the absence of diaphragmatic paralysis.

Percussion on the Left Side

Traube's Space

Surface anatomy: Draw two parallel vertical lines, one from the left 6th costochondral junction and another from the 9th rib in mid axillary line. Then connect the two lines above from the left 6th costochondral junction to the 9th rib in mid axillary line and below along the left costal margin. It forms a semilunar space and is tympanitic on percussion.

Boundaries of Traube's space
Right side   Left lobe of the liver
Left side   Spleen

Above	Left lung resonance
Below	Left costal margin
Content	Fundus of stomach

Traube's space is obliterated in:
1. Left sided pleural effusion
2. Massive splenomegaly
3. Enlarged left lobe of liver
4. Full stomach
5. Fundal growth
6. Massive pericardial effusion.

Traube's space is shifted upwards in:
1. Left diaphragmatic paralysis
2. Left lower lobe collapse
3. Fibrosis of the left lung.

Special Features of Clinical Importance

Percussion Tenderness

It is present in empyema and inflammation of parietal pleura.

Straight Line Dullness

It is present in hydropneumothorax.

Shifting Dullness

This is done to demonstrate the shift of fluid in pleural effusion and hydropneumothorax. In hydropneumothorax shifting occurs immediately, whereas it is very slow in case of pleural effusion. The immediate shift of fluid can be demonstrated by the dull area percussed in the axilla in the sitting posture, becoming resonant on lying down on the healthy side.

"S" Shaped Curve of Ellis

In moderate sized pleural effusion, the uppermost level of dullness is highest in the axilla and lowest in the spine, and tends to assume the shape of the letter "S". Hence the name.

One school of thought is that, this phenomenon is due to capillary suction between the two layers of the pleura, drawing the fluid up maximally in the axillary region.

Another school of thought is that this phenomenon is only a radiological illusion.

Auscultation

General Principles of Auscultation

a. As most normal lung sounds are low pitched, the bell is normally preferred over the diaphragm.

Stretching of the skin under the diaphragm during breathing is apt to produce scratching sound similar to a pleural rub. In order to avoid time consumption and practical difficulty, diaphragm is used
b. The patient should be asked to breathe with his mouth open. This is to prevent sound being produced from a partially closed nose
c. Avoid auscultation within 2-3 cm from the midline in the upper part of the chest, since breath sounds in these areas may normally have a bronchial character
d. If the chest is hairy, moisten the chest wall with water and apply the chest piece tightly to avoid sounds produced by the friction with hair.

Auscultatory Areas

Anterior: From an area above the clavicle down to the 6th rib.

Axilla: Area upto the 8th rib.

Posterior: Above the level of the spine of the scapula down to the eleventh rib.

Technique of Auscultation

a. When abnormal breath sounds are heard, the extent to which the abnormal sound is heard should be mapped from normal to abnormal zone. Note also the area at which the character changes.
b. In case of patient with pleural pain, it is better to test vocal resonance and to avoid frequent deep breathing.
c. Auscultation after coughing is a useful procedure. It helps differentiate coarse crepitation and low pithced rhonchi from pleural rub. Coughing does not alter pleural rub, but may alter the character of rhonchi and crackles.

Importance of Auscultation

a. To assess the character and intensity of breath sounds
b. Presence or absence of any added sounds
c. Character of vocal resonance (voice sounds and whispering sounds)
d. Miscellaneous sounds.

Breath Sounds

Breath sounds are produced by vibrations of the vocal cords due to turbulent flow of air.

Vesicular Breath Sound

It is low pitched, rustling in nature and is produced by attenuating and filtering effect of the lung parenchyma.

Duration of the inspiratory phase is longer than the expiratory phase in a ratio of 3 : 1.

There is no pause between the end of inspiration and the beginning of expiration.

Conditions with diminished vesicular breath sounds
a. Bronchial asthma (silent chest)
b. Tumour
c. Pleural effusion (small)
d. Pleural thickening
e. Collapsed lung with occluded bronchus
f. Emphysema.

Bronchial Breath Sound

It is produced by passage of air through the trachea and large bronchi, heard over an area of diseased, airless or consolidated lung interposed between the bronchi and chest wall.

Character: It is loud and high pitched, with an aspirate or guttural quality. The duration of inspiration is shortened whereas that of expiration is prolonged and sometimes the duration of inspiration and expiration are equal. There is a pause between inspiration and expiration.

Types of Bronchial Breathing

a. Tubular
b. Cavernous
c. Amphoric.

Tubular

They are high pitched and present in:
a. Pneumonic consolidation
b. Collapsed lung or lobe when a large draining bronchus is patent
c. Above the level of pleural effusion (in a partially collapsed lung with a patent bronchus).

Cavernous

They are low pitched and heard in the presence of thick-walled cavity with a communicating bronchus.

Amphoric

They are low pitched, with a high tone and a metallic quality and present in:
a. Large superficial smooth-walled cavity
b. Bronchopleural fistula
c. Tension pneumothorax.

Absent Breath Sounds

a. Pleural effusion (massive)
b. Thickened pleura (fibrothorax)

c. Collapsed lung or lobe when bronchus is occluded
d. Pneumothorax
e. Near fatal asthma (silent chest)
f. Pneumonectomy
g. Agenesis of lung.

Added Sounds

Crackles

They are non-musical, interrupted added sounds of short duration. They are explosive in nature.

Types

1. Fine—They are less loud, short in duration and arise from the alveoli
2. Coarse—They are low pitched, loud and arise from the bronchus and bronchioles.

Crackles may be:
a. Early inspiratory as in chronic bronchitis
b. Mid inspiratory as in bronchiectasis
c. Late inspiratory as in asbestosis, pulmonary fibrosis, pneumonitis, interstitial lung disease, pulmonary oedema.
d. Expiratory as in chronic bronchitis, pulmonary oedema.

Mechanism of Crackles

a. Bubbling or flow of air through secretions in the bronchial level
b. Sudden opening of successive bronchioles and alveoli with rapid equalisation of pressure causing a sequence of explosive sounds.

Crackles without sputum production indicates interstitial lung disease. Crackles with sputum production indicates parenchymal lung disease.

Fine localised crackles are a sign of parenchymal infiltration. If heard over the apices of the lungs, it may be an early sign of pulmonary tuberculosis.

Medium or coarse crackles are a sign of respiratory disorder.

Fine end inspiratory crackles over both lung bases may be an early sign of LVF.

Coarse crackles (death rattle) can occur as a terminal event in gross pulmonary edema.

Rhonchi

They are musical, continuous added sounds.

They may be low pitched (*sonorous*), arising from large airways or high pitched (*sibilant*), arising from small airways.

Types of Wheeze (Fig. 4.21)

Fixed monophonic wheeze: It is a single note of constant pitch, timing and site. It results from air passing through a localized narrowing of airway. It is seen in incomplete obstruction of principal or lobar bronchus, as in:
a. Tumours
b. Foreign body
c. Bronchial stenosis
d. Intrabronchial granuloma.

Random monophonic wheeze: It is a random single note, which is scattered, occurring in inspiration and expiration and varying in duration, site and pitch, e.g. bronchial asthma.

Expiratory polyphonic wheeze: This is a complex musical sound of multiple notes with all its components starting together, continuing to finally end in expiration due to expiratory compression of large central airways, e.g. emphysema.

Sequential inspiratory wheeze: It is due to the opening of distal airways which has become abnormally opposed during previous expiration, e.g. pulmonary fibrosis, fibrosing alveolitis, asbestosis.

Voice Sounds

Vocal Resonance

It is a voice sound heard with the chest piece of the stethoscope.

Types
a. *Bronchophony:* Voice sounds appear to be heard near the earpiece of stethoscope and words are unclear, e.g. consolidation, cavity communicating with a bronchus, above the level of pleural effusion. It is normally heard in proximity to the trachea.
b. *Aegophony:* Voice sound has a nasal or bleating quality. On saying 'E', it will be heard as 'A' (E to A sign), e.g. consolidation, above the level of pleural effusion, cavity.

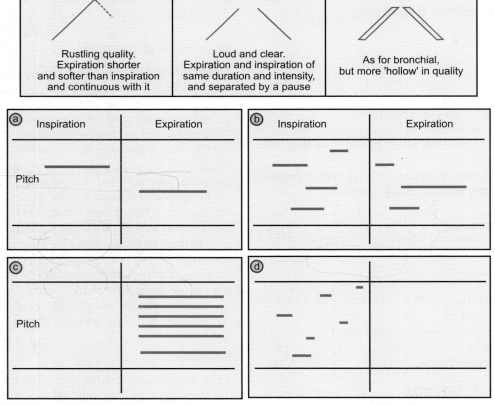

Fig. 4.21: Types of wheeze: (a) Fixed monophonic wheeze, (b) Random polyphonic wheeze, (c) Expiratory polyphonic wheeze, (d) Sequential inspiratory wheeze (squawks)

c. *Whispering pectoriloquy:* The patient is asked to whisper words at the end of expiration, and this whispered voice is transmitted without distortion so that the individual syllables are recognised clearly, e.g. pneumonic consolidation.

Miscellaneous Sounds

Pleural rub: It is a superficial, localised squeaking or grating sound best heard with firm pressure of stethoscope. They are not altered by coughing. They are associated with pain.

Pleuro-pericardial rub: It is present in pleurisy adjacent to the pericardium. It is due to roughened pleural surface adjacent to the pericardium being moved across one another by cardiac pulsation.

Differentiation between Pleural Rub and Crackles

	Rub	Crackle
a.	Superficial and loud	Not superficial or loud
b.	Continuous	Discontinuous
c.	Localised	Heard over a wide area
d.	Unaffected by cough	Intensified or abolished by cough
e.	Pressure with stethoscope over the chest increases the sound	No effect
f.	Associated with pain and tenderness	No pain or tenderness

Other Features of Clinical Significance

Heimlich's manoeuvre: Laryngeal obstruction by a foreign body in an adult can be dislodged by a sudden inward and upward forceful compression of the upper abdomen, by standing behind the patient.

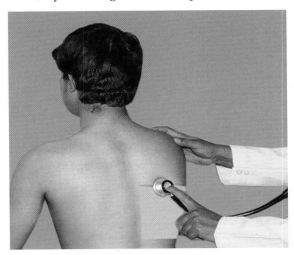

Fig. 4.22: Succussion splash

Post-tussive suction: It is a sucking sound, heard over the chest wall during inspiration, following a bout of cough, over the area of amphoric breath sound. It occurs in the presence of thin-walled superficial, collapsible, communicating cavity.

Succussion splash: Splashing sound heard over the chest either with the stethoscope or unaided ear applied to the chest wall when the patient is shaken suddenly by the examiner (Fig. 4.22).

This is done by asking the patient to lie down laterally with the healthy side in the dependent position. Percuss and determine the air-fluid level in the paraspinal region and keep the stethoscope over that region. Then grasp the non-dependent shoulder and shake it suddenly, when a sound like that of splashing water can be heard (Fig. 4.23).

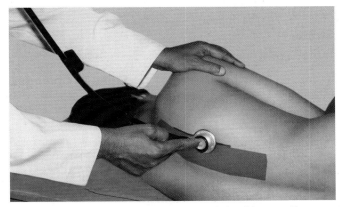

Fig. 4.23: Succussion splash—lateral decubitus position

Succussion splash can be heard in hydropneumothorax (Fig. 4.24), diaphragmatic hernia. It is normally heard over the fundus of stomach filled with air and fluid.

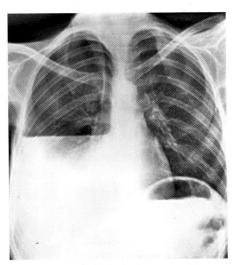

Fig. 4.24: Right hydropneumothorax

The presence of one of the features of severity is sufficient to place a patient in that category.

Management of Nocturnal Asthma

a. Treatment with anti-inflammatory drugs (corticosteroids)
b. Sustained-release theophylline or a beta$_2$-agonist or both
c. Long acting beta$_2$-agonists.

Management of Acute Severe Asthma

a. High concentration oxygen therapy
b. High dose β_2 agonists by nebuliser
c. Systemic corticosteroids
d. If no response with above treatment, ipratropium bromide by nebuliser or IV aminophylline (250 mg over 20 minutes) or IV β_2 agonists
e. Monitor treatment with pulse oximetry
f. Assisted ventilation when needed
g. Treatment with 70-80% helium (balanced oxygen) may be beneficial. This gas mixture reduces airway resistance and improves the effect of aerosolized bronchodilators.

Indications for Assisted Ventilation

1. Coma
2. Respiratory arrest
3. Exhaustion, confusion, drowsiness
4. Deterioration of ABG tensions despite therapy
   PaO$_2$ < 8 kPa and falling (60 mm Hg)
   PaCO$_2$ > 6.5 kPa and rising (50 mm Hg)
   pH   < 7.3 and falling.

Chronic Obstructive Pulmonary Disease (COPD)

COPD is a disease state characterized by airflow limitation that is not fully reversible. The airflow limitation is usually both progressive and associated with an abnormal inflammatory response of the lungs to noxious particles or gases (Fig. 4.28).

A diagnosis of COPD should be considered in any patient who has symptoms of cough, sputum production, or dyspnea, and or a history of exposure to risk factors for the disease. COPD includes chronic bronchitis and emphysema. The diagnosis is confirmed by spirometry. The presence of a post-bronchodilator FEV$_1$ < 80% of the predicted value in combination with an FEV$_1$/FVC < 70% confirms the presence of airflow limitation that is not fully reversible. A low peak flow is

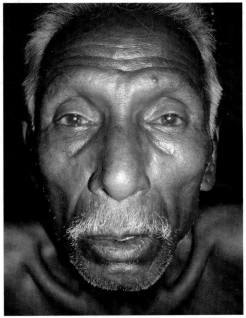

Fig. 4.28: Pursed lip breathing—COPD

consistent with COPD, but it has poor specificity since it can be caused by other lung diseases.

Chronic Bronchitis

This is a condition associated with excessive tracheobronchial mucus production sufficient to cause cough with expectoration on most days for at least 3 months a year for more than two consecutive years. It can be subdivided into:

a. Simple chronic bronchitis (describes a condition with mucoid sputum production).
b. Chronic mucopurulent bronchitis (persistent or recurrent purulent sputum production in the absence of local suppurative disease).
c. Chronic bronchitis with obstruction/chronic asthmatic bronchitis (severe dyspnoea and wheezing in association with inhaled irritants or infections in the setting of bronchitis).

Emphysema

It is defined as distention of the air spaces distal to the terminal bronchiole with destruction of alveolar septa.

Predisposing Factors for COPD

1. Smoking
2. Environmental pollution (dust, smoke)
3. Genetic predisposition

4. Infection (bacterial or viral)
5. α_1 antitrypsin deficiency (for emphysema)
6. Occupational exposure (fumes, etc.)
7. Exposure to dampness, fog and sudden change in temperature.

Pathogenesis

COPD is characterized by chronic inflammation throughout the airways, parenchyma, and pulmonary vasculature. Macrophages, T-lymphocytes (CD8+), and neutrophils are increased in various parts of the lung. Activated inflammatory cells release a variety of mediators—leukotriene B4 (LTB4), interleukin 8 (IL-8), tumour necrosis factor α (TNF- α), and others capable of damaging lung structures. In addition to inflammation, an imbalance between proteinases and antiproteinases and oxidative stress play a role in the pathogenesis of COPD.

Protease—Antiprotease hypothesis holds that destruction of alveolar walls in emphysema is due to an imbalance between proteases and their inhibitors in the lung.

In α_1-antitrypsin deficiency (a major protease inhibitor), emphysema develops at a younger age especially in smokers.

Impaction of smoke particles in bronchioles leads to inflammatory cell aggregation, increased elastase and decreased α_1 antitrypsin resulting in centriacinar emphysema seen in smokers.

Types of Emphysema (Fig. 4.29)

Centriacinar Emphysema: There is destruction and enlargement of central or proximal part of respiratory unit—the acinus. There is predominant involvement of upper lobe and apices. It is commonly seen in male smokers in association with chronic bronchitis.

Panacinar Emphysema: There is uniform destruction and enlargement of acinus. It is predominant in lower basal zones. It is associated with α_1-antitrypsin deficiency.

Paraseptal Emphysema: This involves only the distal acinus. It is found near the pleura and often causes spontaneous pneumothorax.

Irregular: There may be any type of involvement.

Special Varieties of Emphysema

Compensatory Emphysema: Normal lung tissue undergoes hyperinflation as a compensatory mechanism, in response to the damage occurring in part of the same lung or opposite lung. Here, alveolar septae are preserved.

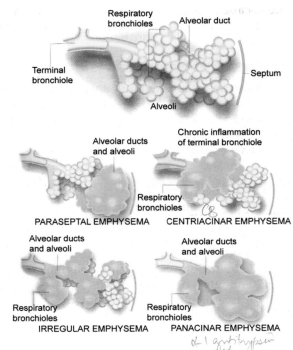

Fig. 4.29: Types of emphysema

Mediastinal Emphysema: This occurs as a result of escape of air rapidly into the mediastinum following rupture of overdistended alveoli. It may occur in the following conditions.
a. Severe bronchial asthma
b. Rupture of emphysematous bullae
c. Rupture of oesophagus.

Differentiating Features between Emphysema and Chronic Bronchitis

Features	Predominant Emphysema (Pink Puffer)	Predominant Bronchitis (Blue Bloater)
1. Age of onset	6th decade	5th decade
2. Cough	After dyspnoea	Before dyspnoea
3. Dyspnoea	Severe	Mild
4. Sputum	Scanty, mucoid	Copious, purulent
5. Infections	Less common	Common
6. Respiratory insufficiency	Often terminal	Repeated attacks
7. Chest X-ray	Hyperinflation $\pm$ bullous changes; small heart	Increased broncho-vascular markings; large heart
8. PaCO$_2$ (mm Hg)	35–40	50–60
PaO$_2$ (mm Hg)	65–75	45–60
9. Pulmonary hypertension	Mild	Moderate to severe
10. Cor pulmonale	Preterminal stage	Common
11. Diffusing capacity	Decreased	Normal to slight reduction

In COPD only quitting smoking & O_2 Rx reduces morbidity & mortality

The escaped air tracks up into the subcutaneous tissues of the neck, manifesting as *subcutaneous emphysema*.

Clinical Features

The hallmark of COPD is expiratory airflow obstruction that is not fully reversible. The main symptoms are cough, sputum production, and exertional dyspnoea. Nocturnal symptoms are unusual in COPD unless associated with cardiac failure. Physical examination reveals prolonged expiration, use of accessory muscles of respiration, chest hyperresonance on percussion, enlarged thoracic volume and decreased breath sounds. Clubbing is not a feature of COPD. Signs of cor pulmonale may be present. Marked tachypnoea, cyanosis, paradoxical abdominal motion may signify the need for assisted ventilation.

Chest radiographs are not sensitive for the diagnosis of COPD. Spirometry is the only reliable means for diagnosis and classification of COPD.

Reid index

The ratio of the thickness of the submucosal glands to that of the bronchial wall is expressed as Reid index.

In normal individuals, it is 0.44 ± 0.09
In chronic bronchitis, it is 0.52 ± 0.08

If the submucosal layer thickness is > 50% of bronchial wall thickness it is highly suggestive of chronic bronchitis.

High index is commonly associated with symptoms.

Complications

Pneumothorax, respiratory failure and cor pulmonale.

Investigations

X-ray Chest

Shows hypertranslucency, low flat diaphragm or bullae. Translucency extends anteriorly up to the 7th rib and posteriorly up to 9th rib. Widened intercostal spaces and tubular heart are seen.

Gold Classification of COPD

$FEV_1/FVC < 70\%$ is diagnostic of COPD except stage 0 At risk

Stages: All stages may or may not have chronic symptoms.
  0: At risk—Normal spirometry—Chronic symptoms like cough and sputum production
  I: Mild COPD—$FEV_1 \geq 80\%$ predicted
  II: Moderate COPD—FEV_1—50 to 80% predicted
  III: Severe COPD—FEV_1—30 to 50% predicted
  IV: Very severe—FEV_1—< 30% predicted or <50% predicted with chronic respiratory failure or clinical signs of right heart failure

Management

Stage 0 At risk—Avoidance of risk factors and influenza vaccination

Assess willingness to quit smoking—advise, assist and arrange to follow up.

- Mild COPD – Add short acting β_2 agonists Fenoterol/ Salbutamol/Terbutaline
- Moderate COPD—Add one or more long acting bronchodilators – Formoterol/Salmeterol and if needed add either short acting (Ipratropium bromide/Oxitropium bromide) or long acting (Tiotropium) anticholinergics.
- Severe COPD—Add inhaled glucocorticosteroids (Beclomethosone/Budesonide/Fluticasone/ Triamcinolone and if the response is not satisfactory, add systemic glucocorticosteroids (Prednisone/ Methyl-prednisolone)
- Very severe COPD—Long-term O_2, Ventilatory assistance, management of cardiac failure, consider surgical management.

All the drugs can be administered in the form of metered dose inhaler or dry powder inhaler or MDI with a spacer device or reservoir or delivery of the drug by a nebulizer.

Methylxanthines (Aminophylline, or theophylline SR) can be added when necessary.

Oxygen should be administered to maintain a PaO_2 >60 mm Hg or $SaO_2 > 90\%$. Patients with chronic respiratory failure need oxygen > 16 hours/day, 2-3 L/ minute and it has been shown to increase survival.

Antibiotics are needed only when there is respiratory infection.

Indications for Noninvasive Positive Pressure Ventilation (NIPPV)

(This mode is advocated only in patients with normal mental status, stable cardiovascular function, fairly cooperative and without respiratory arrest.)

- Severe dyspnoea with the use of accessory muscles and paradoxical abdominal motion
- Acidosis pH < 7.35 and hypercapnia $PaCO_2$ > 45 mm Hg (> 6.0 kPa)
- Respiratory rate > 25/minute.

Indications for Invasive Mechanical Ventilation

- Dyspnoea with the use of accessory muscles and paradoxical abdominal motion
- Respiratory rate > 35/minute
- Hypoxia – PaO_2 < 5.3 kPa (40 mmHg) or PaO_2/FiO_2 < 200 mm Hg
- Severe acidosis – pH < 7.25 and hypercapnia $PaCO_2$ > 60 mm Hg (> 8 kPa)

- Respiratory arrest
- Altered sensorium
- Unstable cardiovascular function—hypotension, shock, failure
- Sepsis, pulmonary embolism, massive pleural effusion, barotraumas
- NIPPV failure.

Surgical Management

- Bullectomy
- Lung volume reduction surgery—resection of damaged portion of lung
  Improves exercise tolerance but does not improve life expectancy
- Lung transplantation $FEV_1 < 35\%$ ($PaO_2 < 60$ mm Hg and $PaCO_2 > 50$ mm Hg).

Bronchiectasis

Persistent and irreversible dilatation and distortion of medium sized bronchi (5th to 9th generation) by more than 2 mm.

Bronchiectasis may be due to bronchial distention occurring as a result of chronic obstruction and recurrent infection.

Factors Predisposing to Bronchiectasis

Congenital

a. Primary
b. Secondary
   Tracheobronchomegaly (Mounier-Kuhn syndrome)
   Bronchomalacia (William-Campbell syndrome)
   Pulmonary sequestration (intralobar, extralobar)
   Kartagener's syndrome (bronchiectasis, sinusitis, situs inversus)
   Young's syndrome (idiopathic obstructive azoospermia)
   Yellow nail syndrome (lymphedema, yellow nails and pleural effusion)
   Cystic fibrosis
   α_1 antitrypsin deficiency
   Immunodeficiency syndromes (hypogammaglobulinaemia).
   Chandra-Khetarpal syndrome—Levocardia, sinusitis and bronchiectasis, but no ciliary abnormality.

Acquired

a. *Infections:* Measles, whooping cough, bronchitis, bronchiolitis, pneumonia, endobronchial tuberculosis.

b. *Bronchial obstruction:* Foreign body, tumour (adenoma/carcinoma), lymph nodes, left atrium, aneurysm [causes may be inside the lumen, on the wall or outside the wall].

c. *Associated immune disorders:* Ulcerative colitis, SLE, rheumatoid disease, ABPA.

Types

1. Cylindrical bronchiectasis
2. Saccular (cystic) bronchiectasis
3. Varicose bronchiectasis
4. Fusiform bronchiectasis.

Clinical Features

Persistent, recurrent cough and large quantity of purulent sputum production; haemoptysis; persistent coarse leathery crackles, with or without bronchial breathing (associated consolidation). Any combination of crackles, rhonchi and wheezes can occur. Clubbing of fingers and toes are present.

Bronchiectasis is common in left lower lobe because the lower lobe bronchus is longer and narrower. Middle lobe and lingual are next frequently involved. Involvement of upper lobe is uncommon.

Sequestration of Lung

It is a region of lung parenchyma that has an incomplete or no connection with the airways and is supplied by an aberrant artery arising from aorta or one of its branches. When it shares common visceral pleural investment with the adjacent normal lung tissue, it is called intralobar sequestration. When it has its own pleural lining, it is called extralobar sequestration.

Upper Lobe Bronchiectasis

This involves posterior and apical segments of upper lobe. It is common in tuberculosis, cystic fibrosis and ABPA.

Dry Bronchiectasis (Bronchiectasis Sicca)

Only hemoptysis is present; there is no sputum production; usually seen in upper lobe involvement in tuberculosis.

Middle Lobe Bronchiectasis (Brock's Syndrome)

This is a term applied to recurrent atelectasis of the right middle lobe (RML) in the absence of endobronchial obstruction. After several episodes of atelectasis, bronchiectasis and chronic fibrosis of the RML may develop. It is usually sequelae to primary pulmonary tuberculosis resulting from obstruction of middle lobe bronchus by TB lymph nodes.

Right middle lobe is involved because:
1. RML bronchus originates as a narrow and often slit-like lumen.
2. RML bronchus is surrounded by a network of lymph nodes draining both middle and lower lobes, which with infection enlarge and compress the bronchus.
3. RML bronchus before bifurcating into medial and lateral segments, runs a longer course (0.75 cm).
4. RML is separated by fissures and by a pleural envelope from the upper and lower lobes and lacks collateral ventilation.

Pseudo (Reversible) Bronchiectasis

It is a temporary bronchial dilatation occurring in an area of lung affected by pneumonic consolidation, tracheobronchitis or lung collapse.

Complications

1. Haemoptysis—may be life threatening.
2. Metastatic abscess (brain, pericardium, etc.)
3. Pneumothorax.
4. Cor pulmonale and right ventricular failure.
5. Amyloidosis
6. Recurrent pneumonia at the same site
7. Pyothorax
8. Lung abscess.

Investigations

Assessment of Ciliary Function

A pellet of saccharine is placed on anterior chamber of nose. The time taken for it to reach the pharynx, so that the patient can taste it, is noted. Normally it should not exceed 20 minutes. It is greatly prolonged in patients with ciliary dysfunction.

Sputum Examination

This is done for identifying the infecting organisms. Classically, a 3 layered sputum is seen (upper layer — frothy and watery, middle layer—turbid and mucopurulent, lower layer—purulent and opaque).

X-ray Chest (Fig. 4.30)

Shows ring shadows, tram track sign, gloved finger appearance, evidence of fibrosis or cor pulmonale.

CT Scan (Fig. 4.31)

It is a non-invasive diagnostic test.
Thick sections—more specific

Thin sections—more sensitive.

Bronchiectasis of proximal airways is suggestive of ABPA. Whereas nodular bronchiectasis suggests *Mycobacterium avium* complex infection.

Bronchography (Fig. 4.32)

It provides excellent visualization of bronchiectatic airways, which helps in confirming diagnosis and for planning surgery.

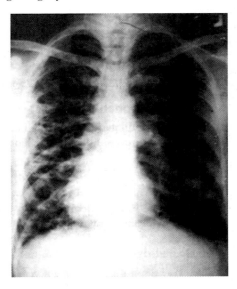

Fig. 4.30: Right sided bronchiectasis

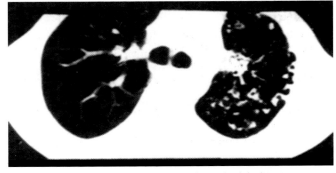

Fig. 4.31: CT scan—bronchiectasis right lung

Management

1. Control of infections by using appropriate antibiotics.
2. Improved clearance of tracheobronchial secretions by adequate hydration, chest physiotherapy with percussion, vibration and postural drainage.

Mucolytics are also tried (adequate hydration, acetyl cysteine, bromhexine). Percussion therapy should not be attempted when the patient has haemoptysis.

3. Serology for *Mycoplasma, Chlamydia, Legionella* and viral infections.
4. Examination of pleural fluid in parapneumonic effusions
5. Chest X-ray shows evidence of consolidation (homogenous opacity) of the affected lobe or segment (Fig. 4.35). May show evidence of pleural effusion. Second X-ray chest is a must in all cases of pneumonias after 7–10 days to assess the response to therapy and to find out if there is development of any complication.

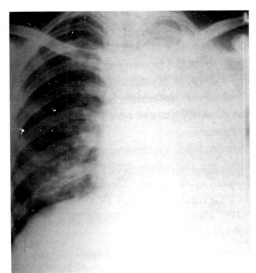

Fig. 4.35: Opaque left hemithorax without mediastinal shift massive consolidation

Bad Prognostic Indicators

1. Old age
2. Tachypnoea (respiratory rate > 30/min)
3. Hypotension (diastolic BP 60 mm Hg or less)
4. Extensive involvement (> one lobe in X-ray)
5. Atrial fibrillation
6. Initial normal leucocyte count
7. Persistent leucocytosis (> 20,000/µL, e.g. empyema)
8. Leucopenia (< 5000/µL)
9. Hypoxemia (PaO_2 < 8 kPa or 60 mm Hg).

Complications

1. Circulatory failure
2. Septicaemia
3. Parapneumonic effusions/empyema
4. Respiratory failure
5. Metastatic infections (meningitis, endocarditis, arthritis)
6. Lung abscess

7. ARDS, renal failure, multiple organ failure
8. Pneumothorax, especially with Staph. aureus
9. Thromboembolic disease
10. Pyrexia due to drug hypersensitivity.

Causes of Unresolved Pneumoniae

1. Incorrect microbiologic diagnosis
2. Inadequate dose or wrong choice of antibiotics
3. Endobronchial obstruction (poor local host defences)
4. Immunocompromised states (disease or drugs)
5. Malignancy.

Causes of Recurrent Pneumoniae in the Same Segment

1. Foreign body
2. Neoplasia (benign or malignant)
3. Sequestration of lung
4. Bronchiectasis.

Special Characteristics of Various Pneumonias

Pneumococcal Pneumonia

Production of rusty sputum is characteristic and the patient may be icteric. It usually involves a lobe and pleuritic reaction is common.

Staphylococcal Pneumonia

This is common in cystic fibrosis and influenza. Multiple, thin-walled staphylococcal abscesses are common (pneu-matoceles). Pneumothorax is a complication. It occurs in extremes of age and in immunosuppressed patients.

Klebsiella Pneumonia

Massive consolidation and excavation of upper lobe with expectoration of chocolate coloured sputum (brick red currant jelly). Lobes characteristically increase in size and it simulates tuberculosis.

Legionella Pneumonia

This is transmitted through infected water from cisterns, vapour or ventilation systems. Patient is toxic with hemoptysis; CNS or renal problems, myoglobinuria may be present. Diagnosis by serology or immunofluorescence.

Viral Pneumonia (Atypical Pneumonia)

Prodromal symptoms precede the onset of pneumonia by one week. Despite extensive radiological findings, respiratory signs and symptoms are minimal. Haemoptysis and parapneumonic effusions are rare. Common viruses causing pneumonia are varicella, H. simplex, CMV, measles, influenza, adenovirus and RSV.

Actinomycosis

A. israelii, an anaerobe can cause suppurative pneumonia when local defences are impaired. Chest wall sinuses and empyema are common with the sinuses discharging pus containing sulfur granules.

Mycoplasma Pneumonia

Presents with dry cough, erythema multiforme, arthralgia, myalgia. Predilection to lower lobe. Cold agglutinins positive.

Pneumonia due to Chlamydia

C. psittaci causes psittacosis or ornithosis. Patient has pneumonia, systemic illness, hepatosplenomegaly. Patchy consolidation is common. Diagnosed by serology.

Nosocomial Pneumonia

Pneumonia developing in a patient who has been hospitalized for > 48 hours. Infection by *Staph. aureus, Pseudomonas* and anaerobes are common.

Factors predisposing to nosocomial pneumonia
1. Aspiration of nasopharyngeal secretions
2. Gastroesophageal aspiration
3. Bacteria introduced by interventions (endotracheal tube, ventilators, nebulizers).

Common Causes of Immunosuppression and Associated Lung Diseases

	Causes	Pathogens involved
Neutropenia	Cytotoxic drugs	Staph aureus
	Agranulocytosis	Gram –ve bacteria
	Acute leukaemia	Candida albicans and Aspergillus fumigatus
T cell defect with or without B cell defect	Lymphoma	Candida albicans
	CLL	Tuberculosis
	Immunosuppressive drugs	Pneumocystis carinii
		CMV
	Bone marrow transplants	Gram –ve bacteria
	Splenectomy	Staph aureus
		Pneumococcus
		H. influenzae
Antibody production	CLL	Pneumococcus
	Myeloma	H. influenzae

4. Reduced host defences (steroid, postoperative state, anaesthesia)
5. Bacteremia (sepsis).

Pneumonia in Immunocompromized Host

This may be caused by *P. carinii, M. tuberculosis*. Onset is less rapid. Symptoms are more than signs. May be bilateral.

Pneumocystis Carinii Pneumonia

Occurs in immunocompromised hosts (AIDS, transplant recipients). It is an interstitial pneumonia. It presents with dry cough, tachypnoea, fever. Diagnosis is by clinical setting, sputum examination (methanamine

Empirical Treatment of Pneumonias

Type of pneumonia	Organism	Antibiotics
Community acquired:		
Mild	S. pneumoniae	Amoxicillin 500 mg-1000 mg x 8th hourly
	H. influenzae	Erythromycin 500 mg x 6th hourly PO
	M. pneumoniae	Fluroquinolone
Severe	As above	Co-amoxicillin or cephalosporin IV e.g. Cefuroxime 1.5 g x 8th hourly IV and erythromycin 1 g x 6th hourly IV
Atypical pneumoniae:	L. pneumophilia	Clarithromycin 500 mg x 12th hourly ± Rifampicin
	Chlamydia species	Tetracycline
	P. carnii	High dose cotrimoxazole
Hospital Acquired:	Gram-negative bacilli	Aminoglycoside IV + Antipseudomonal penicillin or 3rd generation cephalosporin IV
Aspiration:	S. pneumoniae Anaerobes	Cefuroxime 1.5 g x 8th hourly IV + Metronidazole 500 mg x 8th hourly IV
Neutropenic patients:	Gram-positive cocci Gram-negative bacilli Fungi	Aminoglycoside IV + Antipseudomonal Penicillin IV or 3rd generation cephalosporin IV Consider Antifungal drugs

silver stain) and lung tissue histopathology. Chest X-ray may be normal or show ground glass appearance; may spare lower zones.

Management

1. Appropriate antibiotics for 1–2 weeks
   a. *Pneumococcal pneumonia:* Benzyl Penicillin 20 lakh units every 6 hours for 7–10 days. There is total recovery within 1 week.
   b. *Staphylococcal pneumonia:* Flucloxacillin 0.25– 1 g 6th. hourly or erythromycin 2–4 g in divided doses IV. In severe infection sodium fusidate, 500 mg IV 3 times daily should be added. Therapy is continued for 2 weeks.

      Methicillin, vancomycin (for methicillin resistant cases) are the other drugs used.
   c. *Klebsiella pneumonia:* Gentamicin 2–5 mg/kg IV daily tid or ceftazidime 1 gm IV tid or Ciprofloxacin 200 mg IV bid. Therapy should be continued for 2–3 weeks.
   d. *Legionella pneumonia:* Erythromycin 0.5–1 g 6th hourly orally or IV; or Rifampicin 600 mg bid orally or IV in addition in seriously ill patients.
   e. *Actinomycosis:* Benzyl penicillin G 2–4 g IV 6th hourly till there is response (30–60 lakhs 6th hourly).
   f. *Mycoplasma pneumonia:* Tetracycline 500 mg qid or erythromycin 500 mg qid in severe infections.
   g. *Coxiella pneumonia:* Tetracycline 500 mg 4th hourly.
   h. *Viral pneumonia:* Acyclovir 200 mg 5 times daily for 5 days (l/2 dose for children under 2 years) or vidarabine 10 mg/kg for 5 days for varicella infection. There is no specific treatment for other viral pneumonias.
2. Treatment of complications.
3. Ventilatory support when needed.
4. Prevention by pneumococcal vaccine (Pneumovax, 1 dose of 0.5 ml SC/IM repeated after 5–10 years).

Lung Abscess

It is a localized infectious suppurative necrosis of lung tissue of > 2 cm in diameter.

Predisposing Factors

1. Aspiration of infected material (oropharyngeal surgical procedures, dental sepsis, coma, drugs, alcohol, anaesthesia, bulbar palsy, seizures, achalasia cardia).
2. Inadequately treated pneumonia.
3. Bronchial obstruction (tumour, foreign body).
4. Pulmonary infarction.
5. Septic emboli.
6. Spread of infection from adjacent organs, e.g. liver.
7. Infection of congenital or acquired cysts.

   Abscesses vary in size and number. Aspiration abscesses are more common on right, reflecting the more vertical right bronchus. Posterior segment of right upper lobe or apical segment of either lower lobe are commonly involved.

   Chronic abscesses are often surrounded by a reactive fibrous wall.

Common Organisms

Anaerobes, staphylococci, *Pseudomonas*, *Legionella* sp., Streptococcus pneumoniae, M. tuberculosis, Nocardia sp.

Clinical Features

Fever, malaise, weightloss, cough with copious, purulent sputum, haemoptysis, clubbing.

Position of the patient	*Site of aspiration*
1. Supine posture	Posterior segment of right upper lobe and apical segment of right or left lower lobe.
2. Prone position	Right middle lobe and left lingular lobe.
3. Sitting upright	Posterior or lateral basal segment of either lower lobe.

In epilepsy, any lobe can be involved because of bizarre posturing.

Differential Diagnosis

1. Cavitating lung cancer
2. Infected bulla or cyst
3. Pulmonary hamartoma
4. Cavitating pneumoconiosis
5. Infected hydatid cyst
6. Tuberculous, fungal, actinomycotic infections
7. Hiatus hernia.

Investigations

1. *Chest X-ray:* Shows thick-walled cavity with fluid level which moves in decubitus film.
2. Sputum examination and culture.
3. Radioactive Indium-111 labelled leucocyte uptake.

Management

1. Appropriate antibiotics for 4–6 weeks.
2. Physiotherapy and postural drainage.

3. Rigid bronchoscopy for adequate suction of secretions from bronchial tree. Fibreoptic bronchoscope should be avoided as the suction channel is small and the flood of pus may drown the patient.
4. Intercostal tube drainage—*very rarely*.
5. *Surgery:* If there is failure of medical therapy in spite of bronchoscopic clearance, surgical resection is advised. Presence of obstructing carcinoma is an indication for surgery in addition to the definitive management according to the staging and general condition of the patient.

Pleural Effusion

Pleural effusion is the accumulation of serous fluid in the pleural cavity.

Mechanism of Pleural Fluid Formation

1. Elevation of venous pressure (rare in pure RV failure)
2. Decreased plasma oncotic pressure (except in congenital hypoalbuminaemia)
3. Increased capillary permeability due to local inflammation, toxins or vasoactive substances as occurs in collagen-vascular diseases, pancreatitis, pulmonary emboli and pneumonitis
4. Increase in pleural space oncotic pressure as a result of:
   a. Protein leak through capillaries
   b. Protein exudation due to local pleural inflammation.
   c. Defective lymphatic resorption.
      When pleural space oncotic pressure approaches that of plasma (32 cmH$_2$O), fluid absorption is impaired.
5. Simple transfer of ascitic fluid across diaphragmatic defects and also through transdiaphragmatic lymphatics as occurs in cirrhosis and Meig's syndrome
6. Increased negativity of pressure in the pleural space also results in pleural effusion as occurs in atelectasis
7. Obstruction of lymphatics.
   Pleural fluid, on aspiration in normal persons is 3-20 ml. Normal protein content is below 1.5 gm/dl.

Causes of Pleural Effusion

Transudates

1. Congestive cardiac failure
2. Cirrhosis of liver
3. Nephrotic syndrome
4. Myxoedema
5. Peritoneal dialysis
6. Pericardial disease.

Exudates

1. *Neoplasms:* Metastatic disease, mesothelioma
2. *Infectious diseases:* Bacterial, viral, fungal, parasitic, tuberculous
3. Pulmonary embolism
4. *Collagen vascular diseases* (rheumatoid arthritis, SLE, Wegener's granulomatosis)
5. *Gastrointestinal disease* (esophageal perforation, pancreatic disease, diaphragmatic hernia, intra-abdominal abscess, endoscopic sclerotherapy)
6. Uraemia
7. Meig's syndrome (ovarian fibroma, ascites, right sided pleural effusion)
8. *Drug-induced:* Bromocriptine, amiodarone, nitrofurantoin, dantrolene
9. Chylothorax, haemothorax
10. Ovarian hyperstimulation syndrome.

Features	Exudates	Transudates
Colour	Amber coloured	Colourless
Consistency	Sticky	Non-sticky
On shaking	Froth +	No froth
On standing	Clots	Does not clot
On aspiration	Slow flow	Flows fast
Specific gravity	> 1018	< 1018
Cells	+ +	a few lymphocytes
Light's criteria		
1. Pleural fluid protein/serum protein	> 0.5	< 0.5
2. Pleural fluid LDH/serum LDH	> 0.6	< 0.6
3. Pleural fluid LDH	> 2/3 of upper normal value of serum	< 2/3 of upper normal value of serum
Glucose	< 60 mg/dl	> 60 mg/dl
LDH	> 200 IU/L	< 200 IU/L

Pleural Fluid Analysis

If pleural fluid is found to be an exudate, the following tests should be done.

1. *Glucose level:* If <60 mg/dl, consider the following conditions.
   i. Bacterial infections (parapneumonic effusions).
   ii. Rheumatoid pleural effusion (< 30 mg/dl)
   iii. Malignancy
   iv. Tuberculosis
   v. Haemothorax
   vi. Paragonimiasis
   vii. Churg-Strauss syndrome.
   Patients with malignant disease of pleura and a low sugar level have a positive pleural cytology or biopsy or both and they have a poor prognosis of less than 2 months. Sugar level more than 80 mg % suggests SLE.

2. *Amylase level:* Elevated in:
   i. Pancreatic pleural effusion (pseudocyst of pancreas, pancreatitis)
   ii. Oesophageal rupture
   iii. Malignancy (salivary amylase).
   In malignancy and oesophageal rupture only salivary amylase is elevated and not pancreatic amylase.
3. *Total WBC count:* If TC > 1000/mm^3, the fluid is an exudate. If TC > 10,000/mm^3, consider
   i. Empyema
   ii. Parapneumonic effusion
   iii. Pancreatitis
   iv. Pulmonary embolism
   v. Collagen vascular diseases
   vi. Malignancy
   vii. Tuberculosis.
4. *Differential cell count*
   i. *Increased   Pulmonary infection
      neutrophils*   Pulmonary embolization
                          Intra-abdominal abscess
   ii. *Increased   Tuberculosis
       Lymphocytes*   Malignancy
   iii. *Increased eosinophils*
      a. *With peripheral eosinophilia*
         Hodgkin's disease
         Fungal infection
         Parasitic (paragonimiasis)
         Benign asbestos pleural effusion
         Polyarteritis nodosa
         Tropical eosinophilia.
         Drugs—dantrolene, nitrofurantoin
      b. *Without peripheral eosinophilia*
         Trauma
         Pulmonary infarction
         Rarely in carcinoma.
   iv. *Mesothelial cells:* Presence of mesothelial cells is against the diagnosis of tuberculosis and diagnostic of mesothelioma and adenocarcinoma.
5. *pH of the pleural fluid:* If pleural fluid pH is < 7, tube thoracostomy is indicated. If the pH is low, consider
   i. Complicated parapneumonic effusion
   ii. Systemic acidosis
   iii. Oesophageal rupture
   iv. Rheumatoid pleurisy
   v. Tuberculosis (TB pleuritis)
   vi. Malignancy of pleura
   vii. Haemothorax
   viii. Paragonimiasis
   ix. Lupus pleuritis
   x. Urinothorax.

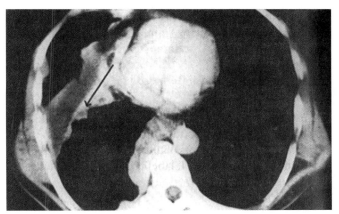

Fig. 4.36: CT scan—irregular, lobulated appearance of pleural mesothelioma

6. High pleural fluid to serum ratio of IgG, IgA, IgM suggests malignancy.
7. Increased gamma interferon is found in tuberculous effusion > 140 pg/ml.
8. Pleural fluid adenosine deaminase (large form) >70 U/L indicates tuberculous effusion and a value of < 40 U/L is against the diagnosis.
   If the small form of ADA is elevated, it is suggestive of lymphoma.
9. Pleural fluid should be sent for Gram's stain and culture, smear for AFB, culture for AFB.
10. Pleural fluid cytology should be done to find out malignant cells.

Clinical Features

Pleuritic chest pain (before effusion develops); dyspnoea (the degree of which depends on the rate and the size of accumulation); tracheal and mediastinal shift to the opposite side; diminished or absent breath sounds and stony dull percussion note; aegophony and bronchial breath sounds just above the level of effusion due to the relaxed lung.

Investigations

X-ray Chest

- Minimal amount of fluid that can be detected in the PA view is 300 ml. Smaller quantities of fluid are detected in lateral decubitus position (in this position, fluid layers along the dependent chest wall).
- Dense uniform opacity in the lower and lateral parts of the haemithorax shading off above and medially into transluscent lung (Ellis 'S' shaped curve).
- Tracheal and mediastinal shift to the opposite side (fluid > 1500 cc). When mediastinal shift does not

when the patient's spontaneous breath rate falls below the selected backup rate.

Synchronised Intermittent Mandatory Ventilation (SIMV): This mode is maintenance as well as weaning mode. Here the required tidal volume and the respiratory rate are set and delivered by the ventilator in synchrony with the patient's own respiratory effort. Potential advantages of SIMV include less respiratory alkalosis, fewer adverse cardiovascular effects due to lower intrathoracic pressures, less requirement for sedation and paralysis, maintenance of respiratory muscle function, and facilitation of long-term weaning.

Pressure Support Ventilation (PSV): This mode augments each patient triggered respiratory effort by specified amount of preset level of positive airway pressure (5-50 cm of H_2O). This mode is primarily to augment spontaneous respiratory efforts during IMV modes of ventilation or during weaning trials.

Continuous Positive Airway Pressure (CPAP): CPAP is used to deliver air via a nasal or oral mask. Nasal continuous positive airway pressure (nCPAP) is the current treatment of choice for most patients with obstructive sleep apnoea-hypopnoea syndrome (OSAHS). nCPAP pneumatically splints open the upper airway and prevents collapse. CPAP is applied in spontaneously breathing patient before weaning from mechanical ventilation. Bilevel positive airway pressure (BIPAP) is more expensive than simple CPAP and can be used to treat patients with OSAHS and in patients who do not tolerate high levels of CPAP. All non-invasive positive pressure or mechanical ventilation devices may induce dryness of the airway, nasal congestion, rhinorrhoea, epistaxis, nasal bridge abrasions, skin reactions to the mask and aerophagia.

Positive End Expiratory Pressure (PEEP): PEEP is defined as the maintenance of positive airway pressure at the end of expiration. It can be applied in the spontaneously breathing patient in the form of CPAP or to the patient who is receiving mechanical ventilation. PEEP usually increases lung compliance by opening the alveoli and oxygenation while decreasing the shunt fraction and ventilation perfusion mismatch. PEEP is used primarily in patients with hypoxic respiratory failure (e.g. ARDS, cardiogenic pulmonary oedema). Low levels of PEEP (3-5 cm of H_2O) is useful in patients with COPD to prevent dynamic airway collapse from occurring during expiration. The main goal of PEEP is to achieve a PaO_2 greater than 55-60 mm Hg with an FiO_2 of 60%. Patients who receive signifivcant levels of PEEP (i.e. > 10 cm H_2O) should not have their PEEP removed abruptly since it can result in collapse of distal lung units. PEEP should be weaned in 3-5 cm H_2O increments while oxygenation is monitored closely.

Inverse ratio ventilation (IRV): It uses an inspiratory-to-expiratory ratio $\geq$ 1:1 instead of the normal 1:2 – 1:3 to stabilize terminal respiratory units (alveolar recruitment) and to improve gas exchange primarily for patients with ARDS. The goals of IRV are:
1. To decrease peak airway pressures
2. To maintain adequate alveolar ventilation
3. To improve oxygenation

Indication for IRV: A PaO_2 less than 60 mm Hg with FiO_2 of greater than 60% and peak airway pressures greater than 40-45 cm of H_2O or PEEP > 15 cm of H_2O.

Most patients need heavy sedation and often muscle paralysis during the implementation of IRV.

Noninvasive Mechanical Ventilation: Noninvasive intermittent positive pressure ventilation (NIPPV) increases pH, reduces $PaCO_2$ reduces the severity of breathlessness in the first 4 hours of treatment, and decreases the length of hospital stay. Intubation rate is reduced by this intervention.

However, NIPPV is not appropriate for all patients.

Indications
1. Moderate to severe dyspnoea with the use of accessory muscles and paradoxical abdominal motion
2. Moderate to severe acidosis (pH < 7.35) and hypercapnia ($PaCO_2$ > 6 kPa, 45 mm of Hg).
3. Respiratory frequency > 25 breaths/minute.

Contraindications
1. Respiratory arrest
2. Cardiovascular instability (Hypotension, arrhythmias, MI)
3. Impaired mental status, somnolence, uncooperative patients
4. High aspiration risk—viscous or copious secretions
5. Recent facial or gastroesophageal surgery
6. Craniofacial trauma, fixed nasopharyngeal abnormalities
7. Extreme obesity

Complications of Mechanical Ventilation
1. Airway malpositioning and occlusion
2. Acute increase in peak airway pressure
   a. Pneumo/haemothorax
   b. Occlusion of patient's airway
   c. Bronchospasm
   d. Accumulation of condensate in ventilator circuit
   e. Worsening of pulmonary oedema

3. Fighting or buckling the ventilator (Asynchronous breathing)
   — inadequate ventilatory support, leak in the ventilatory circuit,
   — inadequate FlO_2 (check the adjustments in the ventilatory system)
4. Barotrauma or volutrauma
   — Subcutaneous emphysema,
   — Pneumopericardium,
   — Pneumoperitoneum,
   — Pneumomediastinum,
   — Pneumothorax,
   — Air-embolism
5. Cardiac arrhythmias
6. Aspiration
7. Pneumonia (nosocomial—>72 hr intubation)
8. Upper GI bleed (gastritis or ulcer)
9. Positive fluid balance and hyponatraemia
10. Oxygen toxicity
11. Tracheal stenosis
12. Hypotension or organ hypoperfusion
13. Mild to moderate cholestasis
14. Acid-base complications (Metabolic/respiratory alkalosis).

Guidelines for Withdrawal of Mechanical Ventilation
1. Mental status of the patient—Awake, alert and co-operative
2. PaO_2 more than 60 mm Hg with FiO_2 less than 50%
3. PEEP < 5 cm H_2O
4. Acceptable $PaCO_2$ and pH
5. Tidal volume > 5 ml/Kg
6. Vital capacity > 10 ml/Kg
7. Respiratory rate < 30/minute
8. Stable vital signs after 1-2 hours spontaneous breathing trial.

Pulmonary Hypertension

Normal pulmonary artery pressures are as follows:
Systolic pressure   15–25 mm Hg
Diastolic pressure   5–10 mm Hg
Mean pressure   10–15 mm Hg

Pulmonary hypertension is present when pulmonary artery systolic pressure is > 30 mm Hg, and pulmonary artery mean pressure is > 20 mm Hg.

Causes of Pulmonary Hypertension
Cardiovascular Causes
1. Cardiomyopathies.
2. Congenital heart diseases (ASD, VSD, PDA, Eisenmenger's syndrome)

3. Valvular heart diseases (mitral heart diseases and LV dysfunction)
4. Persistence of fetal circulation.

Pulmonary Causes
1. Pulmonary parenchymal disorders
   a. COPD
   b. Interstitial lung diseases
   c. Restrictive lung diseases
   d. Granulomatous lung diseases (tuberculosis, sarcoidosis)
   e. Collagen vascular disorders.
2. Hypoventilation syndromes
   a. Sleep apnoea
   b. Central alveolar hypoventilation
   c. Obesity hypoventilation syndrome (Pickwickian syndrome).
3. Pulmonary vascular disorders
   a. Primary pulmonary hypertension (PPH)
   b. Pulmonary thromboembolism
   c. Peripheral pulmonary artery stenosis
   d. Pulmonary veno-occlusive disease
   e. Schistosomiasis.
4. Miscellaneous
   a. Drugs (fenfluramine, diethylpropion, aminorex fumarate)
   b. Systemic sclerosis
   c. Sickle cell anaemia
   d. Liver disorders
   e. High altitude.

Clinical Features

Cough, chest pain, haemoptysis, loud P_2, TR murmur, RVH and features of RV failure later.

Functional assessment of pulmonary hypertension

Class I	No limitation of physical activity—No fatigue, dyspnoea, chest pain or syncope for ordinary physical activity
Class II	Comfortable at rest but symptomatic on ordinary physical activity
Class III	Marked limitation of physical activity—less than ordinary physical activity causes chest pain, undue dyspnea, fatigue or near syncope
Class IV	Unable to carry out any physical activity—Dyspnoeic even at rest with signs of right heart failure

Six-minute walk test: It demonstrates oxyhaemoglobin desaturation on exertion. The distance achieved is lower than expected and it assists in quantifying functional limitations

Investigations

1. *X-ray chest:* In severe pulmonary hypertension, enlargement of RV and pulmonary arteries are seen. It may also show evidence of primary lung or cardiac diseases.
2. *Ventilation-perfusion lung scan:* This shows several segmental or greater-sized perfusion defects in thromboembolism. In contrast, in PPH, perfusion scan is either normal or patchy.
3. *Pulmonary angiogram:* It is indicated when there is suspicion of thromboembolism.

Management

1. Treat the underlying cause
2. Correct hypoxaemia with oxygen
3. Diuretics in RV failure
4. Vasodilators in PPH
   a. Calcium channel blockers
   b. Angiotensin-converting enzyme inhibitors
   c. Epoprostenol and Treprestinil are the drugs approved for the treatment of pulmonary hypertension.
   d. Bosentan-endothelin receptor antagonist and sildenafil – an oral phosphodiesterase -5 inhibitor are also used in the treatment of pulmonary hypertension.

   Caution: Sudden discontinuation of vasodilator/prostacyclin during chronic use can result in rebound PH and death. Calcium channel blockers should be used only in vasodilator-responsive patients and not in nonresponders as it might cause hypotension, RVF and death.
5. Prostacyclin (improves pulmonary hemodynamics, exercise tolerance and survival in PPH when given for more than 12 weeks)
6. Acute inhalation of nitric oxide (in PPH)
7. Creation of a small ASD by balloon septostomy (allows deoxygenated blood to reach LV improving cardiac output)
   Atrial septostomy: It allows decompression of the right heart by creating a hole in the septum when the right heart pressure is greater than the left (right-to-left shunt). It is a palliative procedure and it improves left ventricular filling and cardiac output. This procedure is indicated in severe PPH refractory to maximal medical therapy and this serves as a bridge till the transplantation.
8. Heart-lung transplant
9. Surgical intervention in thromboembolism.

Cor Pulmonale

Cor pulmonale is enlargement of the right ventricle with or without failure, secondary to diseases of the lung, thorax, or pulmonary circulation.

Clinical Features

Features of RV failure and evidence of primary lung diseases.

Investigations

1. *X-ray chest:* prominent RA, RV and pulmonary artery.
2. *ECG:* P pulmonale, right axis deviation, RVH with strain pattern.
3. *Blood count:* secondary polycythaemia.

Management

1. Treat the primary lung disorder
2. Diuretics
3. Vasodilators
4. Bronchodilators
5. Control of infection.

Pulmonary Thromboembolism

Pulmonary thromboembolism is due to detached thrombi from deep veins of leg (80%); of pelvic veins (10%); or other veins and right sided cardiac chambers (5%) and very rare causes air, fat, tumour cells, placental bits, amniotic fluid, and parasites—schistosomes (5%). Ninety percent of deaths occur within the first hour even before a diagnostic therapeutic plan is implemented.

Risk Factors for Deep Vein Thrombosis

1. Deficiency of antithrombin III, Protein C, and Protein S.
2. Presence of lupus anticoagulant
3. Homocystinuria
4. Surgical procedures of more than 30 minutes duration.
5. Prolonged bed rest following medical illness or surgery or fractures involving lower limbs
6. Chronic deep venous insufficiency
7. Malignancy predisposes to DVT
8. Obesity
9. Oral contraceptives
10. Estrogen therapy
- Deep vein thrombosis usually develops in the region of a venous valve.

- Large extensive thrombi can develop within a few minutes.
- Larger leg veins (popliteal and above) are the common source of pulmonary emboli.
- Pulmonary emboli are uncommon in DVT that remains confined to calf veins. Pulmonary embolism is common in the first week of thrombus formation before its fibrinolysis/organization.
- Pain, warmth, and swelling of legs denote deep vein thrombosis.

Investigations

- Doppler ultrasound (duplex) is useful in the diagnosis of DVT.

- Ascending contrast venography is the gold standard test.
- Impedance plethysmography and radiofibrinogen methods are two non-invasive investigatory techniques in the diagnosis of DVT.

Clinical Features

The classical manifestations of pulmonary thromboembolism are unexplained dyspnoea, tachycardia, central chest pain or pleurisy, haemoptysis developing in the second week of postoperative period, especially in patients with a predisposing condition like DVT.

Manifestations of Pulmonary Thromboembolism

	Size of vessels		
	Large (massive)	Medium (segmental)	Microvasculature
Pathology	Reduced cardiac output, sudden loss of cerebral and coronary blood flow, acute right heart failure, altered ventilation perfusion ratio	Pulmonary infarction with or without pleural effusion	Pulmonary hypertension Failure of right heart
Symptoms	Sudden dyspnoea, tachycardia central chest pain sudden syncope	Pleurisy pain Breathlessness Haemoptysis	Dyspnoea and syncope only on exertion
Signs CVS	Shock, raised JVP, tachycardia, hypotension, loud/widely split P2 gallop rhythm	Asymptotic or mild tachycardia mild dyspnoea	Asymptomatic late-loud P2 signs of RV failure
RS	Central cyanosis	Pleural rub, crackles haemorrhagic-pleural effusion	Nil
Urine output	Reduced	Normal	Normal
Fever	———	Low-grade fever	———
Investigations			
X-ray chest	Hilar prominence oligaemic lung fields	Raised hemidiaphragm Wedge shaped or linear opacities Pleural effusion	Prominent Pulmonary trunk And RV Increased TCD
ECG	$(S_I\, Q_{III}\, T_{III})$ S in lead I Q in lead III Inverted T in lead III and chest leads VI toV4 Right axis deviation, AF Right bundle-branch block	———	Right ventricular hypertrophy and strain
Blood gases	Reduced PaO_2 Reduced $PaCO_2$	Reduced $PaCO_2$	Reduced PaO_2 on exertion
Ventilation perfusion (V/Q lung scans)	Larger areas of defective perfusion	Segmental areas	———
CT with contrast MRI, spiral CT	Diagnostic	Diagnostic	———
Pulmonary angiography	Diagnostic	Diagnostic	———
Lung biopsy	Not required	Not required	Confirms diagnosis

The clinical signs and the results of investigations vary depending on the size of pulmonary vessels involved-large (massive), medium (segmental), or pulmonary microvasculature.

Management

1. Administer oxygen (up to 100%)
2. Morphine 10mg IV if patient is distressed
3. Heparin – 10,000 to 20,000 units IV bolus
4. Follow it with heparin standard regimens 4 hours later
   Standard heparin regimens:
   A. Continuous intravenous—1000 units/hour
   B. Intermittent intravenous—5000 units 4th hourly or 7,500 units qid.
   C. Intermittent subcutaneous—5000 units 4th hourly or 10,000 units tid.
   Avoid intramuscular injection of heparin as it causes haematoma. Intramuscular injections must be avoided during heparin therapy. Subcutaneous low molecular weight heparin is equally effective except for the high cost. Heparin therapy is given for 10 days.
5. Thrombolytic therapy with streptokinase or urokinase may be useful in large vein DVT or massive embolism.
6. Pulmonary embolectomy—Rarely indicated
7. Venous interruption—Transvenous placement of filter in the inferior vena cava to protect against emboli greater than 2 mm in diameter.
8. Oral anticoagulants like warfarin to be given for a period of three months afer heparin therapy.

Management of DVT

Use one of the standard heparin regimens or low molecular weight heparin for 10 days. No bolus dose of heparin is required. Follow heparin therapy with oral anticoagulants for 3 months.

Lung Transplantation

Indications

End-stage lung disease
- COPD
- Idiopathic pulmonary fibrosis
- Cystic fibrosis
- Primary pulmonary hypertension
- Alpha-1 antitrypsin deficiency (emphysema)
- Eisenmenger's syndrome.

Types

1. Single lung transplantation (right or left) through a thoracotomy
2. Sequential single lung transplantation (through anterior thoracosternotomy)
3. Heart-lung transplantation (through median sternotomy).

Single lung transplantation is performed for non infectious lung disorders and for Eisenmenger's syndrome (where heart defect is correctable at the time of transplant). There is a definite functional improvement. The lack of available donors to meet the demand makes single lung Tx popular.

Disease	Parameters for Tx	Improvement after Tx
Primary pulmonary hypertension	PHT, RV failure, Class III functional status, No response to vasodilators	Pulmonary artery and right heart pressures normalize
Eisenmenger's syndrome	Near syncope, Chest pressure, Haemoptysis	Lung function tests become normal Functional improvement to class I or II
Cystic fibrosis	FEV$_1$ < 20% Hemoptysis, Weight loss, frequent infections	Lung function tests normalize
Emphysema	FEV$_1$ of 500 cc or less	40–60% after Tx
Interstitial Lung disease	Low D$_L$CO, PHT and RVF, Hypoxaemia during exercise	TLC becomes 70–80%

Complications

Early post Tx period: bleeding, bronchial dehiscence or stenosis, reimplantation pulmonary oedema, acute rejection, infection.

Late complications: infections, renal insufficiency (cyclosporin), obliterative bronchiolitis (warrants sequential bronchoscopy and transbronchial biopsy).

Prognosis

Single lung Tx: 1 year—73%, 2 years—65%, 3 years—62%.

Bilateral, sequential single lung Tx: 1 yr—70%, 2 yr—60%, 3 yr—55% (cystic fibrosis).

Heart lung Tx (Eisenmenger's syndrome): 1 yr—60%, 5 yrs—40%.

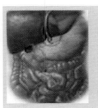

THE HISTORY	THE PHYSICAL EXAMINATION

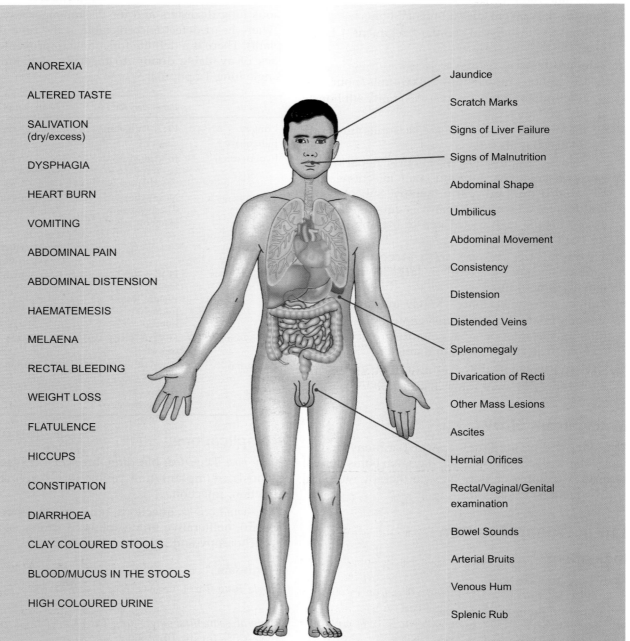

THE HISTORY

ANOREXIA

ALTERED TASTE

SALIVATION
(dry/excess)

DYSPHAGIA

HEART BURN

VOMITING

ABDOMINAL PAIN

ABDOMINAL DISTENSION

HAEMATEMESIS

MELAENA

RECTAL BLEEDING

WEIGHT LOSS

FLATULENCE

HICCUPS

CONSTIPATION

DIARRHOEA

CLAY COLOURED STOOLS

BLOOD/MUCUS IN THE STOOLS

HIGH COLOURED URINE

THE PHYSICAL EXAMINATION

Jaundice

Scratch Marks

Signs of Liver Failure

Signs of Malnutrition

Abdominal Shape

Umbilicus

Abdominal Movement

Consistency

Distension

Distended Veins

Splenomegaly

Divarication of Recti

Other Mass Lesions

Ascites

Hernial Orifices

Rectal/Vaginal/Genital examination

Bowel Sounds

Arterial Bruits

Venous Hum

Splenic Rub

Clinical Examination

Signs and Symptoms

Dysphagia	Difficulty in swallowing
Aphagia	Inability to swallow
Odynophagia	Painful swallowing
Globus pharyngeus	Sensation of a lump lodged in the throat
Phagophobia	Fear of swallowing
Anorexia	Loss of appetite or lack of desire to eat
Sitophobia	Fear of eating because of subsequent abdominal discomfort seen in regional enteritis and in chronic mesenteric vascular insufficiency (abdominal angina)
Nausea	Feeling of imminent desire to vomit, usually referred to the throat or epigastrium
Vomiting (emesis)	Refers to the forceful oral expulsion of gastric contents
Retching	Denotes laboured rhythmic contraction of respiratory and abdominal musculatures that frequently precedes or accompanies vomiting
Hiccough or hiccup or singultus	A phenomenon resulting from sudden spasmodic, involuntary contraction of diaphragm with the glottis remaining closed with the production of short, sharp, inspiratory sounds
Regurgitation	Appearance of previously swallowed food in the mouth without vomiting, e.g. achalasia cardia
Water brash	Sudden filling of mouth with saliva produced as a reflex response to a variety of symptoms from upper GIT
Heart burn or pyrosis	Sensation of warmth or burning located substernally or high in the epigastrium with radiation into the neck and occasionally to the arms
Belching	Chronic repetitive eructations
Aerophagia	Air swallowing
Diarrhoea	An increase in daily stool weight more than 200 gm. Typically the patient may also describe an increase in stool liquidity and frequency of more than 3 bowel movements per day. If consistency is liquid or semi-formed even one episode is considered as diarrhoea.

	Normal bowel frequency ranges from 3 times a week to 3 times a day depending on fibre content, medications, exercise and stress
Pseudo-diarrhoea or hyperdefaecation	Increased frequency of defaecation without increase in stool weight above normal. It is seen in irritable bowel syndrome, hyperthyroidism (increased sympathetic activity) and proctitis
Faecal incontinence	Involuntary release of rectal contents. It is more common when stool is liquid than solid. It reflects weakness of pelvic muscles resulting in abnormal function of anorectal sphincter
Acute diarrhoea	Diarrhoea lasts for 1-2 weeks
Chronic diarrhoea	Diarrhoea lasts for more than 4 weeks
Constipation	Frequency of defaecation less than 3 times a week or the stool is hard or difficult to pass
Haematemesis	Vomiting of blood
Pseudohaematemesis	In patients with upper respiratory bleed, the blood may be swallowed and later vomited as altered blood mimicking an upper GI bleed
Melaena	Passage of stools rendered tarry and black by the presence of altered blood. About 60 ml of blood is necessary to cause melaena. After a single bout of bleeding, melaena persists for about 1 week. Blood must remain in the gut for about 8 hours to produce melaena
Maroon colored stool	Passage of maroon coloured stool occurs when the bleeding site is located in the distal small bowel or right colon
Haematochezia	Passage of frank blood per rectum. It signifies bleeding from a source distal to ligament of Treitz, especially when bleed occurs from anorectum or left colon. Brisk upper GI bleed with rapid intestinal transit may also result in bright red blood per rectum
Jaundice	Yellowish discoloration of skin, sclera and mucous membranes resulting from an increase in serum bilirubin concen/tration more than 2 mg/dl.

3. Striae
4. Divarication of recti.

In ascites, usually flanks are dull and the centre of abdomen is resonant and in ovarian or pelvic tumors, the centre of abdomen is dull and the flanks may be resonant. However, in gross ascites and in large ovarian tumors, both the flanks and the centre of abdomen may be dull on percussion.

Percussion of Cyst (Hydatid Thrill)

Keeping 3 fingers over the cyst, percuss over the middle finger. A thrill is elicited which can be felt by other 2 fingers.

Auscultation

Auscultation of abdomen is done for:

Bowel Sounds

Normal motility of the gut creates a characteristic gurgling sounds every 5-10 seconds which can be heard by unaided ear (Borborygmi).

Bowel sounds are increased in:
a. Simple, acute, mechanical, small bowel obstruction. Increased bowel sounds with colicky pain is pathognomonic of small bowel obstruction. In between colicky pain, bowel is quiet and no sounds are audible
b. Malabsorption
c. Severe GI bleeding
d. Carcinoid syndrome.

Bowel sounds are absent in
a. Paralytic ileus
b. Peritonitis.
   In later stages of paralytic ileus, high pitched, tinkling sounds due to fluid spill over from one distended gas and fluid filled loop to the other can be heard.

Succussion Splash

It is a sound resembling shaking a half filled bottle. It is heard in:
1. Pyloric stenosis
2. Advanced intestinal obstruction
3. Paralytic ileus (with grossly distended loops of bowel)
4. Normal stomach within 2 hours after a meal.

Bruit

- Bruit over aorta can be heard above and to the left of umbilicus in cases of aortic aneurysm. Aortic bruit can also be heard over femoral artery.

- Bruit over mid abdomen is heard in renal artery stenosis.
- Bruit over common iliac artery can be heard in stenosis or aneurysm.
- Bruit over liver may be heard in:
   a. Haemangioma
   b. Hepatocellular carcinoma
   c. Acute alcoholic hepatitis
   d. Hepatic artery aneurysm.
- Bruit can also be heard in coeliac artery stenosis and carcinoma pancreas (due to compression of vessels).

Venous Hum

It is heard between xiphisternum and umbilicus due to turbulence of blood flow in well-developed collaterals as a result of portal hypertension (Cruveilhier-Baumgarten syndrome). It signifies a congenital patent umbilical vein draining into the portal vein.

Friction Rub

It is heard in perisplenitis or perihepatitis due to microinfarction and inflammation.
   Splenic rub is heard in the following conditions:
   a. Chronic myeloid leukaemia
   b. Infective endocarditis
   c. Sickle cell anaemia
   d. After biopsy.

Causes of Hepatomegaly

Infective

a. Along the biliary tree	Cholangitis
b. Along portal vein	Amoebiasis Schistosomiasis Bacterial infections
c. Along hepatic artery Bacterial	Typhoid, brucellosis tuberculosis, syphilis, Weil's disease
Viral	Infective hepatitis-infectious mononucleosis
Protozoal	Malaria, kala-azar
Fungal	Actinomycosis histoplasmosis
Parasitic	Echinococcosis (hydatid cyst)

Congestive

Congestive cardiac failure
Cardiomyopathy
Constrictive pericarditis
Budd-Chiari syndrome.

Degenerative and Infiltrative

Alcoholic fatty liver
Lymphomas
Leukaemias
Multiple myeloma.

Storage Disorders

Niemann-Pick disease
Gaucher's disease
Amyloidosis.

Neoplasia

Hepatocellular carcinoma
Cholangiocarcinoma
Secondaries.

Toxins

Alcohol, arsenic
Phosphorous, drugs.

Causes of Painful Hepatomegaly

Congestive cardiac failure
Viral hepatitis
Hepatic amoebiasis
Pyemic abscess
Hepatoma
Actinomycosis
Secondaries
Budd-Chiari syndrome.

Causes of Pulsatile Liver

Tricuspid regurgitation (systolic)
Tricuspid stenosis (diastolic)
Aortic regurgitation.

Causes of Splenomegaly

Mild (up to 5 cm)

Congestive cardiac failure
Acute malaria
Typhoid
Infective endocarditis
Septicaemia
Systemic lupus erythematosus
Rheumatoid arthritis
Thalassaemia minor
Miliary tuberculosis

Leptospirosis
HIV.

Moderate (5-8 cm)

Viral hepatitis
Cirrhosis
Lymphomas
Leukaemias
Infectious mononucleosis
Haemolytic anaemias
Splenic infarcts
Splenic abscess
Amyloidosis
Haemochromatosis
Polycythaemia.

Massive (> 8 cm)

Chronic myeloid leukaemia
Myeloid metaplasia
Myelofibrosis
Hairy cell leukaemia
Gaucher's disease
Niemann-Pick disease
Sarcoidosis
Thalassaemia major
Chronic malaria
Kala-azar
Congenital syphilis
Extrahepatic portal vein obstruction
Schistosomiasis
Diffuse splenic haemangiomatosis
Lymphoma
Polycythaemia.

Causes of Hepatosplenomegaly

Infections

Malaria
Kala-azar
Infective hepatitis
Disseminated tuberculosis
Bacterial endocarditis
Infectious mononucleosis.

Haematological Disorders

Anaemia (chronic haemolytic anaemia)
Myeloproliferative disorders
　　Chronic myeloid leukaemia
　　Myelofibrosis
Non-Hodgkin's lymphoma
Hodgkin's lymphoma.

Clinical Conditions Producing Stress Ulcer

a. Elderly patients in ICU with concomitant heart and lung disease have a high postoperative prevalence of stress ulcer.
b. Patients in medical ICU who require respirators.

Treatment

1. Treatment of underlying illness
2. Hourly antacid administration to keep the intragastric pH above 4
3. H$_2$ blocker (IV infusion is better than IV bolus).
   Raising the pH above 4 leads to bacterial colonisation of stomach and pharynx, which may lead to development of pneumonia.

NSAID and Peptic Ulcer

These causes mucosal injury and ulceration anywhere in the GIT from esophagus to duodenum.

Complications of NSAID (Apart from PUD)

1. Erosive colitis
2. Pancreatitis
3. Liver damage.

Mechanism of Action

1. Direct mucosal injury
2. Inhibition of PG (aspirin and NSAID act by inhibition of cyclo oxygenase).
   (Steroids produce ulcer either by itself when administered for more than 30 days or when the total dose of prednisolone exceeds 1 gm or when given with NSAID, when the risk of ulceration increases).

Diagnosis

Upper GI Radiography (Barium Meal Series)

1. Barium is seen within the ulcer niche, surrounded by smooth mound of oedema.
2. Secondary changes (folds radiating from ulcer crater and deformities in the region secondary to spasm, edema and scarring).

Differentiation of Benign from Malignant Ulcer

This depends on the site, size, location and presence or absence of duodenal ulcer.

Site and Location

• Benign gastric ulcer can occur anywhere, but more frequently found on the lesser curvature at the incisura.

• Malignant gastric ulcer can also occur anywhere in the stomach, but a high suspicion of malignancy must be entertained when it is located in the greater curvature of the stomach.
• Malignant ulcer is commonly associated with chronic atrophic gastritis, adenomatous polyp, pernicious anaemia and post surgery for PUD.

Size

The larger the ulcer, the more likely that it is malignant.

Coexistence of Duodenal Ulcer

If gastric ulcer is present along with a duodenal ulcer, it is highly unlikely to be malignant.

Endoscopic Differentiation between Benign and Malignant Ulcer

Signs of Malignancy (Fig. 5.18)

1. Presence of an ulcer within a definitive mass.
2. Effaced, interrupted, fused or nodular mucosal folds as they approach the margin of the crater.
3. Irregular filling defects in the ulcer crater.
4. Friability of ulcer and easy tendency to bleed.

Signs of Benign Ulcer (Fig. 5.18)

1. The mucosal folds, as they approach the edge of the ulcer crater, are seen to be smooth and symmetrical.
2. A smooth mound of edema surrounding the ulcer.
3. Smooth translucent band or collar surrounding the ulcer crater.

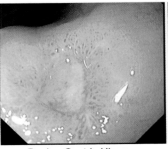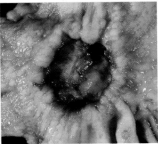

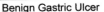

Benign Gastric Ulcer   Malignant Gastric Ulcer

Fig. 5.18: Benign and malignant gastric ulcer

Complications of Peptic Ulcer Disease

1. Upper GI bleed
2. Perforation
3. Gastric outlet obstruction and fluid and electrolyte imbalance
4. Malignancy (with gastric ulcer only)
5. Pancreatitis
6. Gastro-colic fistula.

Treatment of Peptic Ulcer

Drugs	Short-term treatment	Maintenance treatment	Side-effects
Antacids			
1. Magnesium containing antacid	30 ml 1 and 3 hours after a meal and at bedtime	Not recommended	Diarrhoea
2. Aluminium containing antacid	30 ml 1 and 3 hours after a meal and at bedtime	Not recommended	Constipation
H_2 receptor antagonist			
1. Cimetidine	800 mg at night or 400 mg bd	400 mg at night	Delays elimination of warfarin, phenytoin and theophylline and should not be used concurrently with these drugs. Rarely causes confusion in the elderly and gynaecomastia in males. Both effects reversible on stopping the drug
2. Ranitidine	300 mg at night or 150 mg bd	150 mg at night	Reversible confusion
3. Nizatidine	300 mg at night or 150 mg bd	150 mg at night	Sweating, urticaria, somnolence (all rare, none serious)
4. Famotidine	40 mg at night or 20 mg bd	20 mg at night	Headache, dizziness, dry mouth (all rare, none serious). Negative cardiac inotropic effect
Anticholinergics Pirenzepine	50 mg bd	Not recommended	Dry mouth, blurred vision
*Site-protective drug Sucralfate	2 grams bd	Not recommended	Reduces absorption of warfarin, phenytoin, tetracycline, digoxin
Cytoprotective drug			
1. Misoprostol	200 mg 4 times daily	Not recommended	Abortifacient activity. Avoid use in women of child bearing age. Diarrhoea may occur
2. Enprostil	35 mg 2 times daily	Not recommended	—do—
Proton pump inhibit or Omeprazole	20 mg once daily for 4-8 weeks	Not recommended	Delays elimination of diazepam, phenytoin, warfarin. Induces significant hypergastrinemia, bacterial overgrowth
Lansoprazole	30 mg once daily for 4-8 weeks	Not recommended	
Pantoprazole	40 mg/d	Not required	
Rabeprazole	20 mg/d	Not required	

*It is known as a site protective agent as it forms a protective covering over the ulcer and promotes its healing
Sucralfate should not be combined with antacids, as it is active only in acidic medium.

Management of NSAID induced PUD

Clinical setting	Recommendations
Active ulcer NSAID discontinued NSAID continued	H_2 receptor antagonists / PPI PPI
Prophylactic therapy	Misoprostol PPI Selective cox -2 inhibitors
H. pylori infection	Eradicate if active ulcer or past history of PUD

Misoprostol is contraindicated in pregnancy.

Zollinger-Ellison Syndrome

- This is a condition in which there is an association of peptic ulcer with a gastrin secreting pancreatic adenoma (or simple islet cell hyperplasia).
- Gastrin excites excessive acid production which can produce multiple ulcers in the duodenum and stomach.
- 50-60% of the gastrin producing pancreatic tumours are malignant.
- 30% of cases are associated with multiple endocrine neoplasia (MEN type 1).
- It is seen in 0.1% of patients with peptic ulcer disease, especially those refractory to treatment.

- This condition must be suspected in those with multiple peptic ulcers resistant to therapy, particularly if there is associated diarrhoea and steatorrhoea.
- On investigation, there is a raised fasting serum gastrin level (> 100 pg/ml) with a raised basal gastric acid output of > 15 mmol/hour (Normal BAO is 1.5-2.0 mmol/hr).
- Gastrinomas may be localized by measuring the uptake of a somatostatin analogue, [111]Indium—Pentriotide (Octreoscan).
- This condition is treated with a potassium-hydrogen ATPase inhibitor like omeprazole. The drug is started with a dose of 60 mg/day and then gradually tapered to 20 mg/day as symptoms subside.
- Since the long-term effects of omeprazole use are still unknown, it is worthwhile trying to excise the tumour, which is the definitive treatment for this condition.
- If the tumour turns out to be malignant, then the prognosis is poor, 5-year survival being only 20%.

Endoscopy

Upper Gastrointestinal Endoscopy

Indications

1. Dysphagia
2. Caustic or foreign body ingestion
3. Dyspepsia
4. Persistent nausea and vomiting
5. Need to obtain small intestine biopsy
6. Acute or chronic gastrointestinal bleeding
7. Inflammatory bowel disease (as this may be associated with duodenal lesions mimicking a duodenal ulcer)
8. Chronic abdominal pain
9. Suspected polyp or cancer.

Contraindications

1. Perforated viscus suspected
2. Patient in shock
3. Combative or uncooperative patient
4. Severe inflammatory bowel disease or toxic megacolon (colonoscopy).

Preparation of the Patient

1. Patient should be fasted for 6 or more hours to ensure an empty stomach.
2. For emergency, nasogastric suction should be done before endoscopy procedure.

Therapeutic Oesophagogastro-duodenoscopy

1. In case of upper gastrointestinal bleeding, due to a variceal bleed, endoscopic injection of sclerosants (sclerotherapy) of esophageal varices is the most widely accepted therapeutic oesophagogastro-duodenoscopic procedure.
2. It is also used therapeutically for banding of oesophageal varices.
3. Laser therapy through endoscopy to relieve GI obstruction by malignant growth can be done palliatively.
4. Stenting procedure can be done, thereby providing a lumen through the stent for feeding patients with mechanical obstruction to oesophagus causing dysphagia.

Complications of Endoscopy

1. Perforation of viscus
2. Bleeding
3. Cardiac arrhythmias
4. Reaction to medication (sclerosants)
5. Vasovagal reaction
6. Pulmonary aspiration.

Gastrointestinal Bleeding

Haematemesis

It is defined as the vomiting of fresh blood, either bright red or of coffee ground character.

Melaena

It is a tarry black, sticky, foul smelling stool (Other stool darkeners are iron and bismuth).

Special Features

a. Approximately 60 ml of blood is required to produce single black stool.
b. The blood loss > 60 ml produces melena for more than 7 days.
c. To produce melaena the blood must remain in the gut for 8 hrs.

Haematochezia

It is the passage of red or maroon blood from the rectum, usually signifies bleeding from a source distal to the ligament of Treitz. It can also occur from massive upper GI bleed from oesophagus, stomach and duodenum.

Tilt Test

- Tilting the head end of the body upwards at an angle of 75° for 3 minutes leads to accelerated heart rate and a drop in systolic blood pressure
- Increase in heart rate of < 20 beats/min and absence of light headedness, indicates slight or compensated blood loss
- Increase in heart rate of > 30 beats/min and presence of faintness or syncope indicates decompensated blood loss and need for restorative measures.

Assessment of Bleed

Blood loss	Clinical features
a. 500 ml	No systemic signs except in elderly and anaemic patients
b. 1000 ml (20% reduction of blood volume)	Tachycardia, orthostatic hypotension, syncope, light headedness, nausea, sweating and thirst
c. 2000 ml or more (40% reduction of blood volume)	Profound shock and possibly death

- Drop in urine output < 0.5 ml/kg/hr indicates moderate to marked hypovolaemia.
- Early sign of cessation of bleeding and restoration of blood volume is return of the normal heart rate

Aetiology

Duodenal ulcer	35%
Gastric ulcer	20%
Acute gastritis (drugs)	
Erosion/haemorrhagic gastritis	20%
Mallory-Weiss syndrome	5%
Gastric carcinoma	5%
Oesophageal varices	10%
Others	5%

(Leiomyoma, haemophilia, thrombocytopenia, Ehlers-Danlos syndrome, rupture of aorta into stomach, anticoagulants)

Laboratory Findings

1. *Complete blood count*: Mild leucocytosis and thrombocytosis develop within 6 hrs after the onset of bleeding.
2. *Card test*: It is useful for detection of occult blood in stools.
3. *Endoscopy*: It is useful for confirmation and treatment in more than 90% of cases. Risk of rebleeding is higher if a 'visible vessel' is seen in ulcer crater.
4. *Angiography*: It is useful to detect the site of bleeding (>0.5 ml/min).
5. *Radio-labelled RBC*: It is useful in determining low grade bleeding from GI tract and especially when the pathology is out of reach of the endoscope (>0.1 ml/min).

Differentiation between Upper GI and Lower GI Bleed

Features	Upper GI bleed	Lower GI bleed
Site	Above the ligament of Treitz	Below the ligament of Treitz
Presentation	Haematemesis/melaena	Haematochezia
Nasogastric aspiration	Blood	Clear fluid
BUN/creatinine ratio	Increased (> 25:1)	Normal (< 25:1)
Bowel sounds	Hyperactive	Normal

Management

1. Admission of the patient
2. Reassure the patient
3. Establish an IV line
4. Assessment of blood loss by history and vital signs (HR, BP every hour)
5. Introduction of a nasogastric tube for assessment of the quantity and duration of bleed and can also be

Rockall Risk Scoring System for GI bleeds

Score	0	1	2
Age	< 60 yr	60–79 yr	80 yr and above
Systolic BP	> 100 mm of Hg	> 100 mm of Hg	< 100 mm of Hg
Pulse rate	< 100/min	> 100/min	
Co-morbidity	No	IHD/cardiac failure	Renal/liver failure
Diagnosis*	Mallory Weiss tear, no lesions or signs of recent bleed	All other diagnosis	— Upper GI malignancy
Endoscopic evidence of recent haemorrhage	None/dark red spot		Adherent clot/blood in upper GIT/visible vessel

*The score for metastasis liver is 3.
A score of more than 6 is said to be an indication for surgery

Test of Malabsorption

Nutrient tested	Tests		Normal value
1. Fat	a. Measurement of fat in a 5-day collection of stool b. The synthetic bile acid is given orally and its retention is measured at 7 days by whole body counting		Excretion < 7 g/day Retention > 90%. (In severe ileal disease, retention is < 20%)
2. Carbohydrate	a. *Lactose tolerance test*: 50 g of lactose is given orally and blood samples are taken every 20 min for 2 hours b. *Hydrogen breath test*: 50 g of lactose is given orally and breath hydrogen is measured every hour for 4 hours		Rise in blood glucose > 20 mg/dL Less than 10 ppm above baseline in any sample
3. Protein	a. *Faecal clearance of endogenous α_1 antitrypsin*: This normal serum protein is excreted unchanged in the stool when there is any protein loss into the stool and is therefore measured in a 3-day collection of stool		No α_1 antitrypsin in the stool
4. Vitamins	Vitamin B_{12} absorption: 0.5 µg of radiolabelled vitamin B_{12} is given orally followed 2 hours later by 1000 µg of non-radioactive vitamin B_{12} given by intramuscular injection. Urine is collected for 24 hours		More than 16% of radioactivity appears in the urine
5. Small intestinal culture			< 10^5 organisms/ml

Complications

Haemorrhage, perforation, obstruction, fistula formation and malabsorption.

Investigations
Radiology

Plain X-ray of the abdomen
1. Calcified lymph nodes
2. Multiple fluid levels
3. Distended gas filled loops of the intestine or enteroliths.

Barium meal and enema
1. Hypermotility
2. 'Stierlin sign'—a defect characterized by failure of the diseased segment to retain barium which is adequately retained by adjacent areas free of disease.
3. 'String sign'—a thin stream of barium resembling a string may be commonly seen in the terminal ileum.

Ascitic Fluid Examination

a. The ascitic fluid is an exudate.
b. Punch biopsy of the peritoneum reveals tuberculous lesion.

Diagnosis

1. Definite diagnosis by demonstration of organism in the specimen.
2. Radiological features
   a. Thickened mucosa with distortion of mucosal folds

b. Ulcerations
c. Stenosis of the bowel
d. Pseudopolyp formation.

Distinguishing Features between Tuberculosis and Crohn's Disease

Features	Tuberculosis	Crohn's disease
Clinical		
1. Duration	Months	Years
2. Course	Continuous	Remissions and exacerbations
3. Fever	Common	Less common
4. Diarrhoea	Common (constipation may occur)	Very common
5. Lump abdomen	Palpable	Not palpable
6. Ascites	Common	Uncommon
7. Fistulae (internal and external)	Rare	Common
8. Rectal and peri-rectal fistula	Rare	Common
9. Pulmonary lesion	May be present	Not present
Macroscopic		
10. Anal lesions	Rare	Common
11. Miliary nodes on serosa	Common	Rare
12. Length of stricture	Small	Long
13. Ulcers	Annular	Serpiginous
Microscopic		
14. Caseation	Usually Present	Absent
15. Acid fast bacilli	Often present	Absent
16. Fibrosis	Common	Less common

Differential Diagnosis

1. Crohn's disease
2. Tropical sprue
3. Chronic amoebiasis
4. Roundworm infestation
5. Lymphomas
6. Large bowel malignancy.

Treatment

Treat with 3 drug regimen of ATT for 6 months.

Inflammatory Bowel Disease

It refers to idiopathic and chronic intestinal inflammations. Ulcerative colitis and crohns disease are the two main types of IBD.

Differentiation between Ulcerative Colitis and Crohn's Disease

Features	Ulcerative colitis	Crohn's disease
Pain	Crampy lower abdominal pain and relieved by bowel movement	Constant pain; often in right lower quadrant and not relieved by bowel movement
Stool	Usually bloody	Stool usually not grossly bloody
Abdominal mass	No mass palpable	Mass often felt in right lower quadrant
Site of involvement	Affects colon only	May affect small and large bowel; occasionally stomach and esophagus may be involved
Pathology	Mucosal disease (granuloma is not a feature)	Transmural disease (granulomas are sometimes seen)
Nature of involvement	Involvement of bowel continuous from rectum	Usually discontinuous involvement of bowel (skip areas)

Extraintestinal Manifestations of IBD (Common to Both Ulcerative Colitis and Crohn's Disease)

Areas	Conditions
Joints	Peripheral arthritis
	Sacroilitis
	Ankylosing spondylitis
Skin	Erythema nodosum
	Pyoderma gangrenosum
Eyes	Conjunctivitis
	Episcleritis
	Iritis
Liver	Fatty infiltration
	Chronic active hepatitis
	Pericholangitis
	Sclerosing cholangitis
	Bile duct carcinoma
Kidney	Pyelonephritis
	Renal stone
General	Amyloidosis

Special Clinical Features to Crohn's Disease

1. Gallstones
2. Renal oxalate stones
3. Vitamin B_{12} deficiency
4. Obstructive hydronephrosis.
5. Thromboembolic episode
6. Hypercoagulable state
7. Endocarditis
8. Myocarditis
9. Pleuropericarditis
10. Interstitial lung disease

Differential Diagnosis of IBD

1. Bacterial colitis (*Campylobacter, Shigella, Salmonella, E. coli, Clostridium difficile*)
2. Parasitic colitis (amoebiasis and schistosomiasis)
3. Ischaemic colitis
4. Radiation colitis
5. Behcet's colitis
6. Sexually transmitted colitis (*Gonococcus, Chlamydia,* herpes and trauma)
7. Condition simulating Crohn's disease
   a. Lymphoma
   b. *Yersinia* infection
   c. Tuberculosis.

Onset and Course of Symptoms

Both begin in childhood or early adulthood. Patients with ulcerative colitis experience intermittent exacerbations and almost complete remissions between attacks. Patients with Crohn's disease have recurrent symptoms of varying duration with history of growth retardation and failure to develop sexual maturity.

Physical Examination

Thin and under nourished, pallor (due to blood loss), low grade fever, mild to moderate abdominal tenderness (characteristic of ulcerative colitis), tenderness in right lower quadrant (characteristic of Crohn's disease).

Investigations

Laboratory

a. Complete blood count (anemia due to blood loss, leucocytosis)
b. ESR (Increased correlating with disease severity)
c. *Electrolytes*
   • Hyponatraemia
   • Hypokalaemia
   • Acidosis

- Hypocalcaemia and
- Hypomagnesaemia

d. *Stool examination*
- Faecal leucocytes (not common in IBS)
- Ova and parasites
- Stool culture for bacterial pathogens.

Sigmoidoscopy

Ulcerative colitis (Fig. 5.19)

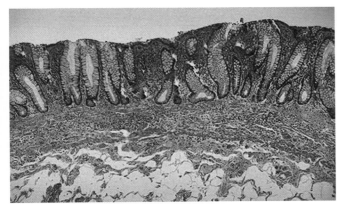

Fig. 5.19: Colitis—microscopic view

- Mucosal surface becomes irregular and granular.
- Mucosa becomes friable and bleeds on touch.
- In chronic condition pseudopolyps may be seen.

Crohn's disease
- Rectal mucosa is normal.

Mucosal Biopsy
Ulcerative colitis
- Infiltration of mucosa with inflammatory cells
- Flattening of the surface epithelial cells
- Decreased goblet cells
- Thinning of mucosa, branching of crypts
- Crypt abscesses.

 All these above findings including the crypt abscess may be seen in Crohn's disease and other colitis.

Crohn's disease
- Granulomas are seen.

Radiography

a. *Plain film of the abdomen*

Ulcerative colitis: Loss of haustral markings and shortening of bowel is seen in severe lesion (Fig. 5.20).

Crohn's disease: Narrowing of bowel lumen is seen.

b. *Barium enema*: It is contraindicated in toxic megacolon.

In Ulcerative Colitis
a. Loss of haustration (pipe stem appearance)
b. Ulcerations
c. Pseudopolyps
d. Shortening of bowel is seen.

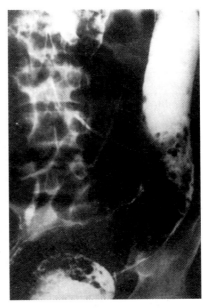

Fig. 5.20: Barium enema—loss of colonic haustrations in ulcerative colitis

In Crohn's disease skip lesions can be seen. Rose thorn appearance (linear fissures throughout bowel), string sign (tubular narrowing of terminal ileum), cobble stone appearance (ulcero nodular pattern), omega sign (concentric lesions) are also seen.

c. *Ultrasonogram*: USG shows Bull's eye appearance in transverse section of two thickened loops in Crohn's disease.

Colonoscopy and Upper GI Endoscopy

- Colonoscopy is useful in assessing progression of proctitis or colitis. It is also useful for screening for development of cancer and early detection of precancerous lesions.
- Upper GI endoscopy is useful in differentiating Crohn's disease of duodenum from peptic ulcer disease, which it may mimic symptomatically.

Liver Function Tests

a. Increased alanine transaminase (chronic active hepatitis)
b. Increased alkaline phosphatase (sclerosing cholangitis).

Treatment Protocol for IBD

Ulcerative Colitis: Active diseases

	Mild	Moderate	Severe	Fulminant
Distal	5-ASA oral and/or enema	5-ASA oral and/or enema Glucocorticoid enema Oral glucocorticoid	5-ASA oral and/or enema Glucocorticoid enema Oral or IV glucocorticoid	Intravenous glucocorticoid Intravenous CSA
Extensive	5-ASA oral or enema	5-ASA oral and/or enema Glucocorticoid enema Oral glucocorticoid	5-ASA oral and/or enema Glucocorticoid enema Oral or IV glucocorticoid	Intravenous glucocorticoid Intravenous CSA

Ulcerative Colitis: Maintenance therapy

Distal	5-ASA oral and/or enema 6-MP or azathioprine
Extensive	5-ASA oral and/or enema 6-MP or azathioprine

Crohn's Disease: Active disease

Mild-Moderate	Severe	Perianal or fistulizing disease
5-ASA oral or enema Metronidazole and/or ciprofloxacin Oral glucocorticoids Azathioprine or 6-MP Infliximab	5-ASA oral or enema Metronidazole and/or ciprofloxacin Oral or IV glucocorticoids Azathioprine or 6-MP Infliximab TPN or elemental diet Intravenous cyclosporine	Metronidazole and/or ciprofloxacin Azathioprine or 6-MP Infliximab Intravenous CSA

Crohn's Disease: Maintenance therapy

Inflammatory	Perianal or fistulizing disease
5-ASA oral or enema Metronidazole and/or ciprofloxacin Azathioprine or 6-MP	Metronidazole and/or ciprofloxacin Azathioprine or 6-MP

Note: CSA—cyclosporine; 6-MP—6-mercaptopurine; TPN—total parenteral nutrition

Oral 5 ASA preparations:	GM/day:	
	Acute phase	Maintenance phase
Sulphasalazine	4-8	2- 6
Olsalazine	1-3	
Balsalazine	2.25 -6.75	
Delayed release preparations:		
Asacol	2.2-4.8	1.6-4.8
Claversal	1.5-3	0.75-3
Sustained release preparation:		
Pentasa	2-4	1.5-4

Treatment

Medical

Diet and Nutrition

1. Avoid high fibre diet in presence of diarrhoea/dysentery

2. Diet should be nutritious
3. Supplemental fat soluble vitamins, medium chain triglycerides and parenteral vitamin B_{12}
4. In severe inflammation
   a. Nothing by mouth
   b. Total parenteral nutrition.

Drugs

1. Sulfasalazine started with 1 gm/day and increased to a maximum of 4 gm/day in advanced cases of ulcerative colitis and in Crohn's disease with colonic involvement.
2. *Corticosteroids*
   a. In ulcerative colitis, it is indicated only when sulfasalazine is not effective.
   b. In Crohn's disease, it is the first drug of choice. Dose is 40-60 mg/day and is gradually tapered and withdrawn after improvement.
      Steroid enema is given when proctitis and distal colitis are present.
      Parenteral glucocorticoids can be administered as hydrocortisone 300 mg/day or methylprednisolone 40-60 mg/day. ACTH is occasionally preferred for glucocorticoids.
3. *Immunosuppressants*:
   a. Azathioprine: 50-100 mg/day
   b. 6 mercaptopurine
   c. Cyclosporine
   d. Methotrexate—for remission 25 mg/week
      For maintenance 15 mg/week.
4. *Antidiarrhoeals*: If no improvement of diarrhoea with steroids and sulfasalazine, codeine and lomotil may be used.
5. *Metronidazole*: It is an alternative to immuno-suppressants and helps in reducing steroid usage. Dose 200 mg 4 times/day.
6. Bile acid binding resins and medium chain triglycerides are used in terminal ileum involvement in ulcerative colitis.
7. Antibiotics are indicated in toxic megacolon and severe ulcerative colitis.
8. Newer drugs:
   a. Infliximab – Anti-TNF antibody
   b. Tacrolimus
   c. Mycophenolate mofetil
   d. Thalidomide
   e. Natalizumab—α 4 integren specific humanized monoclonal antibody.

Psychotherapy

Surgery

Ulcerative Colitis

Indications
a. Acute UC not responding to medical treatment
b. Relapsing and remitting disease
c. Responding poorly to drug therapy
d. Complications

- Perforation
- Abscess
- Uncontrollable haemorrhage
- Unrelieved obstruction
- Fulminating disease
- Carcinoma.

e. Toxic megacolon—If medical management is not effective in 10 days, total colectomy is indicated.

Procedure: The most common operation is pancolectomy with ileostomy.

Indications in Crohn's disease
Perforation
Abscess
Unrelieved obstruction
Unresponsiveness to medical treatment
Intractable disease
Fistulae.

Irritable Bowel Syndrome

Irritable bowel syndrome is the most common of all digestive disorders, affecting nearly everyone at one time in their life.

Clinical Features

Diagnostic criteria for diagnosing irritable bowel syndrome is at least three months of continuous or recurrent symptoms of abdominal pain or discomfort which is
a. Relieved with defaecation and/or
b. Associated with change in frequency of stool and/or
c. Associated with a change in consistency of stool.

The above symptoms may be described by the patient as follows:
a. Altered bowel frequency (> 3 bowel movements a day or < 3 bowel movements a week)
b. Altered form of stool (lumpy/hard or loose/watery stool)
c. Altered passage of stool (straining urgency or feeling of incomplete evacuation)
d. Passage of mucus
e. Bloating or feeling of abdominal distension.

Investigations

All Patients

1. Stool for occult blood series
2. If diarrhoea is present, stool for leukocyte, ova, parasites, bacterial pathogens

3. Sigmoidoscopy
4. Barium enema examination.

Selected Patients

1. Upper GI and small-bowel endoscopy
2. Ultrasound of gallbladder
3. Abdominal CT scan
4. Serum amylase level
5. Lactose tolerance test
6. Mucosal biopsy of small bowel or colon.

Nocturnal and bloody diarrhoea are against diagnosis of irritable bowel syndrome.

Management

For all patients:
1. Reassurance and emotional support
2. Stress reduction
3. Avoid tranquilizers and antidepressants.
4. Low dose tricyclic antidepressants may be tried.

Patients with abdominal pain and constipation:
1. Increase the dietary fibre
2. Avoid laxatives
3. Anticholinergics or antispasmodics.

Patients with diarrhoea:
1. Antidiarrhoeal agents
2. Increase the dietary fibre.

Ischaemic Colitis

This is due to occlusion of the inferior mesenteric artery leading to ischaemia of the left colon.

Patient presents with colicky lower abdominal pain, nausea, vomiting and diarrhoea with the passage of blood and mucus. On examination, there is tenderness and guarding in the left iliac fossa. This episode may be transient or persistent leading to stricture formation. Some patients may present with shock and generalised abdominal pain simulating peritonitis.

A plain radiograph of the abdomen shows thumb printing at the splenic flexure and descending colon which are indentations of the bowel wall from sub-mucosal haemorrhage and oedema. A double contrast barium enema demonstrates the distribution of maximal involvement.

Most cases resolves with conservative management. Surgery is necessary when there are signs of peritonitis or when symptomatic stricture develops.

Carcinoid Tumours

Carcinoid tumours are of argentaffin cell origin and occur at many sites in the gastrointestinal tract but are most common in the appendix, the ileum and the rectum. In small intestine they are multiple. Twenty per cent of these show low-grade malignancy with metastases to the abdominal lymph nodes and the liver (rarely gallbladder, bronchus or gonads).

Carcinoid syndrome refers to the systemic manifestations produced by the secretory products of the neoplastic enterochromaffin cells (serotonin (5HT), 5-HIAA, kinins).

Clinical Features

1. Symptoms are due to local invasion of the bowel or hepatic metastases
2. Flushing* (after alcohol, coffee, various foods or drugs)
3. Diarrhoea
4. Right heart valvular lesions** (tricuspid incompetence, tricuspid stenosis, pulmonary stenosis)
5. Hepatomegaly due to metastases
6. Edema
7. Asthma (due to bronchospasm).
Note: *There are 4 kinds of flushes
a. Paroxysmal erythema
b. Facial telangiectasia
c. Prolonged flushes, e.g. for 48 hours (suggests bronchial carcinoid)
d. White and red patches (suggests gastric carcinoid).
**Left heart valvular lesions can occur when there is a large bronchial carcinoid as the venous effluent enters the left heart without getting inactivated in the lung.

Investigations

1. The estimation of urinary 5-HIAA in a 24-hour collection of urine is more than 15 mg.
2. CT and laparotomy are useful for localization.
3. A gulp of whisky may help diagnostically by inducing the flush.

Management

Medical Treatment

1. Methysergide 2 mg/8 hours per oral (blocks 5 HT); may cause retroperitoneal fibrosis.
2. Cyproheptadine 4 mg/8 hour per orally prevents diarrhoea.
3. Phenoxybenzamine 20-200 mg/24 hours per orally prevents flushing.

Surgical Treatment

The treatment of carcinoid syndrome is usually palliative because hepatic metastases occurs earlier. In the absence of metastases, surgical removal of the tumour may be done.

Prognosis

Median survival is 5-8 years and 30 months if metastases are present.

Gastric Ulcer and Malignancy

- Both ulcer and malignancy are common in the lesser curvature of the stomach.
- Presence of an ulcerating mass or a large ulcer > 3 cm in diameter suggests the probability of malignancy.
- Gastric ulcer with pentagastrin fast achlorhydria indicates malignancy.
- Improper preservation or refrigeration or ingestion of contaminated food leads to bacterial conversion of dietary nitrates to carcinogenic nitrites.
- Biopsy must be performed in the management and follow up of patients with isolated gastric ulcer.

Gastrointestinal Malignancies

Sites, incidence and types	Predisposing factors	Clinical features	Investigations	Management
Oesophagus Upper; least common; squamous cell carcinoma	Tobacco (smoked or chewed)	Progressive dysphagia, sticking of solid food, or upper GI bleed	Barium swallow; Oesophagoscopy	Radiation therapy Oesophagogastrectomy
Middle; less common; squamous cell carcinoma	Alcohol, achalasia			
Lower; common; adenocarcinoma	Paterson-Kelly Syndrome; Barrett's epithelium (smoking)			
Stomach Pylorus or antrum; 60%; adenocarcinoma Body; 20-30%; adenocarcinoma	Food preservatives (nitrites) pernicious anaemia *H. pylori*	Anaemia, asthenia, anorexia, dyspepsia, vomiting, weight loss	Barium meal; OGD; biopsy	Gastrectomy Chemotherapy
Small Intestine Duodenum or jejunum	Coeliac disease; Crohn's disease; multiple polyposis syndromes	Abdominal pain, weight loss, bleeding, obstruction or intussusception	Barium meal series	Surgical
Large Intestine Ascending colon; adenocarcinoma	Ulcerative colitis Familial polyposis (Adenomatous polyp)	Most common malignancy of GIT (western) anaemia (occult bleeding) cachexia altered bowel habits and late obstruction	Rigid sigmoidoscopy, double contrast barium enema	Surgical
Descending colon; adenocarcinoma		Frank blood in the stool and obstruction early	Colonoscopy	Surgical
Rectum; adenocarcinoma	Rich lymphatics predisposes to early spread of carcinoma	Early bleeding and mucous discharge; tenesmus	Proctoscopy and sigmoidoscopy	Surgical
Pancreas Head; 60%; adenocarcinoma	Smoking, high dietary fat, occupational exposure in chemical and metal industries	Epigastric pain (common) Gastrointestinal haemorrhage, diarrhoea, jaundice, abdominal mass	Raised serum alkaline phosphatase, barium meal ERCP, USG, duodenoscopy	Surgical
Body and Tail; 20%; adenocarcinoma				

Hepatology and Pancreas

Hepatic Segments

The liver is divided into a functional right lobe and the left lobe by an imaginary line drawn between the gall bladder fossa and middle hepatic veins. For the purpose of functional anatomy, the liver has been divided into 8 segments. Each of these segments can be considered as functional units, each with a branch of hepatic artery, portal vein, bile duct and drained by a branch of hepatic vein (Fig. 5.21).

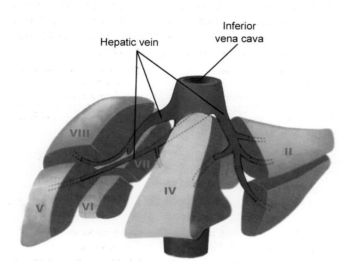

Fig. 5.21: Segmental anatomy of the liver

Liver Function Tests

Serum Enzymes

Serum enzymes are markers of hepatocellular injury and necrosis.

a. *AST (SGOT) and ALT (SGPT)*: Serum transaminases are normally present in the blood (less than 40 units). There are indicators of liver cell damage. Their serial determination reflects the clinical activity of the liver disease. In jaundiced patients, values greater than 300-400, suggest acute hepatocellular disease. Values more than 1000 units are observed in viral hepatitis, toxic or drug-induced liver disease, prolonged circulatory collapse. Lesser degree of elevation is found in mild viral hepatitis, diffuse and focal chronic liver disease (chronic active hepatitis, cirrhosis, secondaries). Sometimes serial estimations may be needed.

AST/ALT (SGOT/SGPT) ratio is most useful in detecting patients with alcoholic liver disease. AST/ALT ratio is greater than 2 in them due to decreased concentration of ALT in the hepatocyte cytosol. Serum of alcoholic patients are deficient in pyridoxal-5' phosphate, a coenzyme necessary for the synthesis of transaminases especially ALT.

Uraemia depresses the aminotransferase levels. Higher degree of elevation of transaminases has a bad prognostic value.

b. *Lactic dehydrogenase (LDH)*: LDH-5 corresponds to the liver but the elevation of LDH-1 is more sensitive for myocardial infarction and haemolysis.

Tests of Biosynthetic Function

a. *Serum proteins*: Liver produces all the serum proteins (especially albumin, prothrombin, fibrinogen) except gamma globulin. A serum albumin value of less than 3 (normal 3.5-5.0 gm/dl) and serum globulins greater than 4 gm/dl (normal 2.0-3.5 gm/dl) suggest a chronic or progressive liver disease.

Increased globulin is as a result of increased stimulation of the peripheral reticuloendothelial compartment due to shunting of antigens past the liver and impaired clearance by Kupffer cells.

Deficiency or absence of alpha 1 globulin is found in alpha 1 antitrypsin deficiency. Increase in albumin value of 2-3 gm towards normal with treatment implies improvement in hepatic function and a more favourable prognosis.

b. *Prothrombin time (PT)*: The liver synthesizes all the clotting factors except factor VIII. The one stage PT which reflects the activities of prothrombin, fibrinogen and factors V, VII and X is dependent on both hepatic synthesis of these factors and availability of vitamin K. Factor VII is the rate limiting factor in this pathway. Prolongation of PT (normal 11.5-12.5 seconds) by 2 seconds or more is considered abnormal.

Prolonged PT may also be present in congenital deficiencies of coagulation factors, consumption coagulopathy, drug intake and hypovitaminosis K. Prolongation of PT by more than 5-6 seconds heralds the onset of fulminant hepatic necrosis.

Prolongation of PT with no response to vitamin K therapy indicates poor long-term prognosis.

Prothrombin time is also prolonged in:
   i. Vitamin K malabsorption
  ii. Poor dietary intake of vitamin K
 iii. Antibiotic therapy (destruction of vitamin K producing commensals).

Tests of Cholestasis

Enzymes

i. *Serum alkaline phosphatase* (normal value 3-13 KA units or 30-120 IU/L): This is derived from three sources
1. Hepatobiliary system
2. Bone
3. Intestinal tract.

The hepatobiliary enzyme is differentiated from others by simultaneous estimation of 5' nucleotidase, gamma-glutamyl transpeptidase or leucine amino-peptidase. Values more than 3-10 times the normal level are suggestive of hepatobiliary diseases (extrahepatic and intrahepatic biliary obstruction, drug induced cholestasis, primary biliary cirrhosis).

Other causes of isolated alkaline phosphatase elevation:
1. Primary or metastatic tumor of liver or bone
2. Granulomatous liver disease
3. Hodgkin's disease
4. Non-Hodgkin's lymphoma
5. Liver abscess
6. CCF
7. Hyperthyroidism
8. Diabetes mellitus
9. Bone disease (Paget's disease, osteomalacia)
10. Partial extrahepatic bile duct obstruction
11. Sclerosing cholangitis
12. Pregnancy.

Persistent elevation of serum alkaline phosphatase > 30 KA units or 300 IU/L indicates obstructive jaundice.

ii. *5'-Nucleotidase* (normal value is 0.3-3.2 Bodansky units or 2-17 U/L): This enzyme is primarily located in the liver. Serum values are elevated in hepatobiliary diseases. In screening for liver metastases, it has a high predictive value. It is done to confirm the hepatic origin of an increased alkaline phosphatase level in children and pregnant women when there is coexisting bone disease.

iii. *Leucine aminopeptidase* This is also useful in the diagnosis of biliary obstructive, space occupying and infiltrative diseases of the liver.

iv. *Gamma-glutamyl transpeptidase*: (Normal value—5-24 U/L) This enzyme is found in liver, pancreas and kidney. Elevated values are seen in liver, pancreas, cardiac, renal, pulmonary and biliary tract diseases. The values are elevated in alcoholic liver disease or in patients taking barbiturates or phenytoin. A GGT/AP value greater than 2.5 is suggestive of alcohol abuse. GGT is a potential marker of alcoholism.

GGT correlates with Alkaline phosphatase levels and it is one of the most sensitive indicators of biliary tract disease.

Serum Bilirubin

Serum bilirubin is measured by van den Bergh's diazo reaction. Unconjugated bilirubin requires the presence of alcohol for the diazo reaction and gives an indirect van den Bergh reaction. Conjugated bilirubin reacts directly without alcohol. Total serum bilirubin is measured with the diazo reaction carried out in alcohol, where both the conjugated and the unconjugated bilirubin react with the reagent. The conjugated bilirubin is then measured from the diazo reaction carried out without alcohol. The difference represents the concentration of the unconjugated bilirubin.

Tests	Obstructive liver disease	Parenchymal liver disease
1. AST and ALT	Mild increase	Moderate to marked increase
2. Alkaline phosphatase	Markedly increased	May be mildly increased
3. Serum albumin	Normal	Decreased
4. Prothrombin time	Normal	Increased
5. Bilirubin	Normal or increased	Normal or increased
6. GGT	Increased	Normal or increased
7. 5' nucleotidase	Increased	Normal

Jaundice

Yellowish appearance of skin and mucous membranes resulting from an increase in bilirubin concentration in body fluids when serum bilirubin concentration exceeds 2 mg/dl. In latent jaundice, serum bilirubin level is between 1 and 2 mg/dl. Scleral tissue is rich in elastin and has a high affinity for bilirubin. Therefore presence of scleral icterus is a highly sensitive index for detecting jaundice. It is best appreciated in natural light.

Yellowish discoloration of carotenemia spares the sclera.

Metabolism of Bilirubin

Eighty per cent of the circulating bilirubin is derived from heme of haemoglobin which is in turn derived from senescent RBCs. Ten to twenty per cent of bilirubin comes from myoglobin, cytochromes and other haem containing proteins.

Haem is oxidized to biliverdin which is then reduced to bilirubin. Bilirubin is insoluble in aqueous solutions.

In blood bilirubin is bound to albumin at a 1:1 ratio. Unbound bilirubin can cross blood-brain barrier and causes kernicterus in neonatal hyperbilirubinaemia.

The processing of serum bilirubin by hepatocyte occurs in four steps namely hepatic uptake, cytosolic binding, conjugation and secretion.

The albumin bound bilirubin dissociates and bilirubin is subsequently transported into the hepatocyte through a saturable protein carrier.

In the hepatocyte, bilirubin binds to two cytosolic proteins ligandin and Z-protein. This limits the reflux of bilirubin back into the plasma.

The conjugation of bilirubin involves its esterification with glucuronic acid forming bilirubin monoglucuronide and diglucuronide, the reaction being catalysed by the enzyme UDP-glucuronyl transferase. Bilirubin is rendered water soluble by this mechanism and hence it is eliminated from the body in bile and urine.

Secretion of conjugated bilirubin into the bile from the hepatocyte is an active process against the concentration gradient involving a specific carrier. It is excreted in bile as a micellar complex with cholesterol, phospholipids and bile salts. It is later deconjugated and converted to urobilinogen by the colonic bacteria. By a process called enterohepatic circulation, a minor portion of bilirubin is reabsorbed. The rest is excreted in the stool (as stercobilinogen) and in urine (as urobilinogen).

Types

1. Hepatocellular jaundice (hepatic)
2. Hemolytic (prehepatic)
3. Obstructive (posthepatic).

Causes

Hepatocellular Jaundice

Viral
Hepatitis—A, B, C, D, E, G and TT virus
Others—CMV, EBV, HSV, and Coxsackievirus
Toxoplasma, Leptospira, Candida, Brucella, mycobacteria and *Pneumocystis*.

Drugs

Halothane
Phenytoin
Carbamazepine
INH, rifampicin
Pyrazinamide
Methyldopa
Captopril, enalapril
Amitriptyline
Imipramine
Ibuprofen
Indomethacin
Ketoconazole
Fluconazole
Zidovudine
Paracetamol

Toxins

Alcohol
Carbon tetrachloride
Yellow phosphorus

Haemolytic Jaundice

1. *Intraerythrocytic*
   Hereditary
   RBC membrane disorders (spherocytosis)
   Disorders of glycolysis (enzyme deficiencies)
   Haemoglobinopathies.
   Acquired
   Dyserythropoietic states (B_{12} and folate deficiency)
2. *Extraerythrocytic*
   Autoimmune
   Isoimmune
   Alloimmune
   Physical trauma
   Prosthetic valve
   Burns
   Chemical trauma (dapsone)
   Infections (malaria)
   Toxic factors
   Inflammations
   Neoplasms.

Obstructive Jaundice

1. Canalicular
   Alcohol
   Viral hepatitis
   Cirrhosis
   Lymphoma
   Bacterial sepsis
   Pregnancy
   Idiopathic
   Drugs
   Erythromycin
   Chlorpromazine
   Chlorpropamide.
2. Biliary
   Calculi
   Carcinoma pancreas

Tumors
    Benign
    Metastatic
Strictures
Biliary cirrhosis.

An Approach to Jaundice

If the physical examination shows

1. Excoriation, consider cholestasis or high grade biliary obstruction
2. Greenish hue (due to biliverdin) suggests long standing liver disease like biliary cirrhosis, sclerosing cholangitis, severe chronic hepatitis or long standing malignant obstruction
3. Fever, epigastric or right hypochondrial tenderness suggests choledocholithiasis, cholangitis or cholestasis
4. Painless jaundice suggests malignant biliary obstruction
5. Enlarged tender liver suggests acute hepatitis, rapidly enlarging hepatic tumor
6. Palpable gallbladder suggests distal biliary obstruction due to malignant tumour
7. Splenomegaly suggests portal hypertension or hemolytic jaundice
8. Palmar erythema, facial telangiectasia, Dupuytren's contracture are seen in chronic ethanol ingestion
9. Evidence of hyperestrogenic state in cirrhosis (gynecomastia, testicular atrophy, spider angiomata)
10. Wasting or lymphadenopathy suggests malignancy
11. Wasting and splenomegaly suggests pancreatic tumor obstructing the splenic vein or a widely metastatic lymphoma
12. Look for increased JVP, KF ring, xanthomata
13. Look for primaries from thyroid, GIT, breast, etc.
14. Hyperbilirubinaemia
    i. Predominantly unconjugated—>70% of total bilirubin
    ii. Predominantly conjucated—> 50% of total bilirubin.

Congenital Jaundice

Crigler-Najjar Syndrome (Type I)

It is an autosomal recessive disorder with severe unconjugated hyperbilirubinemia due to total absence of bilirubin uridine diphosphate—glucuronyltransferase (UDPGT). This results in kernicterus and may cause cerebral damage. This condition is uniformly fatal in the neonatal period. Bilirubin level ranges from 24-25 mg/dl. When patients survive up to 2nd decade, encephalopathy develops.

	Features	Hemolytic	Hepatocellular	Obstructive
1.	Mechanism	Increased bilirubin production	Hepatocellular failure	Bile duct obstruction
2.	Common cause	Haemolysis	Virus, drugs	Ca pancreas, gallstones
3.	Mode of onset	Rapid	Gradual	Gradual
4.	Symptoms	Anaemia, fever	Anorexia, nausea, vomiting, distaste to cigarette, coffee	Recurrent abdominal colic; fluctuating jaundice
5.	Skin	Mild yellow tinged	Orange tinged	Greenish yellow
6.	Urine	Colourless (absent bile pigments)	High coloured	Dark coloured (presence of bile pigments)
7.	Urobilinogen	++	+*	Absent
8.	Pruritus	Nil	+	+++
9.	Bradycardia	Nil	Rare	+
10.	Motion	Normal	**Pale	Clay coloured
11.	Serum bilirubin	Unconjugated	Both (conjugated and unconjugated)	Conjugated
12.	AST and ALT	Normal	Grossly elevated	Slightly elevated
13.	Serum alkaline phosphatase	Normal	Slightly raised	Grossly elevated
14.	Coombs' test	Positive	–	–
	Osmotic fragility	Increased	–	–
15.	Spleen	++	+/–	–
16.	Gallbladder	Not palpable	Not palpable	Palpable

*Urobilinogen is present normally in minimal quantities. In viral hepatitis, the quantum increases initially and disappears during the peak phase due to hepatocellular edema and obstruction; it reappears during the recovery phase;
**Clay coloured stools are passed during the obstructive phase which reverts to normal color in the recovery phase

Treatment

There is no treatment.

Crigler-Najjar Syndrome (Type II)

It is an autosomal dominant disorder due to mild deficiency of UDPGT enzyme. This condition is compatible with normal life. Serum unconjugated bilirubin levels are in the range of 6-25 mg/dl. Kernicterus is uncommon.

Treatment

Phenobarbitone, UV light, liver transplant.

Gilbert's Syndrome

It is an autosomal dominant disorder. There is mild un-conjugated hyperbilirubinaemia due to reduced glucuronyl transferase, mild haemolysis and defective bilirubin uptake. Patients have normal life expectancy. Serum bilirubin ranges from 1.3-3 mg/dl. Patients have normal liver serum tests and histology and there are no systemic symptoms.

Patients when placed on a diet of 300 Kcal without lipids for 24-48 hours, have an elevation of bilirubin by 100% or by 1.5 mg/dl.

Treatment

Occasionally phenobarbitone in a dose of 180 mg/day in divided doses for 2 weeks can be given to enhance the activity of glucuronyl transferase.

Dubin-Johnson Syndrome

It is an autosomal recessive disorder resulting in conjugated hyperbilirubinaemia secondary to a defect in canalicular transport of organic anions. The liver is darkly pigmented. Histologically, a yellow black pigment is seen in lysozomes of hepatocytes. Liver may be slightly enlarged and tender. Serum bilirubin levels may rise up to 30 mg/dl. Urine coproporphyrin I is more than coproporphyrin III (the reverse of normal). Bromsulphthalein excretion is normal at 45 minutes and there is secondary rise at 120 minutes.

Patients have normal life expectancy and usually no treatment is required.

Rotor Syndrome

It is a conjugated hyperbilirubinaemia with nonpigmented liver. There is defective bilirubin uptake and reduced intrahepatic binding. Bilirubin level is usually less than 10 mg/dl. Here also, urine coproporphyrin I is more than III, but not to that extent seen in Dubin-Johnson syndrome.

Bromsulphthalein excretion is abnormal at 45 min and no secondary rise at 120 min.

Patients live normally and no treatment is required.

Viral Hepatitis

Viral hepatitis is caused by five main agents mainly hepatitis A, B, C, D and E viruses (Fig. 5.22).

Differentiating Features of Hepatitis Viruses

Features	HAV	HBV	HCV	HDV	HEV	HGV
Genome	RNA	DNA	RNA	RNA	RNA	RNA
Family	Picorna	Hepadna	Flavi	Viroid	Calci	Flave
Incubation period (days)	15-45	30-180	15-150	30-180	15-60	14-35
Transmission	Faeco oral	Blood, saliva, sexually	Blood	Blood, sexually	Faeco oral	Percutaneous
Clinical						
Age group	Children, young adults	Young adults, babies, toddlers	Any age	Similar to HBV	Young adults	Unknown
Severity	Mild	Occ. severe	Moderate	Occ. severe	Mild	Unknown
Fulminant course	0.1%	0.1-1%	0.1%	5-20%	1-2%	Unknown
Progression to chronicity	None	Occasional (1-10%)	50%	Common	None	Yes
Carrier	None	0.1-30%	0.5-1%	Variable	None	Unknown
Carcinoma	No	+ esp. in neonatal infection	+	±	–	Unknown
Prognosis	Excellent	Worse with age, debility	Moderate	Acute—good; Chronic—poor	Good	Unknown
Prevention						
Active	Inactivated vaccine	Recombinant vaccine	No	Prevention of HBV infection	No	No
Passive	Immune serum globulin	Hyperimmune serum globulin; interferon 40% effective	No Interferon 50% effective	No	No	No

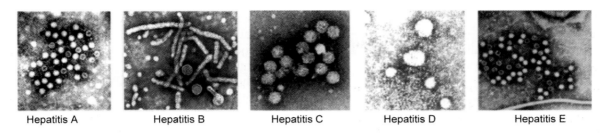

Fig. 5.22: Electron micrograph of viruses

Hepatitis A   Hepatitis B   Hepatitis C   Hepatitis D   Hepatitis E

Clinical Features

Headache, fever, malaise, anorexia, distaste for cigarettes and coffee, jaundice, upper abdominal pain due to stretching of peritoneum over enlarged liver; occasional lymphadenopathy and splenomegaly, arthralgia, skin rashes; mild illness may have an anicteric course.

Investigations

1. Elevation of plasma aminotransferase activity (400–4000 U/L).
2. Plasma bilirubin level (> 2.5 mg/dL up to 20 mg/dL). High bilirubin level of 20–40 mg/dL is common in sickle cell anaemia, G6PD deficiency due to superimposed haemolysis.
3. Serum alkaline phosphatase level rarely exceeds 250 U/L.
4. Prolongation of the prothrombin time (severe synthetic defect).
5. Serological tests for HAV, HBV, HCV, CMV, EB viral infections.
   a. Acute infection of HAV is marked by anti-HAV IgM in serum. Later IgG replaces IgM and persists for years conferring immunity.
   b. HBs Ag appears first and is a marker of active HBV infection, appearing before the onset of symptoms and declining over 3 to 6 months. HBe Ag, HBV-DNA and DNA polymerase are markers of active viral replication. Persistence of HBe Ag indicates continued viral replication and infectivity and progression to chronicity. IgM anti-HBc is usually the first antibody to appear followed shortly by anti-HBe. Appearance of anti-HBe suggests recovery (good prognosis). IgG anti-HBc slowly replaces the IgM over months. Anti HBs persists for years and confers protection against subsequent infection (Fig. 5.23).
   c. HDV can be identified by cDNA probe, radio-immunoassay for HDAg and IgM or IgG anti-HDV.

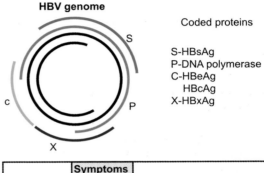

HBV genome

Coded proteins

S-HBsAg
P-DNA polymerase
C-HBeAg
  HBcAg
X-HBxAg

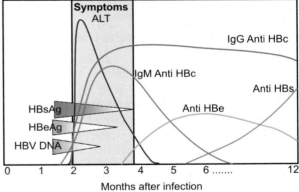

Fig. 5.23: HBV-antigens and antibodies

d. Serological diagnosis of hepatitis C has advanced using newer generation of ELISA's which detect the infection earlier (Fig. 5.24).
   i. First generation assays detect antibodies 1-3 months after the onset of hepatitis. (Antibodies against viral proteins C100-3)
   ii. Second generation assays incorporate recombinant proteins from the nucleocapsid core region of virus (C22-3) and NS 3 region (C33c). These assays are more sensitive and detect anti HCV 30-90 days earlier.
   iii. Third generation immunoassay incorporates proteins from NS 5 region and may detect anti HCV even earlier.

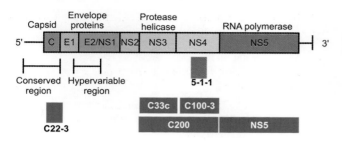

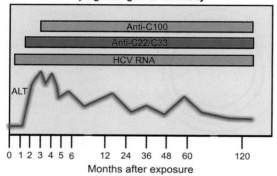

Fig. 5.24: Hepatitis C and its protein

Because of the non-specificity encountered in clinical samples tested for anti HCV, a supplementary recombinant immunoblot assay is also used.

The most sensitive indicator of infection is the presence of HCV RNA, which can be detected by amplification techniques within a few days of exposure.

6. Hypoglycaemia (nausea, vomiting, reduced CHO intake, poor hepatic glycogen) requiring hourly blood glucose estimation.

Complications

• Fulminant hepatic failure
• Cholestatic hepatitis
• Relapsing hepatitis (biochemical/clinical)

• Hyperbilirubinaemia (in Gilbert's syndrome)
• Renal failure
• Henoch-Schonlein purpura
• Chronic hepatitis
• Cirrhosis (HBV, HCV, HDV)
• Hepatocellular carcinoma (HBV, HCV)
• Aplastic anaemia, pancreatitis, myocarditis, atypical pneumonia, transverse myelitis and peripheral neuropathy are rare complications.

Management

1. Bed rest
2. Nutritious diet, glucose and fruit drinks
3. Drugs are best avoided (sedatives, hypnotics, alcohol). Oral contraceptive pills can be resumed after clinical or biochemical recovery.
4. In severe acute hepatitis B treatment with Lamivudine at 100 mg/d orally may tried
5. In acute hepatitis C antiviral therapy with interferon alpha 3 million units subcutaneously thrice weekly helps in reducing the rate of chronicity.

Prognosis

Overall mortality is 0.5%.

Prognostic Indicators

1. HAV and HEV infections have good prognosis; Prognosis is variable in HBV, HCV and HDV infections. HBV and HCV infections are associated with chronicity; HBV and rarely HCV infection may lead to malignancy. HEV can cause a high mortality in pregnancy.
2. Enormous increase of AST/ALT indicate bad prognosis.
3. Bilirubin levels more than 20 mg/dL suggests bad prognosis. However enormous rise more than 40 mg/dL is common in patients with associated G6PD deficiency or sickle cell anaemia.
4. If the liver is not enlarged, it indicates fulminant hepatic necrosis.

Diagnostic Approach in Patients Presenting with Acute Hepatitis

HBsAg	IgM anti HAV	IgM anti HBc	Anti HCV	Interpretation
+	–	+	–	Acute hepatitis B
+	–	–	–	Chronic hepatitis B
+	+	–	–	Acute HAV + chronic hepatitis B
+	+	+	–	Acute hepatitis A + B
–	+	+	–	Acute hepatitis A + B (HBs Ag ↓)
–	+	–	–	Acute hepatitis A
–	–	+	–	Acute HBV (HBs Ag ↓)
–	–	–	+	Acute hepatitis C

Cryptogenic Cirrhosis

The diagnosis of cryptogenic cirrhosis is reserved for those patients in whom no aetiology can be demonstrated. Clinical features, diagnosis and treatment are almost similar to alcoholic cirrhosis.

Biliary Cirrhosis

There are two types of biliary cirrhosis
1. Primary biliary cirrhosis
2. Secondary biliary cirrhosis.

Primary biliary cirrhosis is characterised by chronic inflammation and fibrous obliteration of intrahepatic bile ducts. Secondary biliary cirrhosis is characterised by partial or complete obstruction of larger extrahepatic bile ducts.

Etiology and Pathogenesis of Primary Biliary Cirrhosis

Aetiology unknown. Commonly seen in women of 30–50 years of age.

Primary biliary cirrhosis is associated with auto-immune diseases like CRST syndrome (calcinosis, Raynaud's phenomenon, sclerodactyly, telangiectasia), sicca syndrome, autoimmune thyroiditis. The autoantigen commonly involved is 74-kDa E_2 component of pyruvate dehydrogenase complex.

An increased level of IgG antimitochondrial antibody and increased levels of serum IgM, cryoproteins consisting of immune complexes are seen in 80–90% of patients. Lymphocytes are prominent in the portal regions and surround damaged bile ducts.

Secondary biliary cirrhosis is caused by postoperative strictures and gallstones.

Clinical Features

Patients may be asymptomatic. Earliest symptom is pruritus. Other symptoms include jaundice, fatigue, melanosis, steatorrhea, malabsorption of fat soluble vitamins, elevation of serum lipids resulting in xanthelasma and xanthomas. Later, signs of hepatocellular failure and portal hypertension develop. Fever and right upper quadrant pain (cholangitis/biliary colic) may occur in secondary biliary cirrhosis (Fig. 5.29).

Investigations

1. Two- to five-fold increase in serum alkaline phosphatase and elevation of serum 5' nucleotidase are seen.

2.. There may be an increased titre of more than 1 : 40 of antimitochondrial antibody. It is a specific and sensitive test.
3. Elevated serum cholesterol and lipoproteins are seen.
4. Raised serum bilirubin in terminal stages.
5. Liver biopsy

Stage 1	Necrotizing inflammatory process (acute and chronic inflammatory cells) of the portal triads with destruction of medium and small sized bile ducts
Stage 2	Ductule proliferation
Stage 3	Expansion of periportal fibrosis due to scarring.
Stage 4	Micro or macronodular cirrhosis.

Treatment

No specific therapy for primary biliary cirrhosis.
1. Colchicine in the dose of 0.6 mg orally twice daily.
2. Methotrexate in a low dose and cyclosporine are used to slow the progression or arrest the disease.
3. Ursodiol 13 to 15 mg/kg/day is shown to produce symptomatic improvement and improvement in serum biochemical parameters.
4. Symptomatic treatment includes antipruritic agents and cholestyramine 8 to 12 gm/day for pruritus and hypercholesterolaemia.
5. Low fat diet for steatorrhoea.
6. Vitamin A, D, K supplements parenterally for correction of deficiencies.
7. Secondary biliary cirrhosis is treated by surgical means or endoscopic relief of the obstruction.

Cardiac Cirrhosis

Aetiology

Prolonged severe right sided congestive heart failure may lead to chronic liver injury and cardiac cirrhosis.

Pathogenesis

In chronic right heart failure, retrograde transmission of elevated venous pressure leads to congestion of liver. Hepatic sinusoids become dilated and engorged with blood. Macroscopically the liver is referred to as 'nutmeg liver'.

Clinical Features

Liver is enlarged, firm, nontender and nonpulsatile in spite of TR. Signs and symptoms of right heart failure are seen (Fig. 5.29).

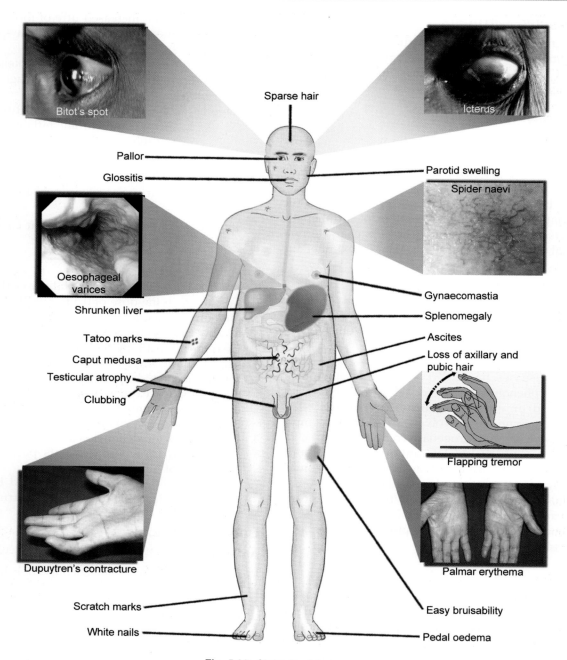

Fig. 5.29: Cirrhosis of liver

Investigations

Mild elevation of serum bilirubin and serum AST levels. Investigations for chronic heart disease (X-ray, ECG, Echo).

Treatment

Treat the underlying cardiovascular disorder.

Complications of Cirrhosis

1. Portal hypertension
2. Ascites
3. Hepatic encephalopathy
4. Spontaneous bacterial peritonitis
5. Hepatorenal syndrome
6. Hepatocellular carcinoma
7. Coagulopathy.

Prehepatic	Intrahepatic			Posthepatic
	Presinusoidal	*Sinusoidal*	*Postsinusoidal*	
a. Portal vein thrombosis b. Splenic arteriovenous fistula c. Constriction of the veins	a. Schistosomiasis b. Sarcoidosis c. Metastatic carcinoma	a. Cirrhosis b. Primary biliary cirrhosis c. Cryptogenic; alcohol-induced cirrhosis	a. Alcoholic hepatitis b. Veno-occlusive disease c. Hepatic vein thrombosis	a. Inferior vena caval web b. Tricuspid insufficiency c. Pericarditis

Portal Hypertension

Normal pressure in the portal vein is 10–15 cm saline or 7–10 mm Hg.

Portal hypertension is present when the sustained elevation of portal pressure is > 10 mm of Hg but the risk of variceal bleeding is greater only when it is > 30 cm saline or > 12 mm of Hg.

Classification

The obstruction to portal blood flow can occur at three levels
1. Portal vein (prehepatic)
2. Intrahepatic (presinusoidal, sinusoidal, postsinusoidal)
3. Hepatic veins (posthepatic).

Clinical Features

Patients may present with any of the complications of portal hypertension namely
1. Collateral circulation and varices
2. Ascites
3. Congestive splenomegaly, hypersplenism
4. Encephalopathy.

Collateral Circulation (Varices)

Extensive portal-systemic venous communications develop in order to decompress the high-pressure portal venous system. Maintenance of portal hypertension after the collaterals are formed, is attributed to a resultant increase in splanchnic blood flow.

Major Sites of Collaterals (Fig. 5.30)

1. Oesophageal and gastric varices (left gastric vein and short gastric vein join with intercostal, diaphragmatic, esophageal and azygos veins of the caval system).
2. Hemorrhoids (Superior haemorrhoidal vein of the portal system to middle and inferior haemorrhoidal veins of the caval system).

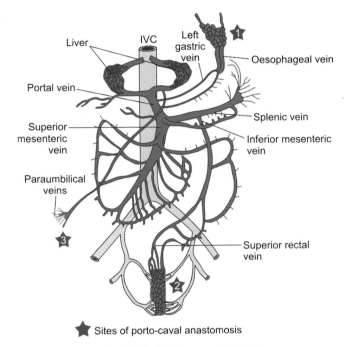

Fig. 5.30: Portal venous system

3. Caput medusae (remnants of the umbilical circulation of the fetus present in the falciform ligament may form a large paraumbilical vein).
4. Other sites of anastomoses are retroperitoneal veins, lumbar veins, omental veins and veins over bare area of the liver.

Investigations

1. *Fibreoptic oesophagoscopy:* Shows the presence of oesophageal and gastric varices.
2. Measurement of portal venous pressure by either percutaneous transhepatic skinny needle catheterization or through transjugular cannulation of the hepatic veins. Wedged hepatic venous pressure is high in sinusoidal and postsinusoidal portal hypertension.
3. *USG abdomen:* Features of portal hypertension such as splenomegaly, collaterals, cause of liver disease

(occasionally) or portal vein thrombosis can be detected. Portal vein size can be assessed. (Normal portal vein size is 1 cm; when portal vein size is 2 cm it is said to be dilated; when it is more than 3 cm it is said to be aneurysmally dilated).

4. *Portal venogram:* Site and the cause of portal venous obstruction can be detected and is also performed prior to surgical therapy.

Complications

- Variceal bleeding
- Congestive gastropathy
- Hypersplenism
- Ascites
- Renal failure
- Hepatic encephalopathy.

Management

1. Beta-blockers like propranolol or nadolol can be used due to their vasodilatory effects on both the splanchnic arterial bed and the portal venous system in combination with reduced cardiac output. Propranolol prevents recurrent bleeding from severe portosystemic gastropathy in cirrhotic patients.
2. Treatment of alcoholic hepatitis, chronic active hepatitis and other diseases results in fall in portal venous pressure and reduction in variceal size.

Variceal Bleeding

Variceal bleeding occurs when portal venous pressure is more than 12 mm Hg. Mostly bleeding arises from oesophageal varices within 3–5 cm of the oesophago-gastric junction or from gastric varices.

Factors Predisposing to Bleeding

- Large varices
- Endoscopic variceal stigma (red spots, red stripes)
- High portal pressure
- Liver failure
- Drugs (NSAIDs).

Usually there are no precipitating factors.

Clinical Features

Symptoms and signs of shock (tachycardia, systolic BP less than 90 mm Hg, urine output less than 30 ml/hour).

Management

Variceal bleeding is a life-threatening emergency.

Modified Child's Classification

Variables	Scores		
	1	2	3
Encephalopathy (degree)	Nil	Slight-moderate	Moderate-severe
Ascites (degree)	Nil	Slight	Moderate-severe
Bilirubin (mg/dl)	< 2	2–3	> 3
Albumin (gm/dl)	≥ 3.5	2.8–3.4	< 2.8
Prothrombin index (%)	> 70	40–70	< 40
Prothrombin time (in seconds)	≤ 14	15–17	≥ 18

Scores are summed to determine Child's class.
Class A 5–7 (suitable for surgery)
Class B 7–10 (marginal risk for surgery)
Class C more than 10 (unsuitable for surgery).

1. Replacement of blood, coagulation factors by fresh, frozen plasma (in coagulopathy).
2. Monitor CVP, PCWP, urine output and mental status.

   Treatment of sequelae of portal hypertension especially variceal bleeding is titrated to reduce the hepatic venous pressure gradient (HVPG) to < 12 mm of Hg or 20% from the baseline (HVPG = Wedged hepatic venous pressure – Free hepatic venous pressure).

   When the HVPG is not feasible or available, reduction of resting pulse rate by 25% -using β-blockers is reasonable.

3. *Vasoconstrictors*
   a. *Vasopressin:* 0.1–0.5 units/minute for 4–12 hours and subsequently reduce the dose and continue up to 48 hours. It reduces blood flow in portal venous system. Side effects are myocardial, GIT, peripheral ischemia, ARF, hyponatremia. Concurrent use of venodilators like nitroglycerin IV infusion, sublingual isosorbide dinitrate may enhance the effectiveness of vasopressin and reduce complications.
   Terlipressin: Terlipressin can be used as a better alternative to vasopressin in the control of acute variceal bleeding because of the beneficial effects in patients with hepatorenal syndrome.
   b. *Somatostatin:* It is a direct splanchnic vasoconstrictor (250 mg bolus followed by constant infusion of 250 mg/hr is as effective as vasopressin).
   c. *Octreotide:* It is a synthetic somatostatin analogue given in a dose of 50 mg IV bolus followed by 50 mg/hour. These drugs can be repeated if the bleeding is severe.

d. Short acting nitrates (nitroglycerin) via transdermal (10 mg every 12 hours), sublingual (0.6 mg every 30 minutes) or IV (40–400 mg/min to maintain systolic BP > 90 mm Hg) routes can be tried. They reduce peripheral vasospastic effects of vasopressin and lower the portal pressure further via direct vasodilation of portal-systemic collaterals.

4. Balloon tamponade of bleeding varices by a triple or four lumen Sengstaken-Blakemore's tube with two balloons (gastric/esophageal). Complications like aspiration pneumonitis, esophageal rupture are common depending on the length of time the balloon is kept inflated. Hence, it has to be deflated after 24 hours. If bleeding has stopped, the tube may be removed in another 24 hours.

5. Endoscopic sclerotherapy can be done using sclerosants like sodium morrhuate, absolute alcohol, tetradecyl, ethanolamine oleate, etc. After control of bleeding, sclerotherapy has to be continued for several weeks to months till the varices are fully obliterated.

    Complications – ulceration, stricture, perforation, pleural effusion, ARDS, sepsis

6. Endoscopic band ligation of varices.

    It is the procedure of choice in non bleeding varices. Complications include superficial ulceration, stricture and dysphagia.

7. *Surgery:* Creation of portal systemic shunt to permit decompression of portal system.
    a. Nonselective shunts to decompress entire portal system, e.g. end to side or side to side portocaval and proximal splenorenal anastomosis. Portal systemic encephalopathy is common.
    b. Selective shunts decompress only the varices allowing blood flow to the liver itself, e.g. distal splenorenal shunt.
    c. Splenectomy—for isolated fundal varices caused by splenic vein thrombosis.

No prophylactic shunt surgery or sclerotherapy should be done on patients with nonbleeding varices.

8. Prevention of recurrent bleeding
    a. Oral beta-blockers, long-acting nitrates
    b. Sclerotherapy
    c. Band ligation
    d. Transjugular intrahepatic portosystemic stent shunting (TIPSS)
    e. Portosystemic shunt surgery.

9. *Liver transplantation:* It is curative for portal hypertension (not in the acute setting of variceal bleed) and should be reserved for patients with advanced liver disease.

Prognosis

Forty to seventy per cent of those bleeding from varices for the first-time die. The prognosis depends upon the various criteria given in modified Child's classification.

Unfavourable Signs

1. Jaundice
2. Ascites
3. Hypoalbuminaemia
4. Encephalopathy.

Ascites

Ascites refers to accumulation of free fluid in peritoneal cavity.

Causes of Ascites

1. Hepatic cirrhosis
2. Malignant disease
    a. Hepatic
    b. Peritoneal
3. Infection
    a. Tuberculosis
    b. Bacterial peritonitis
4. Hypoproteinaemia
    a. Nephrotic syndrome
    b. Protein losing enteropathy
    c. Malnutrition
5. Cardiac failure; constrictive pericarditis (ascites precox)
6. Hepatic venous occlusion
    a. Budd-Chiari syndrome
    b. Veno-occlusive disease
7. Pancreatitis (ascitic fluid amylase > 1000 units/L)
8. Lymphatic obstruction—chylous ascites
9. Uncommon causes
    a. Meig's syndrome
    b. Vasculitis
    c. Hypothyroidism
    d. Renal dialysis.

Features	Transudate	Exudate
Ascitic fluid protein	< 30 gm/L	> 30 gm/L
Serum-ascitic fluid Albumin gradient	> 1.1/dL	< 1.1/dL
Specific gravity	< 1.018	> 1.018

Pathogenesis

Ascites occurs because of the imbalance between the formation and resorption of peritoneal fluid. In cirrhosis of liver, the ascites is due to:

Transudate	Exudate
1. Cirrhosis of liver	1. Bacterial infections
2. Right sided venous hypertension	2. Tuberculosis
3. Hypoalbuminaemia (nephrosis, protein losing enteropathy)	3. Tumour
4. Constrictive pericarditis	
5. Hepatic venous thrombosis	
6. Meig's syndrome	

1. Portal hypertension.
2. Renal changes resulting in increased sodium and water resorption. There is stimulation of renin-angiotensin-aldosterone system, increased ADH release and decreased release of natriuretic hormone or third factor.
3. Imbalance between the formation and removal of hepatic and gut lymph.
4. Hypoalbuminaemia.
5. Elevated plasma vasopressin and epinephrine levels in response to a volume-depleted state, accentuates renal and vascular factors.

Portal hypertension is not associated with ascites unless there is concomitant hypoalbuminaemia.

Ascitic fluid should be analysed in the following ways:
1. Gross appearance: Blood stained fluid is unusual in uncomplicated cirrhosis. It suggests TB/neoplasm.
2. Protein content (given in the table).
3. Differential cell count: If the fluid is a transudate, and contains > 250 WBCs/mL, it suggests tumour

or infection. Detailed cytoanalysis is given in the table below.
4. Cytology for the presence of malignant cells.
5. Gram's stain, smear and culture for AFB.

Spontaneous Bacterial Peritonitis (SBP)

It is defined as infected ascitic fluid in the absence of recognizable secondary cause of peritonitis. It is associated with an ascitic protein of < 1 gm/dL.

Organisms

Coliforms, streptococci, Campylobacter; usually infection is blood-borne.

Cultures are more likely to be positive when 10 ml of ascitic fluid is inoculated into two culture bottles at the bed side.

Clinical Features

Fever, abdominal pain, tenderness.

Criteria for Diagnosis

1. Clinical features + polymorphs > 250/cmm
2. If polymorphs > 500/cmm, even without clinical features.

Management

Inj cefotaxime 1 gm IV tds for 5-7days is the preferred empirical therapy.

Prophylactic maintenance therapy can be done using T. Norfloxacin 400 mg/day or T. Ciprofloxacin 750 mg weekly.

Conditions	Colour of ascitic fluid	Specific gravity	Protein in gm/lit	RBC >10,000/mL	WBC/mL	Other tests
Cirrhosis of liver	Straw coloured/ bile stained	< 1.016 (95%)	< 25	1%	< 250 (mesothelial)	
Neoplasm	Straw coloured Hgic, mucinous, chylous	Variable > 1.016	> 25	20%	> 1000 variable cells	Cytology, cell block. peritoneal biopsy
Tuberculosis hgic, chylous	Clear, turbid, > 1.016	variable	> 25	7% > 70%	> 1000 (70%) lymphocytes	Peritoneal biopsy, stain, culture for AFB
Pyogenic peritonitis	Turbid or purulent	If purulent > 1.016	If purulent > 25	Unusual	Predominantly polymorphs	Positive Gram stain or culture
CCF	Straw coloured	Variable <1.016	Variable 15–53	10%	< 1000 (90%) mesothelial/ mononuclear	
Nephrosis	straw coloured/ chylous	< 1.016	< 25 (100%)	Unusual	< 250, mesothelial /mononuclear	If chylous ether extraction/ Sudan stain
Pancreatic ascites (Pseudocyst)	Turbid/Hgic/ chylous	Variable >1.016	Variable >25	Variable/ bile stained	Variable	- amylase in ascitic fluid/ serum

Chylous Ascites

The fluid is milky, creamy and turbid due to the presence of thoracic or intestinal lymph. Sudan staining of fat globules microscopically and increased triglyceride content (> 1000 mg/dL) by chemical examination clinches the diagnosis.

Causes

Due to lymphatic obstruction from trauma, tumour, TB, nephrosis, pancreatitis, filariasis or congenital lymphatic obstruction.

Mucinous Ascites

Occurs in pseudomyxoma peritonei or colloid carcinoma of stomach or colon with peritoneal implants.

Investigations

1. Ascitic fluid analysis
2. *Plain X-ray abdomen:* Demonstrates haziness of the abdomen with loss of psoas shadow.
3. *Ultrasonogram of abdomen:* It detects as little as 30 ml of ascitic fluid in the right lateral decubitus position. Loculated collections can also be identified.
4. *CT scan abdomen:* In addition to evaluation of intra-abdominal anatomy, it detects small amounts of ascites also.

Management

1. Daily weight chart, I.O. chart, bed-rest
2. Diuretics (spironolactone 25 mg qid with or without frusemide 20–40 mg in divided doses or amiloride 10 mg/day alone or in combination with frusemide or thiazides) are given in
   a. Gross ascites
   b. Tense ascites with umbilical hernia
   c. For facilitating biopsy, scan or venogram
3. Fluid restriction up to 1500 ml/day and salt restriction of 2 gm/day
4. Paracentesis in severe distension causing respiratory embarassment
5. Peritoneal shunt in intractable ascites
6. Albumin can be infused
7. Treat the cause.

Refractory Ascites

In about 10–20% of patients with ascites, medical therapy is a failure. The conditions contributing to refractory ascites resulting in worsening of the primary liver disease are:
a. Active inflammation
b. Portal or hepatic vein thrombosis
c. GI bleed
d. Infection
e. SBP
f. Malnutrition
g. Hepatoma
h. Superimposed cardiac and renal disease
i. Hepatotoxic and nephrotoxic drugs.

Treatment

1. *Peritoneovenous shunt (LeVeen or Denver shunt):* PV shunt routes the ascitic fluid subcutaneously from the peritoneal cavity into the internal jugular vein through a pressure activated one-way valve. The complications are peritonitis, sepsis, DIC, CCF and ruptured esophageal varices. Shunt may get occluded in 30% of the patients and may require replacement. Contraindications to this procedure are sepsis, CCF, malignancy and history of variceal bleeding.
2. *Therapeutic paracentesis:* The procedure involves removal of 4–6 litres of ascitic fluid until the abdomen is completely evacuated. Dietary sodium restriction and diuretics should be continued to prevent rapid reaccumulation of ascitic fluid. The procedure may be repeated every 2–4 weeks. But it may result in protein and opsonin depletion which can predispose to SBP. Albumin infusion is very costly and its replacement after large paracentesis remains controversial.
3. *Liver transplantation:* The 12 months survival of patients with ascites refractory to medical therapy is only 25%. The survival increases to 75% with liver transplantation.

Fulminant Hepatic Failure

It is a rare syndrome in which hepatic encephalopathy results from sudden severe impairment of hepatic function. It occurs within 8 weeks of onset of precipitating illness, in the absence of pre-existing liver disease.

Causes

1. Any viral hepatitis (*HDV + HBV increases risk)
2. *Drugs (paracetamol excess, INH, methyldopa, halothane)
3. Fulminant Budd-Chiari syndrome
4. Acute fatty liver of pregnancy
5. Toxins—carbon tetrachloride
6. Weil's disease
7. Wilson's disease
8. Reye's syndrome.

Note: *Poor prognosis.

Clinical Features

Patients may present with neuropsychiatric changes, stupor, coma, symptoms and signs of cerebral oedema, profuse sweating, haemodynamic instability, tachyarrhythmias, tachypnoea, fever, papilloedema, decerebrate rigidity, deep jaundice, coagulopathy, bleeding, renal failure, acid-base disturbance, hypoglycaemia, acute pancreatitis, cardiorespiratory failure and infections.

Poor Prognostic Indicators

1. Age < 10 or > 40 years
2. If hepatic failure is due to halothane or non-A, non-B hepatitis
3. Duration of jaundice of 1 week before the onset of encephalopathy
4. Serum bilirubin > 18 mg/dL
5. Coma
6. Rapid reduction in liver size
7. Respiratory failure
8. Prolongation of prothrombin time
9. Factor V level < 20%
10. In acetaminophen overdose, blood pH < 7.3, serum creatinine > 3 mg/dL and prolonged prothrombin time.

Treatment

1. Endotracheal intubation
2. Prevent GI bleeding with H_2 receptor blockers and antacids
3. Monitor serum glucose level and administer 10–20% dextrose when needed
4. IV mannitol may be beneficial
5. Liver transplantation should be considered in patients with grade III and IV encephalopathy and other adverse prognostic indicators.

Hepatic Coma
(Hepatic Encephalopathy)

It is a complex neuropsychiatric syndrome characterised by disturbances in consciousness level and behaviour, personality changes, fluctuating neurological signs, asterixis and distinctive electroencephalographic changes.

There are two types of hepatic coma:
1. Acute or subacute—reversible
2. Chronic—progressive leading to irreversible coma and death.

Precipitating Factors

1. Increased nitrogen load (gastrointestinal bleeding, excessive dietary protein, uraemia, constipation).
2. Electrolyte imbalance (hypokalaemia, alkalosis, hypoxia, hypovolaemia).
3. Drugs (narcotics, tranquilizers, sedatives, diuretics).
4. Others (infection, surgery, acute and progressive liver disease).
5. Large binge of alcohol.
6. Large volume of paracentesis.

Pathogenesis

Abnormality in the nitrogen metabolism in which ammonia and/or other amines (octapamine, amino acids) formed in the bowel by the action of urease containing organisms, are carried in the portal circulation to the liver, fail to get detoxified due to hepatocellular disease or portal systemic shunt of blood or both. These substances enter systemic circulation where they interfere with cerebral metabolism.

Clinical Features

- Main feature is the derangement of consciousness, altered sleep rhythm, increased psychomotor activity followed by progressive drowsiness, stupor and coma. Severe brain oedema may occur.
- There may be extrapyramidal signs. There may be exaggeration of deep tendon reflexes and plantars may be extensors.
- There is also dysarthria, mild alexia, with focal or generalized seizures.
- Asterixis or flapping tremor is a characteristic feature of impending hepatic coma.
- Change in hand writing, constructional apraxia and fetor hepaticus, a unique musty odour of the breath due to mercaptans may also be present.

Classification

Hepatic coma can be classified into four stages as follows:

Stage	Mental status	Asterixis	EEG
I	Euphoria or depression, mild confusion, slurred speech, disorders of sleep	+/–	Usually normal
II	Lethargy, moderate confusion	+	Abnormal
III	Marked confusion; incoherent speech; patient is arousable from sleep	+	Abnormal
IV	Coma; patient initially responsive to noxious stimuli, later becomes nonresponsive	–	Abnormal

Diagnosis

It is only by exclusion
1. No pathognomonic liver function abnormality
2. Elevation of serum ammonia
3. CSF analysis is normal
4. CT scan brain does not show any abnormality
5. EEG shows high voltage, slow wave forms (reduced alpha rhythm and increased delta activity; delta waves 3–4 cycles/second). It is the earliest sign in hepatic encephalopathy. There is slowing or flattening of waves with 3 : 1 high-voltage waves.

In the presence of jaundice, portal hypertension or ascites, the cause for coma is most likely to be of hepatic origin.

Treatment

1. Elimination of precipitating factors.
2. Nasogastric aspiration (in case of bleeding) and protection of airway with a endotracheal tube.
3. Avoid constipation and favour bowel emptying by bowel wash, enema or by lactulose (30–50 ml 3 to 4 times daily) or lactitol.
4. Bowel sterilization by neomycin 1 gm qid or ampicillin. Neomycin helps in decreasing ammonia production or its absorption from the bowel.
5. Avoid drugs, especially sedatives and diuretics.
6. Protein must be avoided.
7. IV mannitol as a fast drip for reducing cerebral edema.
8. The use of agents like levodopa, bromocryptine, ketoanalogues of amino acids and intravenous infusion of amino acids in the treatment of acute hepatic encephalopathy is unclear. So also haemoperfusion to remove toxic substances and treatment of cerebral oedema.
9. Liver transplantation.

Hepatorenal Syndrome

It is a progressive functional renal failure occurring in patients with severe liver disease. Mostly patients have decompensated cirrhosis and tense ascites. The kidneys are anatomically, histologically and functionally normal.

Pathogenesis

The hemodynamic alterations in kidneys are as a result of decreased effective blood volume and increased sympathetic tone. Increased intra-abdominal and renal venous pressure and alteration of balance between vasoactive humoral agents such as renin-angiotensin, prostaglandins, thromboxanes, kinins, endotoxins, and renal kallikrein may play a role. Involvement of endothelin-1 and 3 has been implicated in hepatorenal syndrome. Role of nitric oxide has also been suggested as one of the mechanisms.

Criteria for Diagnosis of Hepatorenal Syndrome

Major criteria
1. Chronic or acute liver disease with advanced hepatic failure and portal hypertension.
2. Low GFR indicated by S creatinine > 1.5 mg% or creatinine clearance less than 40 ml/min.
3. Absence of treatment with nephrotoxic drugs, shock, infection or signicificant fluid loss.
4. No sustained improvement in renal function after diuretic withdrawl and volume expansion with 1.5 litres of isotonic saline.
5. Proteinuria < 500 mg% and no USG evidence of obstructive or parenchymal renal disease.

Additional criteria
1. Urine volume   < 500 ml/d
2. U. Na $^+$ < 10 mEq/litre
3. U osmolality   > Plasma osmolality
4. Urine RBC   < 50/hpf
5. S. Na$^+$ < 130 mEq/litre

Management

1. Identification, removal and treatment of any factors precipitating renal failure (diuretics to be stopped, blood volume to be replenished during dehydration or hemorrhage, infections to be treated, avoid nephrotoxic drugs).
2. Saline or salt poor albumin or plasma to be administered till diuresis occurs. If diuresis does not occur, infusion is to be stopped.
3. Drugs like phentolamine, papaverine, aminophylline, dopamine, phenoxybenzamine, prostaglandin E_1 have been tried with no benefit.
4. *Dialysis*: It is indicated in patients with potentially reversible liver disease to allow the liver to regain its function.
5. *Surgery*: Liver transplantation and portacaval shunts have been tried. Liver transplantation is the only definitive treatment.

Hepatocellular Carcinoma (Hepatoma)

Hepatoma is 4 times more common in women. It commonly arises in a cirrhotic liver.

Aetiology

1. Chronic hepatitis B, C infection especially in a cirrhotic liver

2. Aflatoxin B_1 (loss, inactivation or mutation of the P^{53} gene)
3. Haemochromatosis
4. Alpha-1 antitrypsin deficiency
5. Alcoholic cirrhosis; rarely in primary biliary cirrhosis
6. Thorotrast, arsenic (causes angiosarcoma also)
7. Oestrogens, androgens, anabolic steroids (causes adenoma also). Contraceptive steroids used for > 8 years may increase the risk by 4-fold.

Pathology

Macroscopically, there is a single mass or multiple nodules. Microscopically, tumour is made up of well-differentiated cells secreting bile.

Clinical Features

Patients may present with fever of unknown origin, abdominal pain, right upper quadrant abdominal mass, friction rub or bruit over the liver, haemorrhagic ascites or occasionally intra-abdominal bleeding.

Paraneoplastic manifestations are
1. Erythrocytosis (due to erythropoietin like substance)
2. Hypercholesterolaemia
3. Hypercalcaemia (due to PTH like substance)
4. Hypoglycaemia
5. Acquired porphyria
6. Dysfibrinogenaemia
7. Cryofibrinogenaemia.

Investigations

1. Serum alkaline phosphatase: mildly elevated
2. Serum alpha-fetoprotein > 500 µg/l; persistence of levels over 500–1000 µg/l in an adult with liver disease and without obvious GIT tumours or gonadal malignancies suggests hepatocellular carcinoma. Increasing levels suggest progression of the tumour or recurrence after hepatic resection/chemotherapy/chemoembolization
3. *Imaging techniques:* USG abdomen detects tumours of 2–3 cm in size; CT scan of the liver helps in the accurate evaluation of tumour and also to identify enlarged lymph nodes (Fig. 5.31)
4. *Liver biopsy:* Diagnostic biopsy can be taken in an area localized by USG or CT. Risk of tumour cell migration along the biopsy track is small. Since the tumours are vascular, biopsies should be done with caution
5. Detection of des gamma carboxyl prothrombin
6. Cytology of ascitic fluid rarely shows malignant cells
7. Laparoscopy or minilaparotomy can be done to take the biopsy under direct vision

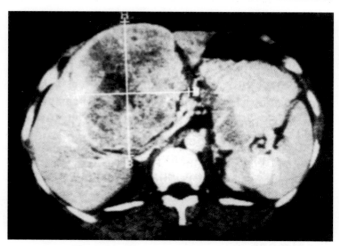

Fig. 5.31: CT scan—hepatoma left lobe

8. Investigations to rule out paraneoplastic syndrome
9. *Angiography:* Celiac axis angiography can determine operability in a patient with hepatoma or solitary metastasis to the liver.

Management

1. Surgical resection (hepatoma or single metastasis confined to one lobe)
2. Hepatic artery embolization with chemotherapy
3. Alcohol ablation via USG guided percutaneous injection
4. USG guided cryoablation
5. Immunotherapy using monoclonal antibodies tagged with cytotoxic agents
6. Gene therapy with retrievable vectors containing genes which express cytotoxic agents
7. *Liver transplantation:* Recurrence/metastasis in the transplanted liver is common.

Prognosis

If untreated, patients usually die within 3–6 months of diagnosis. Monitor course of illness with serial USG, alpha-fetoprotein especially in HBsAg positive patients or patients with cirrhosis due to hepatitis C infection.

Metabolic Liver Disease

Wilson's Disease

Wilson's disease is an autosomal recessive disorder. The genetic defect is on chromosome 13. In 95% of patients, there is also an absence or deficiency of serum ceruloplasmin, the main copper transporting protein in blood, usually associated with the defect in ceruloplasmin gene on chromosome 3.

Clinical Features

It can present as neuro-psychiatric disorder, chronic active hepatitis, fulminant hepatitis, cirrhosis of liver, acquired haemolytic anaemia, ophthalmic problems like sunflower cataracts and Kayser-Fleischer rings (copper deposits laid in the Descemet's membrane around the periphery of cornea).

Renal abnormalities are due to accumulation of copper within the renal parenchyma resulting in decreased GFR, proximal tubular defects resembling Fanconi's syndrome, renal tubular acidosis, hematuria and proteinuria.

Investigations

1. *Serum ceruloplasmin:* Low, often less than 20 mg/dl.
2. *Serum copper level:* Total serum copper often decreased but free copper is elevated. Free copper is calculated by finding the difference between total serum copper and the amount of copper bound to ceruloplasmin (0.047 µmol of copper/mg of ceruloplasmin).
3. *Urine copper excretion:* Levels greater than 1.6 mmol/day is suggestive of Wilson's disease. However, urine copper levels are high in other conditions like cirrhosis, chronic active hepatitis or cholestasis.
4. *Liver biopsy:* It should be done for histology and for hepatic copper estimation. Hepatic copper concentration more than 250 µg/gm of dry tissue is compatible with the diagnosis of Wilson's disease.
5. *Kayser-Fleischer ring:* It is present in all patients with Wilson's disease who have neurological manifestation. It should be sought with slit-lamp examination.

6. Low serum alkaline phosphatase and elevated aminotransferase.
7. *Radiocopper loading test:* In normal persons after giving radioactive copper, it disappears from serum within 4–6 hours. A secondary rise of radioactivity appears after the isotope is incorporated into ceruloplasmin production. In patients with Wilson's disease, the secondary rise is absent since they cannot incorporate radiocopper into ceruloplasmin.

Management

See table below.

Haemochromatosis

It is a disorder in which there is excessive iron absorption either alone or in combination with parenteral iron loading, leading to progressive increase in total body iron stores.

Classification

1. Primary or idiopathic
2. Secondary
   a. Refractory anaemia
   b. Chronic liver injury
   c. Dietary iron overload
   d. Porphyria cutanea tarda
3. Parenteral iron overload
   a. Multiple blood transfusions
   b. Excessive parenteral iron
   c. Haemodialysis

Disease status	1st Choice	2nd Choice
Hepatitis/Cirrhosis without de-compensation	Zinc	Trientine
Hepatic de-compensation Mild Moderate Severe	Trientine and Zinc Trientine and Zinc Hepatic transplant	Penicillamine and Zinc Hepatic transplant Trientine and Zinc
Initial neurologic/psychiatric	Tetrathiomolybdate and Zinc	Trientine and Zinc
Maintenance	Zinc	Trientine
Pre-symptomatic	Zinc	Trientine
Paediatric	Zinc	Trientine
Pregnant	Zinc	Trientine

Zinc acetate – 50 mg of elemental zinc three times daily
Trientine hydrochloride – 500 mg bid an hour before or two hours after food.
Tetrathiomolybdate is not yet commercially available.
Low copper containing diet should be taken. Foods rich in copper, like organ meats, shell-fish, dried beans, peas, whole wheat, and chocolate should be avoided

Idiopathic Haemochromatosis

It is an autosomal recessive disorder with the abnormal gene located in the HLA A6 locus on short arm of chromosome 6.

Clinical Features

Lethargy, weight loss, change in skin color, loss of libido, abdominal pain. arthralgia, symptoms of diabetes mellitus (65%) are common modes of presentation. Patients have hepatomegaly, skin pigmentation, testicular atrophy, loss of body hair, CCF (due to congestive cardiomyopathy) and arthritis (osteoarthritis, pseudogout).

Hepatoma can occur in 30% of patients with cirrhosis. Arrhythmias (atrial and ventricular tachyarrhythmias) and AV blocks are common.

Investigations

1. Serum iron and total iron binding capacity. Serum iron more than 180 to 300 µg/dl and elevated TIBC suggest haemochromatosis.
2. *Serum ferritin:* It is the most specific screening test for increased iron stores. Serum ferritin level is between 600–900 µg/L (normal 10–200 µg/L).
3. Transferrin saturation is 50–100% (normal 22 to 46%)
4. Total iron binding capacity is between 200–300 µg/dL (normal 250–370 µg/dL)
5. *Liver biopsy:* It is helpful in estimating tissue iron by histochemical staining. Hepatic iron concentration by dry weight can also be done and levels > 1000 µg/100 mg of dry weight suggests IHC.
6. *CT scan and MRI:* Increased level of iron in liver is associated with an increased CT density or attenuation coefficient. MRI is sensitive in the detection of moderate iron overload.

Management

1. *Phlebotomy:* There is 250 mg of iron in 500 ml of blood. The body burden of iron in IHC is more than 20 gm, a weekly phlebotomy of 500 ml of blood for 2–3 years may be needed to achieve a haemoglobin of 11 and serum ferritin of 10.
2. *Desferrioxamine:* It is an iron chelating agent given in a dose of 40–80 mg/kg/day, subcutaneously. It removes 10–20 mg of iron/day.

Prognosis

Hepatocellular carcinoma occurs in one-third of the patients with IHC and cirrhosis, despite iron removal.

Causes of Death

Death may be due to CCF, hepatocellular failure, portal hypertension or hepatoma.

Acute Pancreatitis

The pathologic spectrum of acute pencreatitis varies from edematous pancreatitis (mild and self-limiting) to necrotizing pancreatitis.

In haemorrhagic pancreatitis, there is interstitial haemorrhage.

Causes

1. Alcohol ingestion (acute and chronic alcoholism)
2. Biliary disease (gallstones)
3. Postoperative (abdominal, nonabdominal)
4. Post-ERCP
5. Trauma
6. Metabolic
   a. Renal failure
   b. After renal transplantation
   c. Hypertriglyceridaemia
   d. Hypercalcaemia (hyperparathyroidism, drugs)
   e. Acute fatty liver of pregnancy
7. Infections (viral hepatitis, mumps, ascariasis, mycoplasma)
8. Drug induced
   a. *Definite association:* sulfonamides, oestrogens, frusemide, thiazides, tetracycline, valproic acid.
   b. *Probable association:* acetaminophen, ethacrynic acid, procainamide, metronidazole, NSAIDs, ACE inhibitors.
9. *Connective tissue disorders:* SLE, thrombotic thrombocytopenic purpura
10. Penetrating peptic ulcer
11. Obstruction to ampulla of Vater (regional enteritis, duodenal diverticulum)
12. Hereditary pancreatitis, pancreas divisum.

Clinical Features

Abdominal pain (mild to severe and constant), nausea, vomiting, abdominal distension (gastric hypomotility) and chemical peritonitis, low grade fever, tachycardia, hypotension (due to exudation of blood and plasma proteins, vasodilatation due to release of kinin peptides and systemic effects of proteolytic and lipolytic enzymes released into the circulation), jaundice (due to edema of the head of the pancreas), erythematous skin nodules (due to subcutaneous fat necrosis), basal rales, pleural effusion, diminished bowel sounds, palpable pancreatic

These are circumvented by auxiliary liver transplantation, in which an additional segment of liver is implanted to provide temporary support.

Nowadays, a part of the native liver is replaced with an equivalent section of donor organ. This is called auxiliary partial orthotopic liver transplantation (APOLT). This technique has been found useful in Crigler-Najjar syndrome.

Split Liver Transplantation

One cadaver organ can be split between two recipients– adult and one child.

Adult receives right lobe and the child receives left lobe of cadaver liver.

Bioartificial Liver

This newly invented technique has been used in patients with acute liver failure as a bridge until the native liver regenerates or until a donor organ becomes available.

Systems using cultured human hepatocytes, that would have the capacity to remove toxins and provide synthetic functions have been employed.

Extracorporeal liver assist device (ELAD) uses cultured human hepatoblastoma cells grown in the extracapillary space of a hollow fibre dialyser. Venous blood is pumped through the fibres, leading to the ultrafiltration of plasma into the extracapillary space. Return of the ultrafiltrate to the patient allows the delivery of high molecular weight products including clotting factors.

Success Rate

Long-term survival is 60–80%.

Molecular Adsorbent Re-circulating System (MARS)

MARS is based upon the principle of albumin dialysis. It consists of three compartments – blood circuit, albumin circuit and renal circuit. Here the blood is dialysed against an albumin containing solution across a suitable membrane. The albumin bound toxins are potentially taken up by the binding sites of the dialysate albumin and thus removed from the blood.

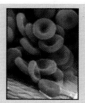

CHAPTER 6

Haematology

SYMPTOMS

SIGNS

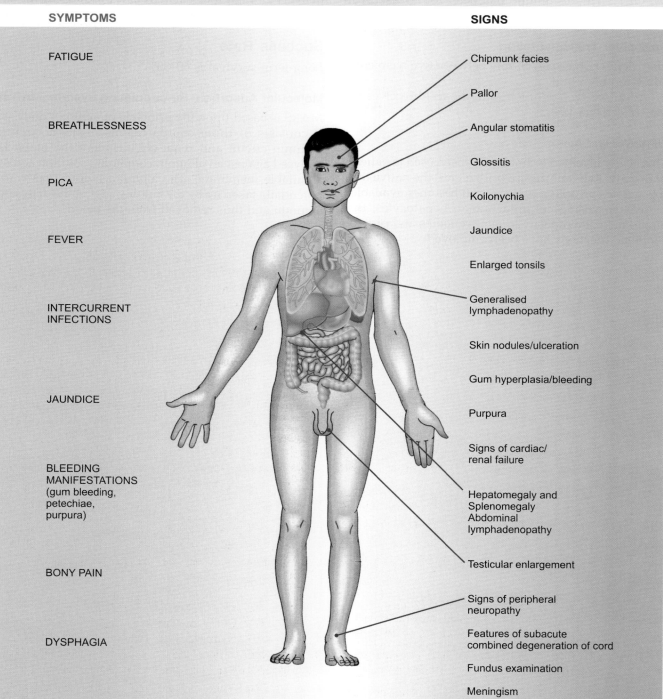

FATIGUE

BREATHLESSNESS

PICA

FEVER

INTERCURRENT
INFECTIONS

JAUNDICE

BLEEDING
MANIFESTATIONS
(gum bleeding,
petechiae,
purpura)

BONY PAIN

DYSPHAGIA

Chipmunk facies

Pallor

Angular stomatitis

Glossitis

Koilonychia

Jaundice

Enlarged tonsils

Generalised
lymphadenopathy

Skin nodules/ulceration

Gum hyperplasia/bleeding

Purpura

Signs of cardiac/
renal failure

Hepatomegaly and
Splenomegaly
Abdominal
lymphadenopathy

Testicular enlargement

Signs of peripheral
neuropathy

Features of subacute
combined degeneration of cord

Fundus examination

Meningism

Haematopoiesis and Haematopoietic Growth Factors

Proliferation of the early haematopoietic cells occurs as the embryo grows and becomes a foetus (10-12 weeks). During early foetal life, after the sixth week of pregnancy upto the second trimester, the liver and the spleen are the major sites for haematopoiesis. The sites of haematopoiesis gradually shift from the liver and spleen to the medullary cavities of the bones. At birth, virtually medullary cavities of every bone contribute to this proliferative process. Pluripotential cells remain in other organs of the reticuloendothelial system as haematopoietic "rest cells." These give rise to extramedullary haematopoiesis when there is a demand.

Haematopoietic Stem Cells

These are a unique clone of cells capable of differentiating into the multiple cell lines of the haematopoietic system (Fig. 6.1). Stem cell proliferation is under direct influence of haematopoietic growth factors present in the reticuloendothelial system.

Haematopoietic Stem Cell Differentiation

Name of the cell	Function
Erythrocytes	Hb present in the erythrocytes helps in the O_2 and CO_2 transport mechanism of blood; it has a minor role in the acid-base balance.
Neutrophils	These are phagocytes capable of ingesting bacteria and fungi by chemotaxis and opsonization. The bacteria are killed by O_2 dependent (H_2O_2 production, myeloperoxidase release) and O_2 independent (lysozyme, lactoferrin release, and reduction of pH in the phagosome) mechanisms. They also produce transcobalamin III, a vitamin B_{12} binding protein which increases in leukaemia. They liberate tissue damaging substances after ingestion of uric acid crystals.
Eosinophils	These are weakly phagocytic and are associated with allergic reactions. They ingest antigen-antibody complexes and can process foreign proteins. They also have a role in the containment of parasitic infestation.
Basophils	These are poor phagocytes and can bind to IgE molecule. Degranulation of basophils can occur with release of histamine (type I hypersensitivity). They also contain heparin which participates in the metabolism of lipids.
Monocytes	These are phagocytic and constitute the monocyte-macrophage system which removes debris as well as micro-organisms by phagocytosis; they help in the collection and presentation of antigenic material to the lymphocytes. They help in the lysis of tumour cells. They also produce IL-I and TNF and other mediators of acute phase reaction. They produce platelet
Lymphocytes	derived growth factor and helps in healing and tissue remodelling. Tissue thromboplastin is produced in response to bacterial endotoxin, thereby activating extrinsic coagulation pathway leading to intravascular coagulation. These arise from committed stem cells of the marrow and migrate to thymus (T-cells). Others become B-cells (bursa of fabricius in birds). A few become null cells. T-cells are involved in cell mediated immunity. B-cells are involved in humoral immunity by producing antibodies.
Thrombocytes (platelets)	They respond quickly to ADP, thrombin and collagen and adhere to vascular subendothelium by becoming spherical. There are three types of storage granules. α granules contain fibrinogen, vWF. Dense granules contain ADP and serotonin. They also have lysosomes which contain acid hydrolases. The release of contents causes platelet aggregation and fibrin deposition on the platelet surface. On activation, platelets release arachidonic acid which results in the formation of thromboxane A_2 which in turn stimulates platelet aggregation.

Haematopoietic Growth Factors

These are heterogenous group of cytokines that stimulate progenitor cells of haematopoietic system and induce proliferation and maturation. These hormones play a critical role in the regulation of all haematopoietic cells in health and disease.

Major Growth Factors

1. *Erythropoietin:* This is synthesised by the peritubular cells of the kidney in response to hypoxaemia and is always present in minute amounts in human urine. About 10% of endogenous erythopoietin is secreted by the liver. The plasma half-life of erythopoietin in anaemic patients is 6-9 hours, and it shortens with continued therapy. The gene coding for erythopoietin is located on chromosome 7 (C_7, q11-22).

   Normal serum level is 10 to 25 IU/L.

2. *Interleukin (IL-3):* T-lymphocytes produce IL-3, and this factor is not lineage specific. IL-3 appears to stimulate production and renewal of the pluripotent stem cell compartment, and for its differentiation into all myeloid cell lines and lymphocytes. The gene coding for IL-3 is located on chromosome 5 (C_5, q23-31).

3. *Granulocyte macrophage colony-stimulating factor (GM-CSF):* GM-CSF is synthesized and secreted by bone marrow stromal cells, fibroblasts, T-cells, and endothelial cells. GM-CSF stimulates the growth of progenitors of granulocytes, monocytes, and erythrocytes, and often causes eosinophilia as well. It activates granulocytes and monocytes/macrophages

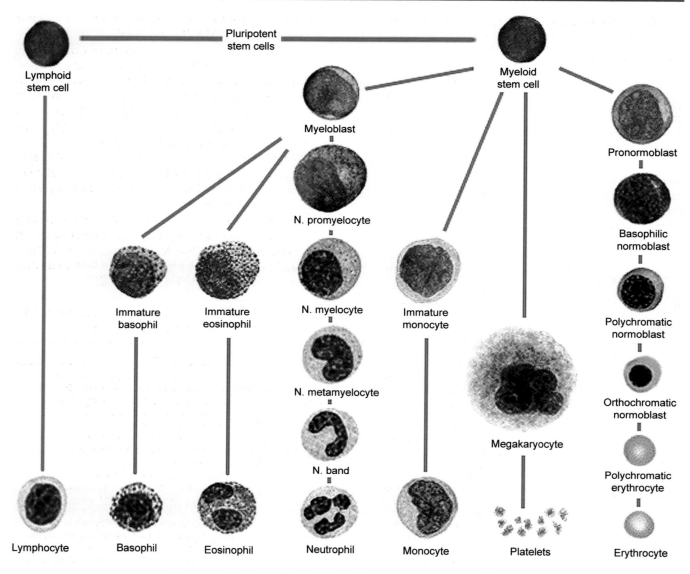

Fig. 6.1: Differentiation of haematopoietic cells

and enhances phagocytosis and other functions of these cells.

4. *Granulocyte colony-stimulating factor (G-CSF):* G-CSF is a potent, low-molecular-weight glycoprotein that stimulates proliferation and maturation of granulocyte precursors. This factor is produced by stromal cells, monocytes, macrophages, and endothelial cells. Within 48 hours after administration, the number of circulating neutrophils dramatically increases. The effect is lineage specific and dose-dependent. The gene coding for G-CSF is located on chromosome 17 (C_{17}, q11-21).

5. *Macrophage colony-stimulating factor (M-CSF):* M-CSF is secreted by stromal cells, macrophages and

fibroblasts. It is a potent stimulator of macrophage function and activation resulting in stimulation and elaboration of other cytokines resulting in increased expression of MHC class II antigen on macrophages and enhanced cytotoxicity. There is a slight to moderate rise in white blood cells after its administration. The gene for M-CSF is located on chromosome 5 (C_5, q33).

6. *Interleukin-2 (IL-2) or T-cell growth factor (T-CGF):* IL-2 is synthesized and secreted by activated T-cells, primarily helper-T cells. IL-2 leads to clonal expansion of antigen-specific T-cells and the induction of the expression of IL-2 receptors (CD_{25}) on the surface membrane of T-cells. It induces non-MHC

10–15% loss—Vascular instability

> 30% loss—Postural hypotension and tachycardia

> 40% loss—Hypovolumic shock, confusion, dyspnoea, diaphoresis, tachycardia, hypotension.

c. *Haemolytic anaemia:* Acute back pain due to intravascular haemolysis, haemoglobinuria, signs of renal failure.

Iron Deficiency Anaemia

Haemoglobin is normally the largest iron compartment of the body. Hb is 0.34% iron by weight. In an adult, total iron content of Hb compartment is about 2 gm.

Haemoglobin at birth is about 20 gm/dl and it gets reduced to 10 gm/dl at 3 months of age. In males, normal Hb level is about 14 gm/dl and in females about 12 gm/dl.

Iron Metabolism

Iron taken in diet is absorbed at all parts of GI tract especially duodenal mucosa. Acid medium favours iron absorption. Acid medium favours formation of soluble macromolecular complexes of iron with vitamin C, sugar, amino acid or bile in the duodenum. Only 10% of the ingested iron is absorbed.

Normal serum iron level is 50 to 150 mg/dl.

Frank iron deficiency increases absorption by 30- 40% and in iron overload, absorption decreases.

Iron absorption is increased in (1) ferrous state, (2) increased erythropoiesis (3) iron deficiency.

Iron absorption is decreased in (1) ferric state, (2) in the presence of phosphates and phytates, (3) bone marrow hypoplasia.

The absorbed iron is stored in the form of ferritin (water soluble form) and hemosiderin (water insoluble form). In men, storage compartment contains about 1000 mg of iron and in women, it ranges from 0-500 mg; In one-third of healthy women, there is no significant iron in storage compartment. The storage organs are liver, spleen, lymph nodes and bone marrow.

Iron is transported after binding with transferrin, a cytoplasmic protein. Transport iron compartment contains 3 mg of iron. Transferrin concentration in plasma is measured by estimating total iron binding capacity or immunologically.

Normally 1 mg of elemental iron is lost from shedding of senescent cells of gastrointestinal tract and genitourinary tract, and from desquamation of skin.

Causes of Iron Deficiency

1. Increased iron utilization (increased demand)

Postnatal growth spurt
Adolescent growth spurt
Erythropoietin therapy

2. Physiologic iron loss
Menstruation
Pregnancy

3. Pathologic iron loss
Gastrointestinal bleeding
Genitourinary bleeding
Pulmonary haemosiderosis
Intravascular haemolysis
Phlebotomy for polycythaemia rubra vera

4. Decreased iron intake
Cereal rich diet
Pica, food fads, malabsorption
Acute or chronic inflammation.

Physiological Causes

In children, iron available during birth is adequate for erythropoiesis till 3 to 4 months and later weaning food rich in iron should be substituted. If weaning is delayed, anaemia develops.

Prematurity and haemorrhage from the cord at birth deprive the infant of normal iron store.

In adolescents, iron deficiency occurs during growth spurt and also occurs because of food fads.

In Adults (Menstruating Women)

Menstruation causes an average loss of 30 mg of iron per month.

In pregnancy, there is no menstrual loss. However, additional iron is needed for the foetus, the placenta, and for the increased red cell mass and for the blood loss during delivery.

Iron requirement in males	1 mg per day
Iron requirement in females	2 mg per day
Iron requirement in pregnancy	3 mg per day

In Postmenopausal Women and Adult Men

Most common cause of iron deficiency in this group is gastro-intestinal bleeding (drug-induced gastritis, gastrointestinal malignancy, peptic ulcers).

At All Ages

Hookworm infestation, schistosomiasis, diet deficient in iron are causes of iron deficiency at all ages, especially elderly.

Stages in Iron deficiency Anaemia

There are three stages in the development of iron deficiency anaemia.

a. Negative iron balance
b. Fe deficient erythropoiesis
c. Iron deficiency anaemia.

Clinical Features

Patients may have angular stomatitis, atrophic glossitis, koilonychia, brittle hair, pruritus, pica, Plummer-Vinson syndrome (postcricoid web) or menorrhagia.

Investigation

1. *Haemoglobin level:* When Hb is greater than 10 gm/dl symptoms of anaemia develop only on exertion or on exposure to hypoxia or high altitude. If Hb level is less than 7 gm/dl, patient is symptomatic even at rest. There is also loss of pigmentation in palmar crease (Fig. 6.3).
2. Microcytic, hypochromic (MCHC < 32%) RBCs in the peripheral smear.
3. Raised platelet count may suggest bleeding.
4. Perl's Prussian blue technique demonstrates empty iron stores in the bone marrow.
5. Serum ferritin level is low (first to reflect iron deficiency). It is often less than 12 mcg/L; values > 80 mcg/L, rules out iron deficiency anaemia (normal ferritin level-15 to 400 mcg/L).
6. *Iron absorption is increased and the total iron binding capacity rises.
7. Chromium labelled red cells may be used to measure blood loss into the gut.
8. RBC protoporphyrin is increased - > 200 μg/dl (normal value –30-50 μg/dl).
9. Serum levels of transferrin receptor protein is increased - (normal- 4-9 μg/dl).

Note: *Serum iron, TIBC and transferrin saturation have a very limited diagnostic value since the results are variable during physiological conditions and during inflammatory diseases.

Differential Diagnosis

1. Anaemia of chronic disease
2. Thalassaemias
3. Hemoglobinopathies (Hb E)
4. Chronic liver disease
5. Chronic renal disease
6. Myelodysplastic disorders (refractory anaemia with ringed sideroblasts)
7. Myeloproliferative disorders
8. Hereditary sideroblastic anaemia
9. Myxoedema
10. Congenital atransferrinemia.

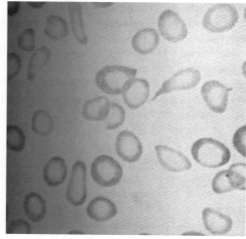

Fig. 6.3: Iron deficiency anaemia—hypochromic microcytes

Management

1. Treat the underlying cause.
2. Iron replacement by ferrous sulphate 200 mg tds orally. 200 mg of ferrous sulphate contains 60 mg of elemental iron. Oral therapy is safest and cheapest. Avoid enteric coated and sustained release tablets. Hemoglobin rises by 1 gm/dl/week or by 1% per day (accompanied by a reticulocytosis). Continue until haemoglobin is normal and for 6-8 months to replenish stores. If there is no response to oral iron therapy, consider the following:
   a. Incorrect diagnosis
   b. Noncompliance
   c. Blood loss exceeding rate of replacement
   d. Marrow suppression by tumour, chronic inflammation
   e. Malabsorption
      Other oral Fe preparations – Ferrous fumarate, ferrous gluconate, polysaccharide iron, Carbonyl iron.
3. *Parenteral iron therapy:* It is given for those who are unable to absorb iron from the GI tract or to those who have intolerance to oral iron.
   100 mg of iron (IM) are required to increase the haemoglobin level by 4% but the total dose of iron should not exceed 2.5 gm.
4. Alternative parenteral Fe preparations:
   a. Sodium ferric gluconate – No test dose is needed. 125 mg in 100 ml of normal saline infused IV over 1 hour and not to exceed 250 mg/day. It is not given as single dose because of adverse reactions like hypotension.

Differential Diagnosis of Microcytic, Hypochromic Anaemia

Features	Iron-deficiency anaemia	β-thalassaemia trait	Anaemia of chronic disease	Sideroblastic anaemia
Serum iron	↓	Normal	↓	↑
TIBC	↑	Normal	↓	Normal
Serum ferritin	↓	Normal	↑	↑
Red cell protoporphyrin	↑	Normal	↑	↑ or Normal
Hb A$_2$	↓	↑	Normal	↓

b. Iron sucrose – 100 mg in 100 ml of normal saline infused IV over 30 minutes and repeated 1-3 times/week.

Iron Requirement

Total dose = Hb deficit (gm/dl) × lean body weight (lb) + 1000 (mg of iron needed for storage).

Each 2 ml of iron dextran contains 100 mg of iron. A test dose of 0.5 ml should be given before therapy.

Iron Dextran-IV (In IM Intolerance)

500 mg of the compound is given with 100 ml of sterile saline; and infused after a test dose of 1 ml and if there is no adverse reaction.

Side effects are fever, chills, arthralgia, lymphadenopathy, splenomegaly, aseptic meningitis, anaphylactic shock, rarely sarcomas at the site of injection, and hemochromatosis.

In conditions simulating iron deficiency anaemia (β-thalassaemia, sideroblastic anemia, anaemia of chronic disease), a therapeutic trial of iron should be given. It is half corrected in 3 weeks and fully corrected in three months in case of iron deficiency anaemia and not in the other conditions.

Oral iron therapy (200 mg tds) raises Hb by 1%

7 days of oral therapy raises Hb by l gm%

Parenteral iron (100 mg), raises Hb by 4%.

If the Hb deficit is 7 gm, oral iron replacement should be continued for at least 7 weeks; Therapy should be continued for 6 to 8 months for replacing iron stores.

Oral iron therapy is safest and cheapest. Avoid parenteral iron therapy unless it is strongly indicated.

Megaloblastic Anaemia

This term refers to abnormal haematomyelopoiesis characterised by dys-synchronous nuclear and cytoplasmic maturation in all myeloid and erythroid cell lines due to aberrant DNA synthesis as a result of single or combined deficiency of either cobalamin (Vit B$_{12}$) or folate.

Similar changes occur in other organs like uterine cervix, aerodigestive tract also and can be mistaken for carcinoma.

A MCV of > 100 fL should prompt the physician to go for further investigations.

Causes of Macrocytosis

1. *MCV > 110 fL*
    Vitamin B$_{12}$ or folate deficiency.
2. *MCV 100-110 fL*
    1. Alcohol
    2. Liver disease
    3. Hypothyroidism
    4. Haemolysis
    5. Pregnancy
    6. Marrow infiltration
    7. Myelodysplastic states
    8. Drugs (zidovudine, azathioprine).

Causes of Vitamin B$_{12}$ Deficiency

1. Inadequate intake: Vegans (rare) pure vegetarians who do not consume milk and milk products.
2. Malabsorption:
    a. Defective release of cobalamin from food
        i.   Drugs that block acid secretion
        ii.   Gastric achlorhydria
        iii. Partial gastrectomy
    b. Inadequate production of intrinsic factor (IF)
        i.   Pernicious anaemia
        ii.   Total gastrectomy
        iii. Congenital absence of IF
        iv.   Functional abnormality of IF
    c. Disorders of terminal ileum
        i.   Tropical sprue
        ii.   Non-tropical sprue
        iii. Regional enteritis
        iv.   Intestinal resection
        v.   Neoplasms
        vi.   Granulomatous lesions
        vii. Selective cobalamin malabsorption
    d. Competition for cobalamin

i. Fish tapeworm (Diphyllobothrium latum)
ii. Bacteria (blind loop syndrome)
e. Drugs – PAS, Neomycin, Colchicine
f. Other rare causes
i. Nitrous oxide
ii. Transcobalamin II deficiency
iii. Congenital enzyme defects.

Metabolism of Vitamin B$_{12}$

1. Sources of vitamin B$_{12}$ are bacteria and animal tissue.
2. Serum level of vitamin B$_{12}$ is 200-600 pg/ml.
3. Requirement of vitamin B$_{12}$ is 1 mcg/day.
4. Total body store of vitamin B$_{12}$ is 5 mg. The storage lasts for 5 years. More than 50% is stored in the liver.
5. The ingested vitamin requires a gastric glycoprotein called intrinsic factor facilitating intestinal absorption, in the terminal ileum (distal 3-4 feet).
6. It is attached to a carrier protein (transcobalamin II) within the ileum and transported into the liver (major site of storage).

Transcobalamin I binds most of serum cobalamin and it has no physiological role.

Transcobalamin III is localized to specific neutrophil granules and the level of this carrier protein is increased in myeloproliferative disorders especially CML.

In pernicious anaemia, serum B$_{12}$ level is < 100 pg/ml.

Causes of Folate Deficiency

1. Dietary cause (poor intake of vegetables, elderly on tea and toasts, junk food anorexia nervosa, haemodialysis patients).
2. Malabsorption (alcoholism, celiac and tropical sprue, Crohn's disease, scleroderma, hypothyroidism).
3. Increased demand of folate-pregnancy, cell proliferation as in haemolysis, neoplasia, hyperthyroidism, ineffective erythropoiesis (pernicious anaemia, sideroblastic anaemia).
4. Drugs (phenytoin, methotrexate, trimethoprim, pyrimethamine, alcohol).

Metabolism of Folate

Normal folate requirement is 100 μg/d. Most dietary folate is available as polyglutamates. Green vegetables especially asparagus, spinach, lettuce, greenbeans are good sources. However, cooking destroys nonprotein bound folates found in these vegetables. Yeast and liver contain protein bound folates resistant to cooking.

Total body storage capacity is upto 5 mg (3-4 months supply).

Serum level of folate is 5-20 ng/ml. Folate is absorbed mainly in jejunum. 5-methyl tetrahydrofolate is the only physiologic form of circulating folate and is loosely bound to albumin. This is converted within the cell to tetrahydrofolate and to various coenzyme forms. All cellular folate coenzymes are polyglutamated forms of this vitamin.

Clinical Features

Pallor (lemon colour), smooth tongue, cardiac "hemic" systolic murmur, hepatomegaly, rarely splenomegaly. Neurologic picture in vitamin B$_{12}$ deficiency ranges from mental inattentiveness to severe mental confusion with or without dorsal and lateral column signs (subacute combined degeneration). However, some signs are not reversible with cobalamin therapy.

Investigations

1. Blood film shows hypersegmented polymorphs (B$_{12}$ deficiency-earliest sign; in folate deficiency > 5 lobes are present) (Fig. 6.4).

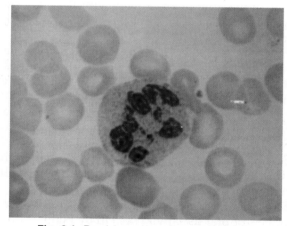

Fig. 6.4: Pernicious anaemia—macrocytosis with multilobed neutrophil

2. Increased ESR (malignancy)
3. Thyroid function tests
4. Serum B$_{12}$ level
5. Red cell folate level
6. Bone marrow biopsy
   a. Megaloblastic—B$_{12}$ or folate deficiency (Fig. 6.5)
   b. Normoblastic—liver damage, myxoedema
   c. Increased erythropoiesis—bleeding or haemolysis
   d. Abnormal erythropoiesis-sideroblastic anemia, leukaemia, aplastic anaemia.
7. *Schilling test:* It helps to identify the cause of B$_{12}$ deficiency. This determines whether a low B$_{12}$ is due

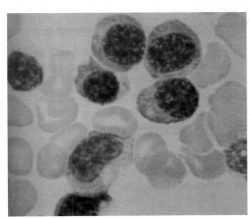

Fig. 6.5: Pernicious anaemia—megaloblasts in bone marrow

to malabsorption or lack of intrinsic factor by comparing the proportion of an oral dose (1 mg) of radioactive B_{12} excreted in urine with and without the concurrent administration of intrinsic factor. The blood must be saturated prior by giving an IM dose of 1000 mg of B_{12}. If intrinsic factor increases absorption, the lack of it is likely to be the cause. If not, look for other causes like blind loops, diverticula and terminal ileal disease.

Beware of diagnosing pernicious anaemia before the age of 40 years and in younger age groups; most common cause would be GI malabsorption.

Useful Clues for Diagnosis

- Serum B_{12} level less than 200 pg/ml.
- Serum folate level less than 4 ng/ml.
- RBC folate level is more diagnostic because it does not fluctuate frequently.
- Both homocysteine and methyl malonoic acid serum values are increased in B_{12} deficiency, but only homocysteine level is increased in folic acid deficiency (MMA normal level).

The presence of antibodies to intrinsic factor is diagnostic of pernicious anaemia.

Management

1. In B_{12} deficiency, hydroxocobalamin 1000 mcg twice during the first week, then 1000 mcg weekly for a further 6 doses. Bone marrow shows a striking change within 48 hours; within 2 to 3 days the reticulocyte count begins to rise (> 50% in 10 days); 1000 mcg of cyanocobalamin per month for life-long should be given.

   Rapid regeneration of the blood depletes the iron reserves of the body and hence ferrous sulphate 200 mg daily should be given soon after the commencement of treatment and the picture will be dimorphic then.

   In combined deficiency, folic acid replacement alone worsens B_{12} deficiency and hence it should not be given alone.

2. In folate deficiency 5 mg of folic acid/day orally is given. 5 mg once a week is given as maintenance therapy.

   Folate supplements 350 mg daily is given for all pregnant women. In methotrexate therapy, to overcome the metabolic block, folinic acid 15 mg daily orally or as a IM/IV injection in a dose of 3 mg/ml are given.

3. Treat the intercurrent infections (UTI or respiratory infections).

4. When Hb level is < 5 gm/dl, transfusion therapy should be given (1 unit of packed red cells over 10-12 hours).

   Hb increases by 1 gm/dL/week on specific therapy; WBC and platelet count should normalize within 1 week of therapy.

5. *Methylcobalamin:* It is the active coenzyme of vitamin B_{12}. Oral methylcobalamin therapy is as effective as conventional injection therapy and useful for long-term management of vitamin B_{12} deficiency and also in the treatment of autonomic and peripheral neuropathy. The dosage schedule can be 1,500 micrograms PO/day for 7days every 1-3 months or 500 micrograms/day for replacement therapy. The higher dose of 1-5 mg/day can be used in the management of diabetic, alcoholic, and chronic renal failure neuropathy.

In case, megaloblastic anaemias are not responsive to B_{12} or folate, think of

1. Antineoplastic agent administration
2. Inborn errors of metabolism (hereditary orotic aciduria, inborn errors of folate metabolism)
3. Myelodysplastic syndromes.

Megaloblastic Disease without Anaemia

1. *Acute megaloblastic disease:*
   - It is seen following nitrous oxide anaesthesia
   - Any patients with serious illness requiring intensive care
   - Resembles immunecytopenias with decreased leukocytes and platelets without anaemia
   - Peripheral smear is normal but bone marrow is megaloblastic
   - They respond with B_{12} and folate
2. *Cobalamin deficiency without anemia:*
   - Seen in elderly due to folate fortification

- Serum transcobalamin II levels decreased
- Serum cobalamin levels may be normal or low
- They respond with B_{12}.

Anaemia of Chronic Disease (ACD) (Sideropenic anaemia, simple anaemia)

This is mild and nonprogressive anaemia, occurring over a period of 3-4 weeks and remains static thereafter.

ACD is most often associated with chronic infections, inflammatory diseases, trauma, and neoplastic diseases.

Causes of ACD

1. Anaemia of chronic inflammation
   a. Infection
   b. Connective tissue disorders
   c. Malignancy

There is disturbed iron metabolism and hypoferremia despite normal body iron stores.

Interleukin-1, TNFα and IFN-gamma are inflammatory mediators, which play a major role in the pathophysiology of ACD by stimulating release of lactoferrin from granulocytes. There is diversion of iron from the dynamic pool to the intracellular storage pool and an insufficient supply of iron for erythropoiesis in the bone marrow.

Interleukin-I: It suppresses erythropoietin production.

TNF –α : It suppresses response to erythropoietin in erythroid cells.

Hepacidin: It is a substance released from liver in the setting of inflammation, which causes decreased iron absorption and utilization.

Hypoferremia and disturbance in iron kinetics is the hallmark of ACD.

Clinical Features

The signs and symptoms are referrable to the underlying disease. Anaemia is usually mild and nonprogressive, rarely less than 9 gm/dl.

Anaemia of chronic inflammation: Anaemia is never severe. If it is severe, search for other causes like bleeding or drug-induced myelosuppression.

Anaemia due to renal disease: This is of normochromic and normocytic type. This is due to lack of secretion of erythropoietin and suppression of its production by toxins. Some patients have evidence of haemolytic jaundice due to defect in hexose monophosphate shunt pathway.

In addition to aluminium toxicity, iron deficiency resulting due to blood loss also aggravates anaemia.

In some forms of acute renal failure the correlation between anaemia and renal function is weaker. Patients with haemolytic uraemic syndrome have increased erythropoiesis in response to haemolysis despite renal failure requiring dialysis. Polycystic renal disease also has a similar degree of erythropoietin deficiency. By contrast, patients with diabetes mellitus have more severe erythropoietin deficiency for a given level of renal failure.

Anaemia due to hypometabolic states (Anaemia secondary to endocrine failure): This may be due to hypothyroidism (associated pernicious anaemia, menorrhagia), Addison's disease, hypogonadism, and panhypopituitarism.

Anaemia of liver disease: This can be normocytic or slightly macrocytic. Stomatocytes (increased membrane due to deposition of cholesterol and phospholipid) and target cells may be seen in the peripheral smear.

In alcoholics, there is direct suppression of erythropoiesis. Ringed sideroblasts may be seen (due to malnourishment). Haemorrhage, gastritis, varices, and duodenal ulcer may worsen anaemia.

Anaemia due to protein starvation: It occurs in elderly and in children with marasmus.

On re-feeding they develop anaemia. They also have deficiency of iron, folic acid and B_{12}.

Investigations

See Table on next page.

Management

1. Anaemia resolves when underlying cause is treated.
2. Anaemia of chronic inflammation is not responsive to haematinics like iron, folate, vitamin B_{12}.
3. Anaemia is never severe and transfusion is rarely indicated.
4. Anaemia of uraemia corrects dramatically after renal transplantation. Anaemia is proportional to azotemia (except in polycystic kidney disease). Recombinant human erythropoietin can be given to maintain haematocrit between 0.32 to 0.37. Hypertension and thrombosis are common after erythropoietin therapy. (See Table on next page).
5. Treatment of anemia secondary to endocrine failure is by giving appropriate hormone replacement.
6. Anaemia of liver disease may improve with improvement in liver function.
7. Anaemia associated with malignancy may improve with cytotoxic drugs.

Diagnosis of Hypoproliferative Anaemias

Tests	Iron deficiency	Inflammation	Renal disease	Hypometabolic states
Anaemia	Mild to severe	Mild	Mild to severe	Mild
MCV (fL)	60–90	80–90	90	90
Morphology	Microcytic	Normocytic	Normocytic	Normocytic
Serum Fe (µg/ dl)	< 30	< 50	Normal	Normal
TIBC	> 360	< 300	Normal	Normal
Saturation (%)	< 10	10–20	Normal	Normal
Serum ferritin (µg/L)	< 15	30–200	115–150	Normal
Iron stores	0	2-4 +	1–4 +	Normal

Guidelines for Erythropoietin/Darbepoietin

Indication	Erythropoietin	Darbepoietin
Chemotherapy induced anaemia/MDS	40,000 U/week	100 µg/week
Anaemia due to renal failure	50-150 U/kg tiw	0.45 µg/kg/week
Anaemia in HIV infection	100-200 U/kg tiw	Not approved
Anaemia of chronic disease	150-300 U/kg tiw	Not approved
Anaemia-unwilling to accept transfusion or Anaemic individual undergoing major surgery	300 U/kg/d × 1-2 wk	Not approved

(tiw – thrice weekly)

Haemolytic Anaemia

Haemolysis is said to occur when the mean RBC survival is less than 120 days. If the bone marrow does not compensate sufficiently, haemolytic anaemia results.

Causes

Congenital

1. Membrane abnormalities (hereditary spherocytosis, hereditary elliptocytosis, acanthocytosis, stomatocytosis, Hereditary pyropoikilocytosis)
2. Haemoglobin abnormalities (thalassaemias, haemoglobin S, C, D)
3. Red cell enzyme defects (G6PD, pyruvate kinase, hexokinase, glutathione reductase deficiency).

Acquired

1. *Immune*
   a. Isoimmune
   b. Autoimmune

   Warm antibody type (Ig G)
   Idiopathic, SLE, lymphoma, chronic lymphatic leukemia, ovarian teratoma, Evan's syndrome, drugs-methyl dopa.

   Cold antibody type (Ig M)
   Cold haemagglutinin disease, paroxysmal cold haemoglobinuria (PCH), mycoplasma pneumonia, lymphoma, infectious mononucleosis, SLE, viral infections, chronic lymphatic leukaemia.

   Drug related
   Drug adsorbed onto RBC surface: penicillin, cephalosporins
   Immune complex mediated: sulphonamides, quinidine.
   c. Alloimmune (antibodies acquired by blood transfusions, or pregnancy, directed against transfused RBCs).
2. *Nonimmune*
   a. Mechanical (artificial valves, burns, march haemoglobinuria)
   b. Infection (malaria, *Clostridium welchii*, bartonellosis)
   c. Drugs (sulfonamide, snake venom-viper, nitrofurantoin)
   d. Dyserythropoietic (paroxysmal nocturnal haemoglobinuria).

Investigations

1. Blood film shows polychromasia, macrocytosis, spherocytes (hereditary spherocytosis), elliptocytes, sickle cells (sickle cell anaemia), target cells (thalassaemias).
2. *Direct Coombs' test:* This test identifies red cells coated with antibody and/or complement and a positive result usually indicates an immune cause for the haemolysis.

Essential Thrombocythaemia (Primary Thrombocytosis)

This is characterised by a very high platelet count of more than $600 \times 10^9/l$. Platelet is abnormal morphologically and functionally and the disease may present with thrombosis or bleeding.

Causes of Thrombocytosis

- Iron deficiency anaemia
- Hyposplenism
- Post-splenectomy
- Malignancy
- Collagen vascular disease
- Inflammatory bowel disease
- Infections
- Haemolysis/haemorrhage
- Polycythaemia vera
- Idiopathic myelofibrosis
- Essential thrombocytosis
- Idiopathic sideroblastic anaemia
- Myelodysplasia (5q – syndrome)
- CML
- Post surgery
- Rebound (cessation of ethanol intake, correction of vitamin B_{12} and folate deficiency).

Clinical Features

Thirty per cent of patients are asymptomatic; others present with GI bleed, arterial clotting, paresthesias, erythromelalgia (burning feet), vascular headaches. Splenomegaly is present in 75% and hepatomegaly is rare (20%). Some patients show Howel-Jolly bodies as an evidence of autosplenectomy.

Diagnostic Criteria

a. Platelet count greater than 600,000/µL on two occasions.
b. Palpable spleen (60-75% of cases).
c. Haemoglobin and hematocrit in normal range (normal red cell mass: men < 36 ml/kg; female < 32 ml/kg).
d. Adequate iron stores in the bone marrow.
e. Absence of Philadelphia chromosome (Ph¹ negative). In addition, the abl/bcr gene rearrangement is not found.
f. Minimal to absent marrow fibrosis (reticulin).
g. No known cause for reactive (or secondary) thrombocythaemia.

Management

Treatment depends on urgency.
1. In an asymptomatic young patient < 40 years, consider aspirin 60 mg/day and observe.
2. Busulphan or hydroxyurea 25 mg/kg/day orally if the platelet count is $> 800 \times 10^9/l$.
3. Bleeding can be controlled with Epsilon aminocaproic acid.
4. Interferon alpha is given for extreme thrombocytosis in a dose of 2-4 mU/m² SC, daily or 3 times a week.
5. When the blood film shows megakaryocytic leukaemia, it is treated like AML.
6. Anagrelide, 0.5-1.0 mg qid PO (causes isolated platelet reduction with minimal toxicity) is under trial.

Primary Myelosclerosis (Myelofibrosis)

There is intense marrow fibrosis with resultant haemopoiesis in the spleen and liver (myeloid metaplasia) causing massive splenomegaly.

Clinical Features

Patients have lassitude, weight loss, night sweats, heat intolerance, aches in muscles, bones and joints. There is marked splenomegaly. The causes of death are MI, GI bleed, leukaemic transformation, infection, major thrombosis.

Exuberant extramedullary haematopoiesis can cause ascites, pulmonary hypertension, intestinal or ureteric obstruction, increased ICT, spinal cord compression and skin nodules. Gout due to hyperuricaemia is also seen.

Investigations

1. Blood film shows macrocytic anaemia, leucoerythroblastic picture, tear drop poikilocytes
2. Neutrophil alkaline phosphatase score is high
3. Raised urate levels
4. Bone marrow biopsy shows an excess of megakaryocytes and increased reticulin and fibrous tissue replacement. Usually there is dry tap.

Diagnostic Criteria

1. Splenomegaly (may be huge)
2. Anaemia (haemolytic and decreased production components)

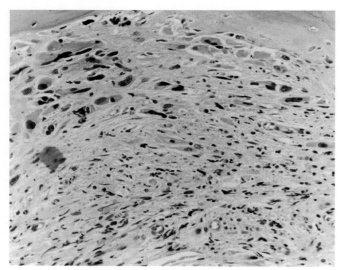

Fig. 6.12: Bone marrow—myelofibrosis

3. Leukocytosis or thrombocytosis may be seen in 60% of patients
4. Leukoerythroblastic peripheral blood picture
5. Tailed (dacrocytes) cells on blood smear
6. Bone marrow fibrosis (reticulin), which may be extensive (Fig. 6.12)
7. Osteosclerosis seen on skeletal X-rays.

Management

1. Blood transfusion
2. Folic acid (50 mg/day)
3. Androgen therapy (oxymetholone 50 mg/day)
4. Corticosteroids (prednisolone 40 mg/day)
5. Cytotoxic drugs (hydroxyurea upto 2 gm/day)
6. Splenectomy (in mechanical embarrassment due to massive splenomegaly, severe haemolysis, hypermetabolism, painful splenomegaly, hypersplenism).

    Splenectomy is contraindicated in active DIC with fibrinolysis, elevated fibrin split products, increased D-dimer, elevated fibrin monomer, hypofibrinogenemia.
7. Radiation to the spleen in small daily doses of 25 to 50 cGy for painful splenomegaly. Focal radiation for controlling extramedullary haematopoiesis.
8. Bone marrow transplantation.

Prognosis

The disease is progressive with steady deterioration.

Myelophthisic Anaemia

It is a term used to define conditions producing marrow fibrosis and the resulting clinical features are similar to primary idiopathic myelofibrosis.

Bone marrow fibrosis is also seen in the following conditions:
1. Other MPDs
2. Hairy cell leukaemia
3. Carcinoma (breast, prostate, ovary) metastatic to bone marrow
4. Radiation therapy for lymphoma and other neoplasms
5. Benzene exposure
6. Miliary tuberculosis
7. Granulomatous diseases
8. Parathyroid disease
9. Paget's disease.

Conditions associated with increased leukocyte alkaline phosphatase score
1. Polycythaemia vera
2. Myelosclerosis
3. Essential thrombocythaemia
4. Hairy cell leukaemia.

Conditions associated with decreased leukocyte alkaline phosphatase score
1. CML
2. Paroxysmal nocturnal haemoglobinuria
3. Aplastic anaemia.

Haematological Malignancies

They can be arising from cells of myeloid or lymphoid series. The myeloid group is further sub-classified into acute myeloid leukaemia and chronic myeloid leukemia.

The WHO has classified lymphoid malignancies into those arising from T cells or B cells and Hodgkin's disease.

Lymphoid Malignancies

B–cell
Precursor B lymphoblastic leukaemia/Lymphoma (Precursor B cell acute lymphoblastic leukaemia)

Mature B Cell Neoplasms
- B cell chronic lymphocytic leukaemia /small lymphocytic lymphoma
- Hairy cell leukaemia
- B cell lymphoma of MALT type (Extranodal – mucosa associated lymphoid tissue)
- Mantle cell lymphoma
- Follicular lymphoma
- Diffuse large B cell lymphoma
- Burkitt's lymphoma/Burkitt cell leukaemia
- Plasma cell myeloma/Plasmacytoma

T–cell
Precursor T lymphoblastic lymphoma/Leukaemia
(Precursor T cell acute lymphoblastic leukaemia)

Mature T Cell Neoplasms
- T cell prolymphocytic leukaemia
- T cell granular lymphocytic leukaemia
- Adult T cell lymphoma/leukaemia (HTLV-1+)
- Aggressive NK cell leukaemia
- Extranodal NK/T cell lymphoma – nasal type
- Mycosis fungoides/Sezary syndrome
- Peripheral T cell lymphoma
- Anaplastic large cell lymphoma.

Hodgkin's Disease

Leukaemias

Leukaemias are malignant neoplasms of the haemato-poietic stem cells, arising in the bone marrow, that flood the circulating blood or other organs. They are classified on the basis of the cell type involved and the state of maturity of leukaemic cells.

Acute Myeloid Leukaemia

The incidence of AML steadily increases with age. Ninety per cent of cases of AML occurs in adults. The incidence is greater after the age of 65.

Etiology
1. Hereditary
   - Down's syndrome, Patau's syndrome, Klinefelter's syndrome
   - Inherited diseases like Ataxia telengiectasia, Bloom's syndrome, Fanconi's anaemia
2. Radiation
3. Chemical and other occupational exposures
   No direct evidence suggests a viral aetiology.

Classification

The categorization of acute leukaemias into biologically distinct groups is based on morphology, cytochemistry, and immunophenotyping as well as cytogenetic and molecular techniques.

According to WHO, the diagnosis of AML is established by the presence of $\geq$ 20% blasts in blood

FAB classification AML (Fig. 6.14)

Class / incidence	Morphology	Comments
M 0 – Minimally differentiated AML (2-3%)	Blasts lack cytological and cytochemical markers of myeloblast. Express myeloid antigens (CD_{13} and CD_{33}), Resembles myeloblasts ultrastructurally	
M 1-AML without differentiation (20%)	Very immature cell but >3%peroxidase positive with few granules or Auer rods, little maturation beyond myeloblast stage	Associated with Inv (3)
M 2-AML with maturation (30–40%)	Full range of myeloid maturation Auer rods positive in most cases	Younger age –myeloid sarcomas, Presence of t(8;21) denotes favourable prognosis
M 3-Acute pro-myelocytic leukaemia (5-10%)	Majority of cells are hypergranular promyelocytes, Many Auer rods /cell – Faggot cells	Patients are younger and develop DIC, t (15;17) is characteristic
M 4–Acute myelomonocytic leukaemia (15-20%)	Myeloid elements resemble M 2 AML Monoblasts stain positive for non-specific esterases	
M 4 Eo – myeloblastic with abnormal eosinophils	Presence of chromosome 16 abnormalities defines this subset with marrow eosinophilia	Excellent prognosis
M 5–Acute monocytic leukemia (10%)	M 5a –Monoblasts with promonocytes predominate in marrow and blood M 5b – Mature monocytes predominate in peripheral blood	Old patients, high incidence of organomegaly, Lymphadenopathy and tissue infiltration
M 6 – Acute erythroleukemia (Diguglimo's syndrome) (5%)	Dysplastic erythroid precursors predominate (> 50%) Myeloblasts as in M 1	Advanced age, 1% denova AML 20% therapy related AML
M 7 – Acute megakaryocytic leukaemia (1%)	Megakaryocytic blasts predominate GP II b / IIIa (CD 41 / 61) positive Often with prominent marrow fibrosis	Least common type

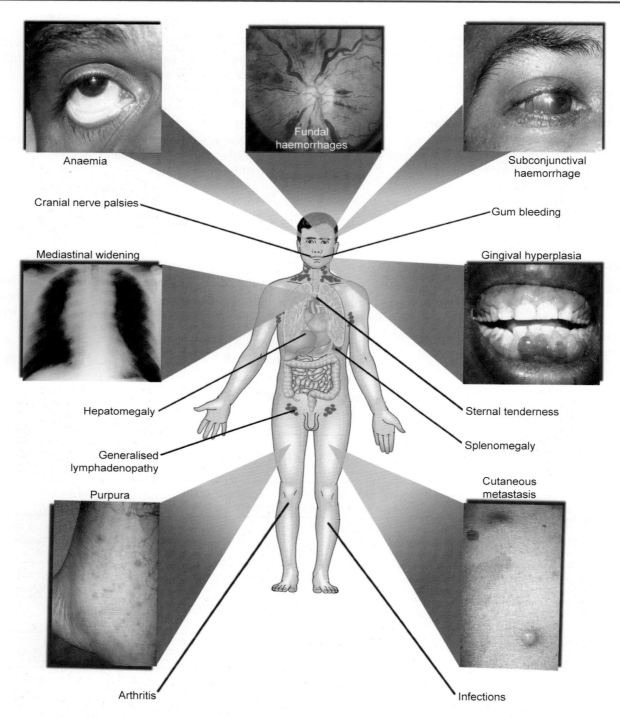

Fig. 6.13: Clinical features in acute leukaemia

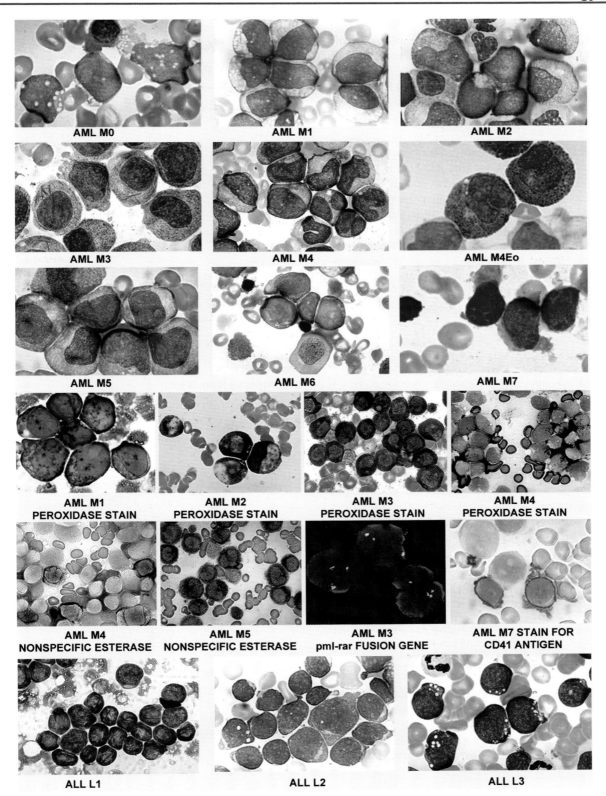

Fig. 6.14: Acute leukaemia (Myeloid and Lymphoid)

Investigations

1. *Platelet count:* Normal count 150-350 × 10^9/l (150,000-350,000/µl). In congenital and acquired thrombocytopenia, the count is low.

2. *Bleeding time:* Normal bleeding time is < 8 min; In thrombocytopenia and in other platelet disorders, bleeding time is prolonged.

   It is a clinical test which assesses platelet endothelial interaction without involving the clotting mechanism.

   Ivy's method for BT: Place a cuff around the upper arm and inflate to 40 mmof Hg. After cleaning the forearm make two puncture marks in the skin with a standard lancet, taking care to avoid damaging superficial veins. Remove the blood oozing from the wound every 15 seconds with filter paper without pressing on the skin until bleeding ceases.

   Normal - < 8 minutes. Take the average of two experiments.

3. *Prothrombin time (PT):* It indicates the integrity of extrinsic coagulation pathway . Normal PT is 12-14 sec. Prothrombin time is prolonged in factors II, V, VI, X deficiency, liver disease, warfarin therapy and DIC.

   When the prothrombin time is used for diagnosis as a screening test, values obtained above the reference range will be further investigated with specific quantitative assays as clinically indicated.

   When the PT is used for therapeutic monitoring of oral anticoagulants, the lack of standardisation is a more serious problem. Therefore, calculation of INR is a method of standardisation to avoid these complications and helps in comparison to standard values.

   INR only has meaning for patients on a stable dose of anticoagulants and on treatment for at least one week.

Guidelines for anticoagulants – Target levels for INR

Disorders	INR
1. Atrial fibrillation	2-3
2. Above knee DVT	2-3
3. Pulmonary embolism	2-3
4. Recurrent embolism	3.5
5. Prosthetic heart valves	3-4.5

Excessive anticoagulation

- INR < 6 Reduce the dose of drug or omit the drug
- INR 6-8 Stop the drug and start when INR < 5
- INR > 8 Stop the drug and give 1-2.5 mg vitamin K

- Major bleed –Stop the drug and give prothrombin complex concentrate
  Or fresh frozen plasma along with vitamin K 5 mg IV.

Duration of therapy – Anticoagulants

1.	Situational DVT	6 weeks to 3 months
2.	Idiopathic DVT	3-6 months
3.	Recurrent idiopathic DVT	12 months
4.	VTE with ongoing risk factors	Long term/Indefinite
5.	Pulmonary embolism	6 months
6.	Massive pulmonary embolism	Long term/Indefinite
7.	Valvular heart disease with poor LV systolic function	Long term/Indefinite
8.	AF/Age > 75 years/ H/O embolism	Long term/Indefinite
9.	MI with LV dysfunction/ LVthrombus	Long term/Indefinite
10.	Cardiomyopathy with LV thrombus	Long term/Indefinite
11.	MI with good LV function	Maximum 3 months
12.	Prosthetic valve	Long term/Indefinite

4. *Activated partial thromboplastin time (PTT):* It indicates the integrity of intrinsic coagulation pathway. Normal PTT is 30-40 sec. PTT is prolonged (60-85 sec) in deficiency of factors II, V, VIII, IX, X, XI, haemophilia A and B, von Willebrand's disease and DIC.

5. *Fibrinogen level:* Normal level is 1.5-3.0 gm/dl. The level is low in congenital hypofibrinogenemia.

6. Clot retraction time.

   Abnormal prolongation of clot retraction time indicates platelet function defects like Glanzmans thrombasthenia, Bernard-Soulier syndrome, etc.

7. *Activated clotting time:* ACT is similar to aPTT except that fresh whole blood is used (rather than citrated plasma used in aPTT) Normal range: 70 –120 seconds. This test is used to monitor heparin anticoagulation. Most patients with lupus anticoagulants that prolong the aPTT have a normal ACT.

8. *Plasma thrombin time:* It tests the time taken for fibrinogen conversion to fibrin. It indirectly measures plasma fibrinogen concentration and it is prolonged in the following conditions.
   - Afibrinogenemia
   - Hypofibrinogenemia
   - Therapeutic or circulating anticoagulants
   - Inherited dysfibrinogenemias.

Bleeding Disorders

Bleeding may occur as a result of qualitative or quantitative defects in platelets.

Qualitative Platelet Disorders

1. *Congenital*
   a. Disorders of membrane glycoproteins (thrombasthenia, Bernard-Soulier syndrome)
   b. Disorders of platelet secretion of ADP/prostaglandins (storage pool disorders)
   c. Defective platelet aggregation (platelets fail to aggregate with ADP, collagen, epinephrine or thrombin).
2. *Acquired*
   a. Drugs
      (i) NSAIDs (aspirin, indomethacin)
      (ii) Antibiotics (penicillins, cephalosporins)
      (iii) Heparin
      (iv) Beta-blockers
      (v) Dextran
   b. Uraemia.

Quantitative Platelet Disorders

Thrombocytopenia: Spontaneous bleeding occurs when the platelet count falls below $30 \times 10^9/l$ unless the function is also compromised, e.g. NSAID intake.

Platelet count	
> 60,000	No bleeding
30,000-60,000	Bleeding with trauma
< 30,000	Spontaneous bleed

Causes

1. Decreased production of platelets
   Marrow failure
   (i) Hypoplasia of the marrow (idiopathic, or drug induced)
   (ii) Megaloblastoses (B_{12} or folate deficiency)
   (iii) Infiltration of the bone marrow (leukaemia, myeloma, carcinoma).
2. Decreased platelet survival:
   a. Immune thrombocytopenic purpura (ITP)
   b. Viral infections (HIV)
   c. DIC
   d. Drugs (quinine, quinidine, methyldopa)
   e. SLE
   f. Lymphoma
   g. Thrombotic thrombocytopenic purpura (TTP)
3. Platelet sequestration (hypersplenism)
4. Defective platelet aggregation (aspirin, heparin)
5. Dilutional (massive blood transfusion).

Immune Thrombocytopenic Purpura (ITP)

It is an autoimmune disorder due to the presence of autoantibodies directed against platelet membrane glycoprotein IIb and IIIa resulting in premature removal of platelets by macrophage monocyte system. Sometimes the reaction is immune complex mediated.

Clinical Features

In children: Typically presents 2-3 weeks after a viral infection with sudden onset of purpura, nasal or oral bleeding.

In adults: ITP involves females more commonly and has an insidious onset. Symptoms and signs of collagen vascular disorders (like rheumatoid arthritis) may be present. The course is chronic with remissions and relapses.

Presence of splenomegaly does not favour the diagnosis of ITP.

Investigations

1. Blood film shows decreased platelet count
2. Bone marrow shows increase in megakaryocytes.

Management

In children, the disease is usually self-limiting within a few weeks.

1. If the platelet count is $< 10 \times 10^9/L$, prednisolone 2 mg/kg/day is given till the count rises (i.e. within 2-3 days)
2. Bleeding from nose, GIT, retinal haemorrhages, intracranial bleeding should be treated accordingly (platelet or fresh blood transfusion)
3. Intravenous immunoglobulin for fresh bleeding persisting for a few days following steroid introduction.

Treatment in adults

1. Prednisolone 1 mg/kg/day till the platelet count rises but the response is less rewarding.
2. Persistent or life-threatening bleeding should be treated accordingly (platelet or fresh blood transfusion).
3. Intravenous IgG (1 gm/kg) should be given if the patient has haemorrhage or if there is life-threatening bleeding. It acts by blocking monocyte-macrophage Fc receptors.
4. Relapse is treated by increasing prednisolone dose.
5. Splenectomy is considered if there are two relapses. Pneumococcal, meningococcal and *H. influenzae* vaccination should be given subcutaneously before splenectomy. Splenectomy is curative in 70% of the patients.

If the patient responds to prednisolone, a large dose should be given preoperatively to raise the platelet count over 50,000/ml.

If he does not respond to steroids, a 5-day course of gamma globulin IV, 0.4 gm/kg body weight/day, can be used to raise platelet count transiently.

If there is no response, a platelet transfusion (2 units/10 kg of body weight) may be given at the time of intubation for anaesthesia.
6. If splenectomy fails, long-term maintenance with prednisolone 5 mg/day should be given.
7. If bleeding persists, despite splenectomy, vincristine 2 mg IV weekly for 3 doses, small dose of steroids, danazol 200 mg PO qid, cyclophosphamide 2 mg/kg/day PO, or immunoglobulin infusions 0.4 gm/kg IV daily for 5 days should be considered.

Thrombotic Thrombocytopenic Purpura (TTP)

TTP is characterised by thromobocytopenia, micro-angiopathic haemolytic anaemia, increased LDH levels, fever, transient neurologic deficits and renal failure. This is due to widespread hyaline microthrombi found in arterioles and capillaries.
Causes include
1. Pregnancy
2. Metastatic cancer
3. HIV infection
4. High dose chemotherapy
5. Mitomycin C
6. Antiplatelet agents like ticlopidine.

The presence of severe Coombs' negative haemolytic anaemia with fragmented RBC in peripheral smear, thrombocytopenia and minimal activation of coagulation confirms the diagnosis.

Patient presents commonly in fourth decade. TTP is treated with corticosteriods, platelet aggregation inhibitors and exchange transfusions. Plasma exchange removing 40 ml/kg body weight of plasma and replacement with an equal volume of fresh frozen plasma daily until platelet count rises to 1,00,000/μL with decrease in LDH.

Splenectomy is performed in those who show minimal improvement.

Microangiopathic Haemolytic Anaemia

The microangiopathic haemolytic anaemias are mechanical haemolytic anaemias in which the red cell fragmentation is due to contact between red cells and the abnormal intima of partly thrombosed, narrowed, or necrotic small vessels.

Causes
• Haemolytic uraemic syndrome
• Thrombotic thrombocytopenic purpura
• Disseminated intravascular coagulation
• Disseminated carcinoma
• Malignant hypertension
• Eclampsia
• Immune disorders-SLE, scleroderma, polyarteritis nodosa, Wegener's granulomatosis, acute glomerulonephritis, renal transplant rejection
• Haemangiomas.

Disorder due to Deficiency of Clotting Factors

HAEMOPHILIA A

Reduction of factor VIII results in haemophilia A.
Incidence : 1/10,000 persons

Factor VIII is synthesised by the liver primarily and also by spleen, kidney and placenta. It is bound to the von Willebrand factor (vWF).

The normal factor VIII gene has been cloned and used for treating patients. Haemophilia is a X-linked disorder. All daughters of haemophiliacs are obligate carriers and sisters have a 50% chance of being a carrier. If a carrier has a son, he has a 50% chance of having haemophilia and a daughter has a 50% chance of being a carrier.

Females can be haemophiliacs when
1. She is born to an affected father and a carrier mother (25%)
2. She has a defective gene with Turner's syndrome (45 XO)
3. When lyonisation (inactivation of normal X-chromosome) has occurred.

Clinical Features

The normal factor VIII level is 50-100% (0.5-1.5 U/mL) and is usually measured by a clotting assay. If factor VIII level is < 2%, patient presents with recurrent, spontaneous haemarthrosis which later leads to osteoarthritis, muscle haematomas involving calf and psoas muscles (it may lead to compression of femoral nerve and paraesthaesia in thigh and weakness of the quadriceps and contraction and shortening of the Achilles tendon).

If factor VIII level is 2-10%, mild trauma or surgery may cause haematomas. If the factor VIII level is 10-50%, major injury and surgery may cause excessive bleeding.

Complications

1. Arthropathy

Classification of von Willebrand's and Laboratory Abnormalities

Features	Type I	Type IIA	Type IIB	Type IIC	Type III
Genetic transmission	Autosomal dominant	Autosomal dominant	Autosomal dominant	Autosomal recessive	Autosomal recessive
Bleeding time	Prolonged	Prolonged	Prolonged	Prolonged	Prolonged
VIII-C	Decreased	Decreased or normal	Decreased or normal	Normal	Markedly decreased
vWF	Decreased	Decreased or normal	Decreased or normal	Normal	Markedly decreased or absent
Ristocetin cofactor	Decreased	Markedly decreased	Decreased or normal	Decreased	Absent
Ristocetin induced platelet aggregation (RIPA)	Decreased or normal	Absent or markedly decreased	Increased	Markedly decreased	Absent
Multimeric structure	Normal in plasma and platelets	Absence of large and intermediate multimers from plasma and platelets	Absence of only large multimers from plasma; normal in platelets	Absence of large multimers from plasma and platelets; triplet structure aberrant	Variable

2. Muscle atrophy (due to haematomas)
3. Mononeuropathy (compression by haematomas)
4. Risk of hepatitis (A, B, C, D) and HIV through blood and blood product administration.

Management

1. Bleeding episodes are treated by factor VIII concentrate infusion (from donor plasma) which can be stored in domestic refrigerators at 4°C. This should be tested for hepatitis and HIV antibodies.

   Development of factor VIII antibodies may result in failure in 20% of patients.

   In those patients, porcine factor VIII, infusions of activated clotting factors, e.g. VIIa, FEIBA (factor eight inhibitor bypassing activity), activated concentrate of factors II, IX and X may stop bleeding.
2. IV desmopressin 0.3 mg/kg, can be given to raise factor VIII level to three to five fold. This can be given to cover minor surgeries like dental extraction and can be repeated 6-8 hours later (tachyphylaxis occurs with subsequent injections).
3. Surgery can be done with adequate doses of factor VIII concentrate and along with a 10 day course of tranexamic acid (a fibrinolytic inhibitor) and an antibiotic.
4. Physiotherapy.
5. Avoid intramuscular injections.

HAEMOPHILIA B (CHRISTMAS DISEASE)

Aberration of the factor IX gene, present on X chromosome, results in a reduction of factor IX level, giving rise to haemophilia B.

Treatment

Factor IX concentrate.

VON WILLEBRAND'S DISEASE

von Willebrand's disease (vWD) is the most common hereditary bleeding disorder. It is characterised by a prolonged bleeding time (BT) and factor VIII-C levels between about 10-40%. Joint bleeding is rare.

The gene for von Willebrand's factor (vWF) is located on chromosome 12 and is inherited as an autosomal disorder. Type I, IIA and IIB are autosomal dominant type. IIC and III are autosomal recessive.

Type I

It is characterised by a reduced quantity of circulating vWF. The synthesis of vWF is not impaired but the release of vWF multimers is inhibited by an unknown mechanism. This is the most common type of presentation.

Type 2

This is less common. Here multimer assembly is defective and hence the large and intermediate multimers, representing the most active form of vWF are missing from plasma.

Clinical Features

Superficial bruising, epistaxis, menorrhagia and GI bleeding are common especially after trauma or surgery.

The diagnostic pattern consist of:
1. Prolonged bleeding time

c. Immunizations
d. Cirrhosis
e. Amyloidosis
f. Reflux nephropathy.

4. OTHER TYPES OF PROTEINURIA

a. *Benign orthostatic proteinuria* is typically found in tall adolescents.

Protein is found in the urine collected on retiring and in the morning after the patient has been ambulant, but not in the overnight specimen collected immediately on rising. There should be no abnormality in the urine sediment, and proteinuria should not exceed 1 gm per day. In half the patients proteinuria disappears within 10 years, however, in a small proportion overt renal disease will develop in later life.

b. *Transient proteinuria* may be associated with conditions like cardiac failure, fever, or heavy exercise. It disappears within hours after cessation of exercise and with resolution of the disease process. Proteinuria after marathon running may be as heavy as 5 gm per liter of urine.

Selective proteinuria is said to occur when the ratio of clearance of IgG (1.6 lakh kd) to transferrin (88,000 kd) is less than 0.1. Minimal change disease in children produces selective proteinuria. Because of lower molecular weight there is selective excretion of albumin in urine.

Microalbuminuria

This indicates an excretion of albumin of 20–200 microgram per minute (albumin excretion rate or AER), or a daily excretion of albumin in the range of 30–300 mg.

Causes

a. Diabetes mellitus with early renal involvement
b. Hypertension
c. Myocardial infarction

Difference between Tubular and Glomerular Proteinuria

	Tubular proteinuria	Glomerular proteinuria
1.	Occurs in injury involving the tubulointerstitial region of kidney	Occurs due to injury of the renal glomerulus
2.	Comprises of a. Low molecular weight proteins (β₂ microglobulin) filtered by the glomerulus and not reabsorbed by the tubules b. Cellular enzymes secreted by renal tubules c. Increased amount of Tamm-Horsfall protein	Comprises predominantly of albumin (low molecular weight protein)
3.	Quantitative excretion of protein is usually < 2 gm/day	Quantitative excretion of protein may be large (> 3–3.5 gm/day)
4.	Urinary protein electrophoretic pattern (UPEP) shows more globulin than albumin.	UPEP shows more albumin than globulin
5.	Albumin : β₂ microglobulin ratio is 100 : 1 (normal ratio is 50–200 : 1)	Ratio > 1000 : 1

d. Acute phase response.
e. Obesity
f. Hyperlipidemia
g. Alcohol intake
h. Physical exercise.

Reducing Substances in Urine

1. Diabetes mellitus (glycosuria)
2. Renal glycosuria (defective tubular reabsorption of glucose)
3. Pregnancy (lactosuria)
4. Ingestion of fruits like grapes, plums, cherries (pentosuria)
5. Inborn error of metabolism (galactosuria, fructosuria)
6. Alkaptonuria (homogentisic acid)
7. Drugs (ascorbic acid, aspirin, cephalosporins, nalidixic acid).

Methods of screening Microalbuminuria

Method	24-hour urine specimen	First morning urine specimen	Microalbumin to creatinine ratio in random / first morning urine specimen
Normal range	< 30 mg/24 hours	< 20 mg/L	< 30 mg/g for women < 20 mg/g for men
Microalbuminuria	30–300 mg/24 hours	20 – 200 mg/L	30-300 mg/g (women) 20-200 mg/g for men
Macroalbuminuria	> 300 mg/24 hours	> 200 mg/L	> 300 mg/g for women > 200 mg/g for men

Creatinine Clearance (Cl$_{Cr}$)

If the serum creatinine is stable, the glomerular filtration rate (GFR) can be estimated by using the Cockcroft-Gault formula for creatinine clearance.

$$Cl_{Cr} (ml / min) = 140 - age \times Ideal\ body$$
$$weight\ in\ Kg / 72 \times serum\ Cr\ (mg/dl)$$

(x 0.85 for women)

Urinary Tract Infection

Definitions

Upper urinary tract infection: Infection involving the kidney.

Lower urinary tract infection: Infection involving the bladder, prostate, and urethra.

Bacteriuria: It is the presence of bacteria in urine. Its presence places the entire urinary system at risk of invasion by bacteria.

Significant bacteriuria: It is defined as the presence of 1,00,000 (10^5) or more colony forming units (CFU) of bacteria per milliliter of midstream urine.

Pyelonephritis: It is a specific or nonspecific inflammation of the renal parenchyma.

Acute bacterial pyelonephritis: It is a clinical syndrome characterized by chills and fever, flank pain, and constitutional symptoms caused by bacterial invasion of the kidney.

Chronic pyelonephritis: It is a renal disease that is caused by a variety of disorders such as chronic obstructive uropathy, vesicoureteral reflux (VUR) (reflux nephropathy), renal medullary disease, drugs and toxins, and chronic or recurring renal bacteriuria.

Cystitis: It is infection confined to the urinary bladder.

Urethritis: It is infection confined to the urethra.

Prostatitis: It is infection confined to the prostate.

Relapse of infection: Relapse is a recurring infection due to the same micro-organism that is often drug resistant. Most relapses occur after treatment of acute pyelonephritis or prostatitis.

Reinfection: It is a recurring infection due to a different micro-organism that is usually drug susceptible. Most recurring episodes of cystourethritis are due to reinfection.

Asymptomatic bacteriuria: It is the presence of bacteriuria, indicating urinary tract infection, in the absence of symptoms. It occurs commonly in pregnant women.

Uncomplicated urinary infection: It is an episode of cysto-urethritis following bacterial colonization of the urethral and bladder mucosa. This type of infection is considered uncomplicated because sequelae are rare.

Complicated urinary infection: These are infections involving parenchyma (pyelonephritis or prostatitis) and frequently occur in the presence of obstructive uropathy or following instrumentation. Episodes may be refractory to therapy, often resulting in relapses and occasionally leading to significant sequelae such as sepsis, metastatic abscesses and rarely, acute renal failure.

Risk Factors Associated with Urinary Tract Infection

1. Obstruction to urine flow
   a. Congenital anomalies
   b. Renal calculi
   c. Ureteral occlusion (partial or total)
2. Vesicoureteral reflux
3. Residual urine in bladder
   a. Neurogenic bladder
   b. Urethral stricture
   c. Prostatic hypertrophy
4. Instrumentation of urinary tract
   a. Indwelling urinary catheter
   b. Catheterization
   c. Urethral dilation
   d. Cystoscopy
5. Sex—Women
   a. Honeymoon cystitis
   b. Pyelitis of pregnancy
   c. Use of diaphragm or spermicide.

Pathogenesis

Bacteria in the enteric flora periodically gain access to the genitourinary tract. Close proximity of the anus to the genitourinary tract in women is a likely factor. Subsequent bacterial colonization of uroepithelial cells sets the stage for persistent bacteriuria.

Opposing colonizations are several host factors, like acid pH, normal vaginal flora, type-specific cervicovaginal antibodies and flushing effect of urine during micturition.

Following periurethral colonization, uropathogens gain access to the bladder via the urethra, to the kidneys via the ureters, and to the prostate via the ejaculatory ducts. The urethra and ureterovesical junction are mechanical barriers that prevent ascension.

Urine adequately supports the growth of most uropathogens. However, the urinary bladder has several protective mechanisms to prevent its colonization and growth.

1. Mucopolysaccharide (urine slime) layer covers the bladder epithelium and prevents colonization.
2. Tamm-Horsfall protein, adheres to *P fimbriae* of the micro-organism and prevents colonization.
3. Urine flow and bladder contraction serve to prevent statis and colonization.

Symptoms of UTI

1. Frequency
2. Dysuria
3. Haematuria
4. Incontinence
5. Retention of urine
6. Fever with chills and rigors
7. Urgency
8. Strangury
9. Pain over loin or suprapubic region.

Investigations

1. Urine specimens for culture, sensitivity and colony forming unit counts.

Common microbial pathogens causing UTI

Escherichia coli	50–90%
Klebsiella or Enterobacter	10–40%
Proteus, Morganella or Providencia	5–10%
Pseudomonas aeruginosa	2–10%
Staphylococcus saprophyticus	2–10%
Enterococcus	2–10%
Candida albicans	1–2%
Staphylococcus aureus	1–2%

2. Localisation of infection with segmented cultures of the lower urinary tract in men.

Positive culture obtained from the first 10 ml of voided urine indicates urethral infection.

Positive culture from midstream sample of urine indicates bladder infection.

Positive culture obtained from the first 10 ml of voided urine obtained after a prostatic massage, indicates prostatic infection. This is done by asking the patient to assume the knee-elbow position, with a full bladder. A prostatic massage is then performed per rectally. The patient is then asked to void urine, which is cultured.

3. Microscopic examination of urine for Gram's stain and sediments.

Causes for sterile pyuria
   1. Inadequately treated UTI

2. Infection (TB, atypical streptococci, corynebacteria, fastidious micro-organisms)
   Fastidious micro-organisms like Chlamydia, ureaplasma urealyticum
3. Calculi
4. Bladder tumour
5. Chemical cystitis
6. Prostatitis
7. Papillary necrosis
8. Interstitial nephritis
9. Polycystic kidneys
10. Appendicitis.

4. *Biochemical tests for bacteriuria:* Two metabolic capabilities shared by most bacterial pathogens of the urinary tract are, use of glucose and reduction of nitrate to nitrite. Significant number of bacteria in urine results in absence of glucose and presence of nitrite detected by dipstick devices.

5. *Radiography:* The principal role of radiographic and urologic studies in patients with UTIs is to detect VUR (vesicoureteric reflux), renal calculi, and potentially correctable lesions that obstruct urine flow and cause stasis.

Infants, boys, and men with first episode and girls and women with relapsing UTIs should have an intravenous pyelogram (IVP) with postvoiding radiographs. For a detailed evaluation of the ureterovesical junction, bladder, and urethra, a voiding cystourethrogram and measurement of the residual urine after voiding may be necessary.

Principles of Treatment of UTI

1. Asymptomatic patients should have colony counts greater than or equal to 10^5 per milliliter on at least two occasions before treatment is considered.
2. Unless symptoms are present, no attempt should be made to eradicate bacteriuria until catheters, stones, or obstructions are removed.
3. Selected patients with chronic bacteriuria may benefit from suppressive therapy.
4. A patient who develops bacteriuria as a result of catheterisation should have treatment to re-establish a sterile urine.
5. Antimicrobials used for treatment should be the safest and least expensive agents to which the causative microorganisms are susceptible.
6. Efficacy of treatment should be evaluated by urine culture one week after completion of therapy.

Relief of clinical symptoms does not always indicate bacteriological cure.

Hepatic cysts and intracranial aneurysms also may be present. Azotemia is usually progressive. Diagnosis is by IVP or ultrasound.

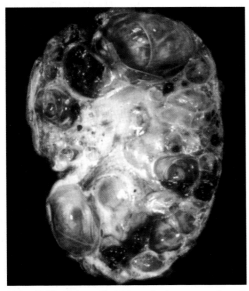

Fig. 7.11: Polycystic kidney (autopsy specimen)

Treatment

1. Control of hypertension (as hypertension accelerates development of renal failure).
2. Treatment of UTI promptly
3. Sodium chloride replacement in patients with inability to conserve sodium.

Medullary cystic disease manifests with polyuria, acidosis, and salt wasting, which precedes slowly progressive renal failure.

Acute Renal Failure (ARF)

ARF is a syndrome characterised by rapid decline in GFR (hours to days), retention of nitrogenous waste products, and perturbation of ECF volume and electrolyte and acid-base disturbances.

This condition comprises of a rapidly rising serum urea, creatinine and K^+, usually (but not invariably) with anuria or oliguria (< 15 ml/hr). Only half of the patients with ARF have anuria or oliguria. A preserved urine output implies a mild disorder and a better prognosis.

Causes of ARF

1. *Prerenal failure*
   a. Hypovolaemia (diarrhoea, vomiting, haemorrhage, overdiuresis, pancreatitis, peritonitis)
   b. Vasodilatation (sepsis, drugs, anaphylaxis)
   c. Cardiovascular (CCF, MI, cardiac tamponade)
   d. Renal hypoperfusion (renal artery stenosis, NSAIDs).
2. *Intrarenal failure*
   a. Hypotension
   b. Sustained prerenal failure
   c. Postoperative and postpartum haemorrhage
   d. Rhabdomyolysis
   e. Drugs (aminoglycosides, NSAIDs)
   f. Contrast dye
   g. Glomerulonephritis
   h. Vasculitis
   i. Interstitial nephritis.
3. *Postrenal failure*
   a. Intrarenal (crystals, calculi, papillary necrosis)
   b. Extrarenal (prostate enlargement, pelvic or bladder neoplasm, retroperitoneal neoplasm or fibrosis, urethral or bladder neck obstruction)

Fractional excreted sodium =
$$\frac{[Urine\ Na\ /\ Serum\ Na]}{[Urine\ Cr\ /\ Serum\ Cr]} \times 100$$

Renal failure index = $\dfrac{Urine\ Na \times Serum\ creatinine}{Urine\ creatinine}$

Characteristic Features of ADPKD and ARPKD

Features	ADPKD * (Adult type)	ARPKD** (Infantile type)
1. Inheritance pattern	Autosomal dominant	Autosomal recessive
2. Prevalence	1/400 to 1/1000	Rare
3. Age of onset	Usually adults	Neonates, children
4. Presenting symptom	Loin pain, haematuria, infection of renal cysts	Abdominal mass, renal failure, failure to thrive
5. Haematuria	Common	May be present
6. Recurrent upper urinary tract infection	Common	May be present
7. Renal calculi	Common	Uncommon
8. Hypertension	Common	Common
9. Method of diagnosis	Ultrasound	Ultrasound
10. Renal size	Normal to very large	Large

* Autosomal dominant polycystic kidney disease (may be associated with cysts in liver, spleen, pancreas, ovaries, uterus, broad ligament, bladder, testis, epididymis, lungs and thyroid; Cardiac anomalies like MVP, MR, AR, TR and intracranial berry aneurysms)

** Autosomal recessive polycystic kidney disease

Urinary Indices Useful in Distinguishing Pre-renal from Renal Causes of Oliguria

Indices	Pre-renal	Renal (acute tubular necrosis)
Urine osmolality (mOsm/kg)	> 500	< 350
Urine sodium (mEq/L)	< 20	> 40
Urine/serum creatinine	> 40	< 20
Urine/serum osmolality	> 1.2	< 1.2
Fractional excreted sodium	< 1	> 1
Renal failure index	< 1	> 1
Urine specific gravity	> 1.020	< 1.010

ATN

This is due to ischaemic or toxic injury acting on renal vessels, glomeruli, and/or tubules causing decreased GFR and increased intratubular pressure.

Ischaemic ATN may be due to abrupt hypoperfusion or any condition causing severe prerenal failure, particulary in elderly patients or when nephrotoxins are present.

Nephrotoxic ATN can result from exogenous or endogenous causes.

Exogenous nephrotoxins include:
1. Aminoglycosides
2. Contrast dye.

Endogenous nephrotoxins include:
1. Myoglobin released after muscle trauma
2. Intravascular haemolysis.

Clinical Features

Patients with prerenal failure usually have volume contraction, hypotension or impaired cardiac function. Diagnosis is confirmed when renal perfusion improves with volume repletion, improvement in cardiac function or repair of renal artery stenosis.

Postrenal failure may be evident from a distended bladder, large prostate, pelvic mass or hydronephrosis. The pattern of urinary flow may indicate total obstruction (anuria) or partial obstruction (polyuria). Crystals or infection may be evident in urinary sediment.

ARF due to intrinsic renal disease may require a renal biopsy for diagnosis. RBC casts and heavy proteinuria suggest GN or vascular inflammatory disease. Interstitial nephritis may cause fever, skin eruption and pyuria with eosinophils in the urinary sediment.

The ischaemic ARF consists of three phases.
1. *Initiation Phase:* It takes hours to days. It is the initial period of renal hypo-perfusion during which ischaemic injury is evolving.
2. *Maintenance phase:* It takes one to two weeks. It is the phase in which renal injury is established with low urine output resulting in uremic complications.
3. *Recovery phase:* This phase is characterized by repair and regeneration and gradual return of GFR to normal. It results in marked diuresis.

Course

ATN begins with diminishing urine output within a day of the insult and may cause anuria.

Oliguria lasts for 10–14 days. If oliguria persists > 2–3 weeks, other diagnoses should be considered.

The daily increments in BUN and creatinine average 10–20 mg/dl and 0.5–1.0 mg/dl respectively, but may be higher in catabolic states.

Complications

1. Sodium and water overload
2. Hypertension
3. CCF
4. Hyperkalaemia (due to decreased excretion)
5. Metabolic acidosis with an anion gap (due to retention of acids)
6. Hyperphosphataemia (due to decreased excretion)
7. Hypocalcaemia
8. Hypermagnesemia
9. Hyperuricaemia
10. Anaemia
11. Infection
12. GI bleeding
13. Paralytic ileus
14. Pericarditis.

Recovery

During the recovery phase, urine volume increases progressively. BUN and creatinine level-off and then begin to fall. Major complications of ARF may first appear during this stage in the form of fluid and electrolyte depletion.

Management of ARF

1. Search for and correct prerenal and postrenal causes.
2. Search for evidence of ischaemic or nephrotoxic injury or renal parenchymal disease.
3. In ATN, if patient is volume overloaded, high dose of furosemide IV (20 times the serum creatinine value) can be given. In patients who are not volume overloaded 500 to 1000 ml of normal saline is infused over 30 to 60 mts.

4. Conservative therapy
   a. Urinary catheter to accurately detect urine output (however, it should not be kept for a long-time due to danger of UTI)
   b. Strict intake and output chart
   c. Daily weight measurement
   d. Limits fluids to 500 ml + previous day's losses
   e. Avoid nephrotoxic drugs
   f. Treat hyperkalemia and acidosis
5. Dialysis for volume overload, pericarditis, GI bleeding, symptomatic uraemia, severe hyperkalaemia or acidosis.
6. Pigment induced renal injury occurring during haemolysis or rhabdomyolysis is treated with alkalinisation of urine.

Indications for Urgent Dialysis

1. Potassium persistently high (> 6.0 mEq/L)
2. Acidosis (pH < 7.2)
3. Daily rise in level of blood urea more than 30 mg/dL or a total rise of blood urea more than 300 mg/dL.
4. CO_2 combining power < 13 mEq/L
5. Serum creatinine > 7 mg/dl
6. Pulmonary oedema not responding to diuresis.
7. Pericarditis
8. Cardiac tamponade
9. High catabolic state with rapidly progressive renal failure.

Chronic Kidney Disease

Chronic kidney disease is due to several aetiologies lasting for more than 3 months leading to reduction in nephron number and function as evidenced by either structural abnormalities or proteinuria and frequently leading to end stage renal failure.

CKD – Risk factors:
• Family history of heritable renal disease
• Hypertension
• Diabetes mellitus
• Autoimmune disorders
• Older age
• Past episode of ARF
• Current evidence of kidney damage
   In stages 1 and 2–Patients are asymptomatic.
   In stages 3 and 4–Patients are symptomatic with positive clinical signs and laboratory parameters.
   In stage 5–Patients require dialysis or renal replacement therapy.

Stages of Chronic Kidney Disease

Stage	Features	GFR(ml/min)
1	CKD with normal or increased GFR	≥ 90
2	Mild CKD	60 - 89
3	Moderate CKD	30 - 59
4	Severe CKD	15 - 29
5	ESRD	<15

Chronic Renal Failure (CRF)

CRF refers to the permanent loss of renal function, which culminates in signs and symptoms termed uraemia. Unlike ARF, from which recovery is frequent, CRF is not reversible and may lead to a vicious cycle with progressive loss of remaining nephrons.

Common Causes

1. Diabetic nephropathy
2. Hypertension
3. Chronic glomerulonephritis
4. Polycystic kidney disease
5. Chronic pyelonephritis
6. Interstitial nephritis.

Symptoms, Signs and Consequences of CRF (Fig. 7.12)

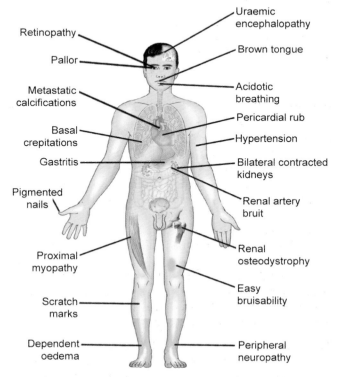

Fig. 7.12: Clinical features in chronic renal failure

b. Chronic respiratory failure (chronic obstructive airway disease).

The arterial findings in respiratory acidosis are:
1. PCO_2 always raised
2. In acute respiratory failure.
   a. pH low
   b. $[HCO_3^-]$ high normal or slightly raised, as compensatory changes take sometime to occur.
3. In chronic respiratory failure
   a. pH normal or low, depending on chronicity (time for compensation to occur)
   b. HCO_3 raised.

II. ALKALOSIS

1. Metabolic Alkalosis

In metabolic alkalosis the primary abnormality in the bicarbonate buffering system is a rise in $[HCO_3^-]$. There is little compensatory change in PCO_2. It is less common than metabolic acidosis.

It is characterised by
  (i) Increase in plasma bicarbonate
  (ii) Rise in pH
  (iii) Small compensatory rise in $PaCO_2$.

Conditions producing metabolic alkalosis are:
  (i) Vomiting or gastric aspiration
  (ii) Diuretics (thiazides, furosemide)
  (iii) Hypokalemia (due to movement of $[H^+]$ into the cell)
  (iv) Primary and secondary hyperaldosteronism
  (v) Cushing's syndrome
  (vi) Administration of liquorice, carbenoxolone
  (vii) Administration of exogenous alkali (oral or IV bicarbonate).

Clinical Features

Acute alkalosis may cause tetany due to acute fall in plasma ionised calcium and enhanced release of acetylcholine. Confusion and drowsiness may occur.

Treatment is of the underlying cause.

2. Respiratory Alkalosis

In respiratory alkalosis the primary abnormality is a fall in PCO_2. The compensatory change is a fall in $[HCO_3^-]$. A primary fall in PCO_2 is due to abnormally rapid or deep respiration, when the CO_2 transport capacity of the pulmonary alveoli is relatively normal.

Causes of respiratory alkalosis are:
  (i) Hysterical overbreathing
  (ii) Raised intracranial pressure or brainstem lesions
  (iii) Hypoxia
  (iv) Pulmonary oedema
  (v) Lobar pneumonia
  (vi) Excessive artificial ventilation.

The fall in PCO_2 slows the carbonate dehydratase mechanisms in renal tubular cells and erythrocytes. The compensatory fall in $[HCO_3^-]$ tends to correct the pH.

The arterial blood findings in respiratory alkalosis are:
  (i) PCO_2 always reduced
  (ii) $[HCO_3^-]$ low normal or low
  (iii) pH raised or normal.

Treatment is of the underlying cause.

Approach to Acid Base Disorders

Introduction

Normal pH of blood is maintained between 7.35-7.45 inspite of 40-60 millimoles of H^+ ions added to body fluids due to daily metabolism. This is achieved by 3 systems.
1. Chemical buffering system
2. Respiratory regulation of $PaCO_2$
3. Renal regulation of HCO_3

Acid base disorders can arise as a result of either primary respiratory abnormality or primary metabolic abnormality or mixed problem.

Basic Concepts

Acidosis	: pH < 7.35
Alkalosis	: pH > 7.45
Respiratory acidosis	: $PaCO_2$ > 45 mm Hg
Respiratory alkalosis	: $PaCO_2$ < 35 mm Hg
Normal HCO_3 21-30 milli equi/litre	

A primary respiratory pathology is reflected as an alteration in $PaCO_2$, whereas a primary metabolic problem will be reflected as an alteration in HCO_3 level.

Hypoxic index: In conditions with primary lung pathology the oxygenation mechanism is defective and will be reflected by inappropriate PaO_2 for the given FIO_2. (FIO_2 is the percentage of oxygen in the inspired air. Patient breathing room air FIO_2 is 21%). Hypoxic index will help us to find out whether the oxygenation is sufficient for the given FIO_2.

Hypoxic index = PaO_2/FIO_2
Normal value is 400-450. Low value suggests primary lung pathology.

Algorithm for ABG Analysis

I . Assessment of history and clinical examination will give clue regarding interpretation of ABG.

II.

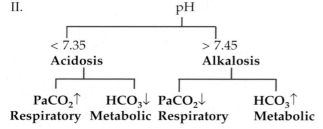

Primary Respiratory

In case of respiratory acidosis, we have to look for metabolic compensation. It is calculated by the formula,

The expected pH decrease for the increase in $PaCO_2$

In acute respiratory acidosis = $0.08 \times (PaCO_2-40)/10$

In chronic respiratory acidosis = $0.03 \times (PaCO_2-40)/10$

If actual pH > expected pH => Respiratory acidosis + Metabolic alkalosis

If actual pH < expected pH => Respiratory acidosis + Metabolic acidosis.

Primary Metabolic

In case of metabolic acidosis, we have to look for respiratory compensation. It is calculated by the formula,

Expected $PaCO_2$ = (1.5 × HCO_3) + (8 ± 2)

If the actual $PaCO_2$ > expected $PaCO_2$ => metabolic acidosis + respiratory acidosis

If the actual $PaCO_2$ < expected $PaCO_2$ => metabolic acidosis + respiratory alkalosis

In the presence of metabolic acidosis, anion gap has to be assessed. It is given by the formula,

AG = Na^+ - (Cl^- + HCO_3^-)

Normal value = 12

Anion gap is elevated in
1. Diabetic ketoacidosis
2. Lactic acidosis
3. Toxins
4. Uraemic acidosis

Anion gap is normal in
1. Renal tubular acidosis
2. Ureterosigmoidostomy
3. Diarrhoea

In case of metabolic alkalosis, we have to look for respiratory compensation. This is calculated by the formula,

Expected $PaCO_2$ = HCO_3 + 15

If the actual $PaCO_2$ > expected $PaCO_2$ => metabolic alkalosis + respiratory acidosis

If the actual $PaCO_2$ < expected $PaCO_2$ => metabolic alkalosis + respiratory alkalosis.

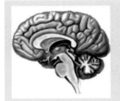

SYMPTOMS

HEADACHE

VOMITING

SEIZURES

ALTERED SENSORIUM/
LOSS OF CONSCIOUSNESS

BEHAVIOURAL
ABNORMALITIES

VISUAL
DISTURBANCES

VERTIGO

SPEECH DISORDER

DYSARTHRIA

DYSPHAGIA

WEAKNESS OF
LIMBS

SENSORY
DISTURBANCES
(positive and negative)

UNSTEADY GAIT

ABNORMAL
MOVEMENTS

SYNCOPE

FALLS

DROP ATTACKS

SIGNS

ASSESSMENT OF
CONSCIOUS LEVEL

PUPILS
EXTRAOCULAR MOVEMENTS

DYSARTHRIA

HANDWRITING

APRAXIA

AGNOSIA

CRANIAL NERVE DYSFUNCTION

WEAKNESS OF LIMBS
(bilateral/unilateral
distal/proximal
UMN/LMN type)
Reflexes

SENSORY SYSTEM
ABNORMALITIES

ROMBERG'S SIGN

GAIT ABNORMALITIES

CEREBELLAR SIGNS

INVOLUNTARY MOVEMENTS

FUNDUS CHANGES

MENINGEAL SIGNS

SPINE AND CRANIUM EX.

FEATURES OF PARKINSONISM

NEUROCUTANEOUS MARKERS

Higher Functions

Definitions

Consciousness

It is defined as the state of awareness of self and the environment.

Confusion

It is lack of clarity and coherence of thought, perception, understanding or action. It is often the first feature of cognitive impairment.

Coma

It is a state of unconsciousness in which the patient does not respond to any type of external stimuli or inner need.

Stupor (or) Semiconsciousness

It is a state of disturbed consciousness from which only vigorous external stimuli can produce arousal.

Glasgow Coma Scale (GCS)

Eye Opening

Spontaneous	4
To speech	3
To pain	2
No response	1

Best Verbal Response

Fully oriented	5
Mild confusion	4
Moderate confusion (inappropriate)	3
Severe confusion (incomprehensible)	2
No response	1

Best Motor Response

Obeys commands	6
Localizes pain	5
Withdrawal to pain	4
Abnormal flexor response (decorticate posture)	3
Extensor response (decerebrate posture)	2
No response	1

GCS is useful in assessing level of consciousness in a patient with head injury.

Best total score is	15
Mild injury	13 to 15
Moderate injury	9 to 12
Severe injury	8

This gives an indication of the patient's state of consciousness and is not a substitute for neurological examination.

Abbreviated Coma Scale (AVPU)

A **a**lert
V responds to **v**ocal stimuli
P responds to **p**ain
U **u**nresponsive.

Coma Vigil (vegetative state)

Patient is comatose, but the eyelids are open giving the appearance of being awake. Patient may perform random limb and head movements, but there is complete inability to respond to command or to communicate.

Akinetic Mutism

This refers to a partial or fully awake patient who is immobile and silent. This state may be seen in hydrocephalus, mass in the region of third ventricle or large bilateral hemispherical lesions.

Abulia

This is a mild form of akinetic mutism, in which patient is hypokinetic, but is able to communicate. This is seen in lesions in the periaqueductal region or lower diencephalon.

Locked-in Syndrome (Pseudo Coma)

Patients are awake, alert and selectively de-efferented. They are non communicable with intact lid movements, eye movements in the vertical plane and quadriplegia with involvement of lower cranial nerves. The site of lesion is either ventral pons or bilateral medulla with intact tegmentum (which contains fibres of Reticular Activating System). Infarction of ventral pons transects all descending corticospinal and corticobulbar tracts, but spares ARAS, which maintains arousal.

i.e. patient can open eyes & look up & down.

Causes

1. Demyelination (central pontine myelinolysis)
2. Ventral pontine infarction (basilar artery occlusion)
3. Bilateral infarction of lateral 2/3 of cerebral peduncle
4. Peripheral disorders associated with locked in syndrome
   a. Severe polyneuropathy
   b. Myasthenia gravis
   c. Neuromuscular blocking agents.

Catatonia

Patient appears awake and blink spontaneously. There is a waxy flexibility (limbs maintain the posture implemented by the examiner). This is seen in schizophrenia.

Delirium

This is synonymous with acute confusional state characterised by periods of agitation, heightened mental activity, increased wakefulness, hallucinations, motor hyperactivity and autonomic stimulation. There is an associated impairment of attention.

Causes of Delirium

Head injury
CVA
Cerebral infections
Epilepsy
Hypoglycaemia, DKA (diabetic ketoacidosis)
Hypoxia
Renal or hepatic failure
Electrolyte or acid-base imbalance
Wernicke's encephalopathy
Septicaemia, malaria, SBE, pneumonia
Heat stroke, hypothermia
Toxins
    Alcoholic intoxication
    *Alcohol and drug (Barbiturates and narcotics) withdrawal
Psychiatric disorders
    Acute mania
    Extreme anxiety
    Schizophrenia (auditory hallucinations)
    Hysteria.

Note: *Alcohol withdrawal causes delirium tremens which is characterised by delirium, tremors and visual hallucinations.

Dementia

It is a syndrome of acquired global or multifocal impairment of cognitive function involving decline in intellect, memory or personality in the presence of normal consciousness.

Causes of Dementia

1. Primary dementias
   a. Alzheimer's disease (diffuse cortical atrophy)
   b. Pick's disease (circumscribed cortical atrophy, early frontal and temporal)
   c. Frontal lobe degeneration.

2. Secondary dementias
   a. *Degenerative disorders*
      Parkinson's disease
      Hereditary ataxias
      Progressive supranuclear palsy (Steele-Richardson syndrome)
      Motor neuron disease
      Huntington's chorea
      Multiple sclerosis.
   b. *Conditions with raised intracranial tension*
      • Primary & secondary tumours
      • Hydrocephalus
      • Chronic subdural hematoma
        Carcinomatous meningitis.
   c. *Vascular dementia*
      • Multi infarct dementia
        Lacunar infarct
        Thalamic infarct
        Diffuse atherosclerosis
      • Vasculitis: SLE, Polyarteritis nodosa, Behcet's disease.
   d. *Chronic infections*
      • Syphilis, GPI
      • Tuberculosis
      • Fungal, protozoal infections
        Slow viral diseases:
        * Subacute sclerosing panencephalitis
        * Creutzfeldt-Jacob disease
        * Papova virus
        * HIV.
3. Dementia due to Diffuse Brain Damage
   Anoxia
   Encephalitis
   Acute head injury
   Pugilistic dementia (boxers).
4. Endocrine Disorders
   • Chronic hypoglycaemia
   • Hypothyroidism
   • Hypo and hyperparathyroidism
   • Adrenal insufficiency
   • Cushing's syndrome.
5. Vitamin Deficiencies
   • Vitamin B_{12} deficiency
   • Thiamine deficiency
   • Niacin deficiency.
6. Toxins
   • Alcohol
   • Drug and narcotic poisoning
   • Heavy metal intoxication
   • Dialysis dementia.
7. Dementia in Adolescents and Young Adults
   • Wilson's disease

Progressive myoclonic epilepsy
Tuberous sclerosis
Leukodystrophies
Storage diseases.

Note: • Treatable Causes

Presenile Dementia   It occurs before 65 years of age (Pick's disease, Alzheimer's disease)

Senile Dementia   It occurs after 65 years of age

Cortical Dementia   It occurs in Pick's disease and Alzheimer's disease

Subcortical Dementia   It occurs in Huntington's disease, multiple sclerosis and HIV.

Differences between Alzheimer's Disease and Pick's Disease

Features	Alzheimer's disease	Pick's disease
1. Portion of brain affected	Diffuse cortical involvement (esp. hippocampus & temporal lobes)	Confined to frontal and temporal lobes (lobar sclerosis)
2. Pathology	Neurofibrillary tangles, senile plaques seen	Pick's bodies seen
3. Age of onset	Presenile or senile	Presenile
4. Clinical features	Features of diffuse cortical involvement seen: Frontotemporal features less prominent	Prominent fronto temporal features seen

Amnesia

It is a disorder of memory characterized by inability to remember past events and to learn new information despite normal consciousness and attention.

As a result of head injury, memory disturbance occurs for events before (*retrograde amnesia*) and after the time of injury (*post-traumatic amnesia*). (anterograde)

Anterograde Amnesia

Impairment in learning new material which accompanies post traumatic amnesia.

Duration of post-traumatic amnesia indicates the severity of head injury; the ability to learn new material often being the last cognitive deficit to recover.

Transient Global Amnesia

It is a syndrome in which a previously normal person suddenly becomes confused and amnesic. It is usually of spontaneous origin but also may be due to immersion in cold or hot water, emotional stimuli, exertion, intercourse or travel in motor vehicles.

There is severe impairment of recall of recent and sometimes most distant events. Immediate memory is intact. There is no other neurological sign. It is usually benign. Rarely it may be due to temporal lobe tumour, migraine or temporal lobe epilepsy.

Examination of Higher Mental Functions

Consciousness

Find out the level of consciousness of the patient (whether the patient is comatose, stuporose or delirious).

Causes of Coma

Trauma

Cerebral contusion, concussion and laceration
Subdural haematoma
Extradural haematoma.

Cerebrovascular Disease   usually

Subarachnoid haemorrhage → due to berry aneurysms
Intracerebral haemorrhage
Massive cerebral infarction
Brainstem infarction or haemorrhage
Cerebellar infarction or haemorrhage
Cerebral venous sinus thrombosis.

Infections

Meningitis
Encephalitis
Cerebral abscess
Cerebral malaria.

Seizure Disorders and Raised ICT

Epilepsy
Space occupying lesions.

Endocrine and Metabolic Disturbances

a. Diabetes mellitus: Hypoglycaemia, ketoacidosis, hyperosmolar coma
b. Myxoedema
c. Hypocalcaemia
d. Hypercalcaemia
e. Hypoadrenalism
f. Hypopituitarism
g. Hepatic failure
h. Respiratory failure

i. Cardiac failure
j. Uraemia
k. Metabolic acidosis
1. Metabolic alkalosis
m. Electrolyte disturbances (hypo and hypernatremia).

Cardiovascular Disorders

Congestive cardiac failure
Hypertensive encephalopathy
Shock
Arrhythmias.

Physical Agents

Hyperpyrexia
Hypothermia
Electric shock
Lightning.

Toxins and Others

Acute poisoning
Alcohol
Thiamine deficiency.

Tropical Coma

Cerebral malaria
Typhoid fever
Trypanosomiasis
Rabies.

Approach to Coma

A comatose patient has to be approached systematically to derive maximum information. The aim of physical examination is to arrive at following conclusions.
1. Localisation of coma
2. Etiology of coma (structural vs metabolic)

Approach to the Patient

I. *History and general examination.*
    A meticulous history and detailed general examination will give clue regarding the etiology of coma.

II. *Neurological examination.*
    The neurological examination of a comatose patient serves 3 purposes.
    a. To aid in determining the cause of coma
    b. To help determine the prognosis of coma
    c. To provide a base line.

For localization of structural lesion and to assess the prognosis, the following examinations are the most helpful
    1. State of consciousness
    2. Respiratory pattern
    3. Pupillary size and reactivity
    4. Ocular motility
    5. Skeletal muscle motor response.

1. State of Consciousness

Auditory, visual and noxious stimuli of progressively increasing intensity should be applied to the patient. The maximal state of arousal, intensity of stimuli required for that and the response of the patient has to be noted. Any asymmetry in the response to stimuli points towards structural lesion.

All patients in coma should be asked to open their eyes and look up and down. Because in locked in syndrome only these voluntary movements are spared. Patient will be alert and aware, but quadriplegic with lower cranial nerve paralysis, thus mimicking coma.

2. Respiration

Respiratory patterns that are helpful in localizing level of involvement are the following (Fig. 8.1).

A. Cheyne-Stokes breathing.
    i. Rate of respiration will be around 30 per minute
    ii. There is waxing and waning of respiration.
    iii. Waning of respiration is followed by apnoea for about 15 sec.

Causes
    i. Bilateral hemispheric damage
    ii. Diencephalic insults
    iii. Bilateral damage anywhere between forebrain and upper pons
    iv. Prolonged circulation time as in cardiac failure.

Prognosis
    i. Stable pattern of Cheyne-Stokes respiration is a good prognostic sign
    ii. Emergence of Cheyne-Stokes breathing in a patient with unilateral mass lesion may be a sign of herniation.
    iii. Change in pattern from Cheyne Stokes to other patterns described is ominous.

B. Central neurogenic hyperventilation.
    i. Refers to rapid breathing (40-70 per minute)

Types of Agnosia

Modality	Subtypes	Neuroanatomical correlates
Vision	Visual object agnosia	Bilateral occipitotemporal
		Left occipitotemporal
	Associative prosopagnosia	Bilateral occipitotemporal
	Apperceptive prosopagnosia	Right occipitotemporal and occipitoparietal
Audition	Environmental sound agnosia	Bilateral posterior superior Temporal
	Phonagnosia	Right inferior parietal
	Amusia	Right posterior temporal and inferior parietal
Somatosensory	Tactile object agnosia (complete)	Right and left parietal operculum, posterior insula
	Tactile object agnosia (nonmanipulable stimuli)	Right superior mesial parietal
Perception of disease	Anosognosia	Right parietal and bilateral ventromedial frontal

B. Visual Agnosia

It is the inability to recognize what is seen with the eyes in the presence of intact visual pathway. At the same time they can describe the colour, size, and shape of the object without recognizing it.

C. Prosapagnosia

It is the inability to identify a familiar face which occurs in parieto-occipital lesion.

D. Anosognosia

In right parietal lobe lesion, there is lack of awareness to recognize the paralysed limb.

Sleep

Sleep is an elemental phenomenon of life and an indispensable phase of human existence. Sleep represents one of basic 24-hour circadian rhythms. Most adults sleep for 7 to 8 hours/day.

Age	Duration of sleep
Newborn	16–20 hours
Child	10–12 hours
10 years	9–10 hours
Adolescence and adults	7–8 hours
Late adult life	About 6.5 hours

States and Stages of Sleep

It comprises of 2 distinct physiological states namely REM and Non REM Sleep.

1. REM (Rapid eye movement sleep/dreaming/desynchronized/D-sleep)
2. Non REM Sleep (orthodox/synchronized/S-sleep).

Non REM Sleep has 4 stages, two of which are known as 'slow-wave' or deep sleep because they are associated with low frequency synchronized waves on EEG.

Stage 1: Transition from wakefulness is characterised by disappearance of regular α pattern and emergence of a low amplitude mixed frequency pattern the theta range (2–7 Hz). It is associated with slow rolling eye movements.

Stage 2: There is occurrence of K complexes and sleep spindles superimposed upon a background activity similar to that of stage 1 (low amplitude).

Stage 3: There is predominance of delta EEG activity in 20 to 50% of the record (increased amplitude and decreased frequency).

Stage 4: More than 50% of the record is dominated by delta EEG activity.

Types of waves in EEG	Rate
α	7–13/Sec
β	> 13/Sec
θ	4–6/Sec
δ	< 4/Sec

REM Sleep

This comprises of low amplitude, mixed frequency waves.

REM sleep develops after progression through various stages of NREM sleep, usually within 90 minutes. It is the stage in which most dreaming occurs. During a night's sleep, there is a cycle of Non-REM and REM sleep with episodes of REM becoming relatively longer.

Tonic muscle activity is minimal during REM sleep. Eye movements are rapid and conjugate in all directions. Gross body movements occur every 15 min or so in all stages of sleep, but are maximal in the transition between REM and NREM sleep.

REM sleep has phasic and tonic components. During the phasic period in addition to eye movements, the pupils dilate and constrict alternately and BP, pulse, and respiration increase and may become irregular. During the nonphasic period there is flaccidity, atonia of upper airways, intercostal muscles and abdomen which may pose a threat to life in infants with excessive respiratory difficulty and in patients with kyphoscoliosis, muscular dystrophy, and paralytic poliomyelitis.

About 20 to 25 % of total sleep time in young adults is spent in REM sleep, 3 to 5 % in stage 1, 50 to 60% in stage 2 and 10 to 20% in stage 3 and 4 combined. Stage 3 and stage 4 sleep decreases with age and in elderly over 70 years, there is no stage 4 sleep virtually.

Most adults sleep 7–8 hours/night usually. At the extremes of age, infants and the elderly have frequent interruptions of sleep.

Adults with habitual sleep durations of less than 4 hours or greater than 9 hours have increased mortality rates as compared to those who sleep for 7–8 hr/night.

Rapid onset of REM sleep in adults may suggest:
Endogenous depression
Narcolepsy
Circadian rhythm disorders
Drug withdrawal.

During sleep there is:
a. Fall in body temperature, mainly during NREM period
b. During REM sleep glucose metabolism is increased in comparison with the waking state
c. In urine, absolute sodium and potassium excretion decreases
d. Secretion of cortisol and TSH are decreased at the onset of sleep. Cortisol secretion increases at awakening
e. Melatonin (from pineal gland) is secreted at night and ceases upon retinal stimulation by sunlight
f. During stages 3 and 4, growth hormone is secreted till middle and late adult life

g. Prolactin secretion increases at night in both men and women
h. Sleep associated secretion of LH occurs in pubertal boys and girls.

Physiologic mechanism governing NREM and REM sleep lie in the pontine reticular formation.

Neuroanatomy of Sleep (Sleep Centre)

Generation of sleep is from medullary reticular formation, the thalamus and basal forebrain. Generation of wakefulness or EEG arousal is maintained by brainstem reticular formation, the midbrain, the subthalamus, the thalamus and the basal forebrain. Current hypothesis suggests that the capacity for sleep and wake generation is distributed along an axial 'core' of neurons extending from the brainstem rostrally to the basal forebrain. There is no specific sleep centre.

Function of Sleep

Sleep is thought to be useful for body restitution, facilitation of motor function and for consolidation of learning and memory.

Effect of Sleep Deprivation

Deprivation of sleep (REM, NREM) for about 60–200 hours causes increased sleepiness, fatigue, irritability and difficulty to concentrate. Performance of skilled motor activity decreases. Self care is neglected. Later, stages of microsleep occurs leading to all types of errors and accidents. Illusions, hallucinations (visual and tactile) may occur.

Patient may have nystagmus, impairment of saccades, loss of accommodation, slight tremor of hands, ptosis, expressionless face, thickness of speech, mispronunciation, etc. Seizure threshold is reduced. Concentration of 17-OH corticosteriods increases and catecholamine output rises. Rarely, psychotic episodes of screaming and sobbing may occur. During recovery, patients go straight into stage IV NREM at the expense of stage II and REM sleep. The next day, REM sleep occurs with a longer duration.

International Classification of Sleep Disorders

Dyssomnias

Intrinsic Sleep Disorders

1. Psychophysiologic insomnia
2. Idiopathic insomnia

3. Narcolepsy
4. Recurrent or idiopathic hypersomnia
5. Post-traumatic hypersomnia
6. Sleep apnoea syndromes
7. Periodic limb movement disorder
8. Restless leg syndrome.

Extrinsic Sleep Disorders

1. Inadequate sleep hygiene
2. Environment sleep disorders
3. Altitude insomnia
4. Adjustment sleep disorders
5. Sleep onset association disorders
6. Food allergy insomnia
7. Nocturnal eating/drinking syndrome
8. Drug/alcohol dependent sleep disorders.

Circadian Rhythm Sleep Disorders

1. Time-Zone changes (jet lag) syndrome
2. Shift work sleep disorder
3. Delayed sleep phase syndrome (patient goes to bed late (2–3 am) and gets up late (11 am)
4. Advanced sleep phase syndrome (patient goes to bed early (8–9 pm) and gets up early (4–5 am)
5. Non-24 hours sleep wake disorders.

Parasomnias
Arousal Disorders

1. Confusional arousal
2. Sleep walking
3. Sleep terrors.

Sleep Wake Transition Disorders

1. Rhythmic movement disorders
2. Sleep talking
3. Nocturnal leg cramps.

Parasomnias Associated with REM Sleep

1. Nightmares
2. Sleep paralysis
3. Impaired sleep related penile erection
4. Sleep related painful erection
5. REM sleep related arrhythmias
6. REM sleep behaviour disorders.

Others

1. Sleep bruxism
2. Sleep enuresis
3. Nocturnal paroxysmal dystonia.

Sleep Disorders Associated with Medical or Psychiatric Disorders
Associated with Mental Disorders

Schizophrenia, anxiety, affective illness, obsessive-compulsive neurosis, chronic alcoholism, depression.

Associated with Neurological Disorders

a. Cerebral degenerative disorders
b. Parkinsonism
c. Fatal familial insomnia
d. Sleep related epilepsy
e. Sleep related headaches.

Associated with Other Medical Disorders

1. Sleeping sickness
2. Nocturnal cardiac ischaemia
3. COPD, cystic fibrosis
4. Sleep related asthma
5. Sleep associated gastroesophageal reflux, peptic ulcer disease
6. Chronic renal failure, liver failure
7. Hyperthyroidism
8. Drugs (theophylline, adrenergic agonists, glucocorticoids can disrupt sleep)
9. Chronic pain.

Insomnia

It is a complaint of inadequate sleep. It can be
a. Sleep onset insomnia—difficulty in falling asleep.
b. Sleep maintenance insomnia (frequent or sustained awakenings).
c. Nonrestorative sleep—persistent sleepiness despite sleep of adequate duration.

Sleep Apnoea Syndromes

There is respiratory dysfunction during sleep. Cough reflex is depressed. There is falling back of tongue or epiglottis. The cessation of breathing may be due to either occlusion of the airway (obstructive sleep apnoea) absence of respiratory effort (central sleep apnoea) or a combination of these (mixed sleep apnoea). These are common in obese men and elderly, often associated with hypertension.

Parasomnias

These are behavioural disorders occuring during sleep that are associated with brief or partial arousals but not without marked sleep interruption. There is no impairment of daytime alertness.

The two most important parasomnias are sleep walking and night terror both of which occur in slow wave sleep.

Somnambulism (Automatic Motor Activities During Sleep)

Patients may walk, urinate inappropriately or exit from the house while remaining unconscious or uncommunicative. Arousal is difficult. It occurs in stages 3 and 4 of NREM sleep. It is common in children and adolescents. Diazepam can be tried in severe cases.

Sleep Terrors (Pavor Nocturnus)

It occurs in young children during first several hours of sleep (stage 3 or 4 of NREM). Child screams with autonomic arousal (sweating, tachycardia, hyperventilation) and usually does not remember the episode.

Nightmares occur during REM sleep and cause full arousal with memory for the dream associated unpleasant episode. It occurs following withdrawal of alcohol or sedatives or may be due to barbiturate intoxication. Autonomic changes are less frequent. As an isolated event they can occur following fever, indigestion, reading blood curdling stories or exposure to terrifying movies.

REM Sleep Behaviour Disorders

It is common in men of middle or old age. There is previous history of GBS, degenerative disorders, dementia, subarachnoid haemorrhage or stroke. Commonly there is injury to the bystander. Upon waking patient reports vivid dreams. It has to be differentiated from nocturnal seizures after a polysomnogram.

One-third of patients will go onto develop Parkinsonism.

Narcolepsy and Cataplexy

There is excessive daytime sleepiness with involuntary daytime sleep episodes, disturbed nocturnal sleep and cataplexy (sudden weakness or loss of muscle tone often elicited by emotion). It consists of a clinical tetrad of
a. Excessive daytime somnolence
b. Cataplexy
c. Hypnogogic hallucinations
d. Sleep paralysis.

Associated symptoms are automatic behaviour during wakefulness, amnesia lasting for a few seconds to hours, sudden burst of words without meaning or relevance terminating the attack.

The cause of this disorder is unknown. Rarely it may follow cerebral trauma, multiple sclerosis, craniopharyngioma, tumours of third ventricle or brainstem and diabetes insipidus.

Treatment

1. Strategically placed 15–20 minute naps
2. Use of stimulant drugs (dextroamphetamine sulphate, methylphenidate, pemoline)
3. Tricyclic antidepressant for the control of cataplexy
4. Modafinil 200-400 mg/day single dose is a novel weight promoting agent for the treatment of excessive daytime somnolence in narcolepsy.

They should be warned of the danger of sleep attacks and analogous lapses of consciousness while driving or during engagement in other activities that require constant alertness.

Sleep Bruxism

This is a involuntary, forceful grinding of teeth during sleep that affects 10–20%. The typical age of onset is 17–20 years. Spontaneous remission may occur by the age of 40 years.

Malocclusion of teeth and central neural mechanisms may be involved in the pathophysiology. Severe cases are treated with rubber tooth guard and stress management should be given.

Sleep Enuresis (Bed Wetting)

This occurs during slow wave sleep in the young. It is normal before 5 or 6 years. The condition improves at puberty and is rare in adulthood.

Primary enuresis: Failure to attain continence since birth.

Secondary enuresis: Patient fully continent for 6 to 12 months and then becomes incontinent. It may be due to
a. Emotional disturbances
b. UTI
c. Cauda equina lesions
d. Epilepsy
e. Sleep apnoea
f. Urinary tract malformations.

Treatment

1. Bladder training exercises
2. Behavioural therapy
3. Stress management
   a. Oxybutynin chloride
   b. Imipramine
   c. Intranasal desmopressin. (ADH)

Sleep Disorders with Neurologic Disorders

This may be due to
1. Pain (cervical spondylosis)
2. Dementia (nocturnal wandering, exacerbation of symptoms at night)
3. Epilepsy may present during sleep.

Nocturnal epilepsy occurs soon after the onset of sleep or during the lst hour after awakening, mainly at stage 4 NREM or REM sleep. Deprivation of sleep on prior days may be conducive to a seizure. Sleeping epileptics attract attention to their seizures by cry, violent motor activity or laboured breathing. They fall into a state from which they cannot be aroused. Sometimes, disheveled bed clothes or a few drops of blood on the pillow, urinary incontinence, bitten tongue or sore muscles indicate seizures. Rarely they may die during an attack or due to arrhythmias.

4. Movement disorders (Parkinson's disease, hemiballismus, Huntington's chorea, Gilles de La Tourette syndrome—patients have extrapyradimal symptoms and coprolalia) are associated with disturbed sleep.
5. Headache syndromes may show sleep associated exacerbations (migraine, cluster headache).
6. *Fatal familial insomnia:* It is a hereditary disorder. There is bilateral degeneration of anterior and dorsomedial nuclei of the thalamus. Later autonomic dysfunction, dysarthria, myoclonus, coma and death may occur.

Circadian Rhythm Sleep Disorders

These are disorders of sleep timing rather than sleep generation.

It can be organic if the defect is in the circadian pacemaker or it can be environmental.

Jet-Lag Syndrome

It is associated with excessive daytime sleepiness, sleep onset insomnias, frequent arousals or GI discomfort; it occurs up to 2–14 days depending on the number of time zones crossed, the direction of travel, age and phase shifting capacity of the traveller. Those who spend a lot of time outdoors can adapt quickly. East bound travellers fall asleep late and face an early sunrise. West bound travellers face late sunset, a long night sleep and adapt early.

Shift-Work Sleep Disorders

Sleep deprivation and misalignment of circadian phase produce decreased alertness and performance and cause increased safety hazards among night shift workers. There is improvement if the following criteria are followed.

(i) Work schedule should favour a clockwise rotation of shift.
(ii) Minimize the frequency of shift rotation (Alteration in shift timings should be done every 2–3 weeks).
(iii) Consecutive night work days should be restricted to 4–5 days only per week.

Speech and Language

Definitions

Aphasia: Disturbance in the comprehension or production of language in written or spoken forms.

Dysphasia: It means difficulty in speech. The disorder is usually incomplete.

Language: This refers to the selection and serial ordering of words according to learned rules by which a person can use spoken or written modalities to communicate with others and to express cerebral activities involved with thinking and learning.

Anarthria: Total loss of articulation.

Dysarthria: Difficulty in articulation usually related to poor pronunciation of consonants.

Agraphia: Inability to write.

Dysgraphia: Faulty writing skills due to disturbances of motor skills in writing.

Alexia: Inability to read.

Dyslexia: Difficulty in reading.

Word deafness: It means difficulty in understanding the meaning of words heard.

Word blindness: It means difficulty in understanding the meaning of words seen.

Paraphasia: Simple syllabic or word elements are missing and are replaced by substitutions so that desired response is only approximated.

Paraphasia may be
a. Literal   incorrect letters (Grass is greel)
b. Verbal   incorrect words (Grass is blue)
c. Neologisms nonsense words (Grass is grumps).

Aphonia: Total loss of production of voice.

Dysphonia: This means difficulty in phonation (voice). It is due to disease of larynx or its innervation causing

proliferation of glial tissue. The entire architecture of optic nerve head is lost resulting in indistinct disc margins (Fig. 8.15).

   a. Papillitis
   b. Papilloedema
   c. Vascular lesions.

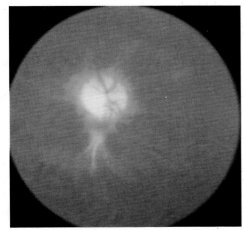

Fig. 8.15: Secondary optic atrophy

3. Consecutive optic atrophy (consecutive to retinal disease)
   a. Cerebro macular degeneration
   b. Toxic retinopathy (quinine)
   c. Retinitis pigmentosa (Fig. 8.16).

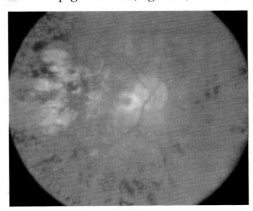

Fig. 8.16: Retinitis pigmentosa

   d. Ischaemic retinal infarction (central retinal artery obstruction)
   e. Diffuse chorioretinitis
   f. Extensive photo-coagulation.

Aetiologic Classification of Optic Atrophy

a. *Hereditary*
   Congenital or Infantile
   1. Infantile hereditary recessive type (profound visual loss)

2. Infantile hereditary dominant type (no blindness)
   Leber's Optic atrophy
   Friedreich's ataxia
   Marie's ataxia
   Behr's hereditary optic atrophy
   Lipidoses (cerebromacular degeneration).

b. *Consecutive*
   Chorioretinitis
   Pigmentary retinal dystrophy
   Cerebromacular degeneration
   Extensive photocoagulation
   Toxic (quinine) retinopathy
   Myopic chorioretinal degeneration.

c. *Circulatory*
   Central retinal artery occlusion (Figs 8.17 and 8.18)
   Carotid artery disease
   Cranial arteritis
   Post-haemorrhagic (GI Hge).

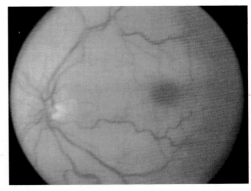

Fig. 8.17: Central retinal artery occlusion

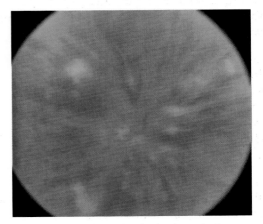

Fig. 8.18: Central retinal vein occlusion

d. *Metabolic*
   Thyroid ophthalmopathy
   Cystic fibrosis

Juvenile diabetes mellitus
Nutritional amblyopia.

e. *Toxic Amblyopia*
Ethambutol
Sulphonamides
Chloramphenicol
INH
Arsenic
Streptomycin
Lead.

f. *CNS Diseases*
Multiple sclerosis
Devic's disease
Herpes zoster
Charcot-Marie-Tooth disease
Tabes dorsalis/GPI.

g. *Pressure or Traction Atrophy*
Glaucoma (Fig. 8.19)
Papilloedema
Tumours of optic nerve
Arachnoiditis
Exophthalmos
Aneurysm.

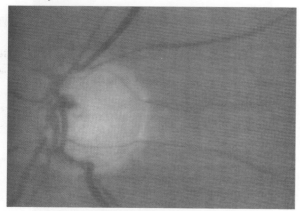

Fig. 8.19: Glaucomatous optic disc with secondary atrophy

h. *Post-inflammatory*
Optic neuritis
Perineuritis (post-meningitis, orbital cellulitis).

C. Papillitis

It is the edema of the optic disc < 3 Dioptres. It is a painful condition of the eye. Patient experiences pain in the eye on moving the affected eyeball and there is a sudden loss of visual acuity.

Differentiation between Papilloedema and Papillitis

Papillitis	Papilloedema
1. Painful condition	Painless
2. Central scotoma	Peripheral constriction of visual field
3. Sudden loss of vision can occur	No visual loss
4. Swelling of disc < 3 dioptres	Swelling of disc > 3 dioptres
5. Due to demyelination	Causes listed above
6. Steroids (prednisolone 60 mg per day given early may shorten course of illness)	Treatment of the underlying cause

D. Retrobulbar Neuritis

The optic disc is normal even though patient is blind. The media of the eye is also normal. "Neither the doctor, nor the patient sees anything". *Usually followed by MS after 2 years.*

E. Examination of the Macula

The abnormalities of the macula that may be noticed are

1. Macular 'fan' (extension of oedema from optic disc to macula)
2. Macular haemorrhage (hypertension)
3. Cherry red spot (central retinal artery occlusion; Tay-Sach's disease).

Amaurosis fugax: It is a transient monoocular blindness, lasting for a few seconds and occasionally for a few hours.

Features of Primary, Secondary and Consecutive Optic Atrophy

Features	Primary	Secondary	Consecutive
Disc	Papery white	Grey white	Waxy pale
Margin	Clear cut	Blurred margin	Normal
Physiological cup	Seen well	Filled up	Present
Lamina cribrosa	Prominent	Not seen	Not seen
Vessels in and around the disc (normally 9–10 vessels are seen)	Minimally seen on disc (Kestenbaum sign)	Sheathing of vessels close to disc	Vessels attenuated
Peripheral fundus	Normal; Vessels normal	Vessel changes seen (Haemorrhage and exudates may be seen)	Altered (pigment/degeneration)

Clinical Aspects of III, IV and VI Cranial Nerves

Name	Muscle supplied	Eye movements	Other functions	Signs of lesion
Oculomotor (III)	Superior rectus	Elevation (on abduction)	Elevated upper eyelid	Ptosis (ptosis may be bilateral in nuclear lesion); Dilated pupil;
	Inferior rectus	Depression	Pupillary constrictor	Abducted eye (divergent
	Medial rectus	Adduction	Ciliary muscle	squint); The contralateral SR
	Inferior oblique	Elevation (on adduction)		and ipsilateral IO and IR are affected
Trochlear (IV)	Superior oblique	Depression (on adduction)		Oblique diplopia on gazing down and inwards (on looking down and reading or while climbing downstairs); Intorsion of the conjunctival vessels on action of the SO muscle is noted
Abducent	Lateral rectus	Abduction		Horizontal diplopia on lateral gaze; Convergent squint

Causes

1. Migraine
2. Microembolism of central retinal artery with platelet or cholesterol emboli from ipsilateral carotid artery
3. Idiopathic.

The Oculomotor (Third), Trochlear (Fourth), and Abducent (Sixth) Cranial Nerves

These three nerves and their central connection are usually considered together, since they function as a physiological unit in the control of ocular movements (Fig. 8.20).

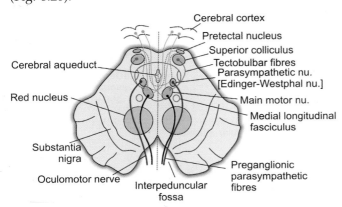

Fig. 8.20: Oculomotor nucelus and its connections

Anatomical Peculiarities

The oculomotor nuclear complex is located in the midbrain at the level of superior colliculus. It consists of one unpaired and four paired nuclear columns. The unpaired column constitute Edinger-Westphal nucleus and subnucleus for levator palpebrae superioris. The paired nuclei constitutes subnuclei for superior, inferior and medial recti and inferior oblique.

Trochlear nerve passes posteriorly and the fibres from the right and left trochlear nuclei decussate on the dorsum of mid brain. This is the only cranial nerve that emerges dorsally from the brainstem. The left trochlear nucleus sends fibres to the right superior oblique muscle, and vice versa.

Abducent nerve has a very long intracranial course and supplies the lateral rectus muscle.

Because of its long intracranial course, it is affected in conditions producing raised intracranial tension, thereby producing a false localizing sign.

External Ocular Muscles and Their Actions (Fig. 8.21)

Upwards to the left	Upwards	Upwards to the right
Left SR Right IO	Left & Right SR Left & Right IO	Right SR Left IO
To the left	Straight ahead	To the right
Left LR Right MR	General contraction of all extraocular muscles	Right LR Left MR
Downwards to the left	Downwards	Downwards to the right
Left IR Right SO	Left & Right IR Left & Right SO	Right IR Left SO

- The eyes normally move 30° upwards, 50° downwards, 50° medially and 50° laterally.
- The recti are adductors and the obliques are abductors, in addition to their respective actions.
- In the abducted position, the recti are pure elevators or depressors. In the adducted position, the obliques are pure elevators or depressors.

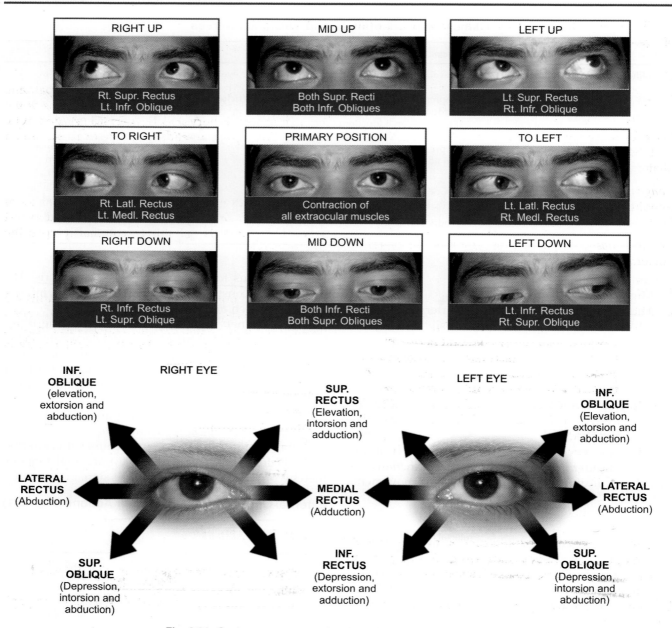

Fig. 8.21: Ocular movements and actions of individual ocular muscles

- The obliques, due to their oblique placement, have an opposite action (SO causes depression and IO causes elevation of the eyeball).
- The superior oblique and superior rectus are internal rotators (*superiors are internal rotators*).
- Inferior oblique and inferior rectus are external rotators (*inferiors are external rotators*).

Pseudo von Grafe's Sign

This sign occurs as a result of aberrant regeneration of the III nerve and may occur after trauma, aneurysm, congenital III nerve palsy or migraine.

The clinical signs include abnormal upper eyelid movement (lid elevation) on attempted ipsilateral adduction/depression of the eye.

There will be lid depression on attempted abduction of eyeball.

Examination of III, IV and VI Cranial Nerves

Inspection of the Eyes

1. Size of Palpebral Fissures

Look for narrowing of the palpebral fissures (*Ptosis*).

Ptosis may be congenital or acquired, unilateral or bilateral, partial or complete.

Congenital ptosis: It is due to bilateral congenital hypoplasia of the third nerve nuclei, and results in bilateral ptosis.

Acquired ptosis: Acquired ptosis may be unilateral or bilateral.

Causes for Unilateral Ptosis

a. Third nerve lesion
   (i) Compression of third nerve by the uncus of temporal lobe during cerebral herniation
   (ii) Compression of third nerve by aneurysm of posterior communicating artery, posterior cerebral artery, or internal carotid artery
   (iii) Cavernous sinus thrombosis (usually the fourth and sixth cranial nerves are also involved)
   (iv) Third nerve palsy can occur without involving the pupillary fibres in the following conditions
      • Diabetes mellitus
      • Hypertension
      • Atherosclerosis
      • Collagen vascular disease.
   NB: The pupillary fibres are peripherally located in the optic nerve. So in compressive lesions there is early pupillary loss and ischaemic lesions there is pupillary sparing.
b. Lesion of cervical sympathetic pathway (Horner's syndrome) *Sup-tarsal m.*
c. Trauma
d. Lesions of the upper eyelid.

Causes for Bilateral Ptosis

a. Myopathies
b. Myasthenia gravis
c. Bilateral Horner's syndrome
d. Bilateral ptosis occurs when there is a lesion of the third nerve nucleus, supplying the levator palpabrae superioris in the midbrain (as a single nucleus in the midbrain supplies the levator palpabrae superioris of both eyes)

e. Snake bite
f. Botulism.

Partial Ptosis

This occurs with lesion of the cervical sympathetic pathway (Horner's syndrome) due to weakness of the tarsal muscles, innervated by cervical sympathetic nerves. The upper eyelids can however be raised voluntarily.

Complete Ptosis

This occurs with third nerve lesions due to paralysis of the levator palpabrae superioris, innervated by the third nerve. The patient is not able to voluntarily open the affected eye.

2. Size of Pupils

Normal size of pupil varies from 3 to 5 mm. Pupils < 3 mm size in average condition of illumination are called miotic and pupils > 5 mm are called mydriatic. Pin point pupil is said to be present when the pupillary size is less than or equal to 1 mm.

Causes for Miosis

a. Old age
b. Horner's syndrome
c. Drugs or toxins
   • Neostigmine
   • Morphine
   • Organophosphorous poisoning
d. Pontine haemorrhage.

Causes for Mydriasis

a. Infancy
b. Lesion of third cranial nerve (midbrain lesion)
c. Drugs like atropine and pethidine
d. Blindness due to optic nerve damage (optic atrophy).

Pupillary Reflexes

a. Light Reflex

Light reflex pathway: The light reflex is carried by the visual pathway up to the optic tracts, after which the fibres carrying this reflex are relayed to the Edinger-Westphal nucleus, bilaterally, and from here through the ciliary ganglion to the sphincter pupillae by the ciliary nerves (Fig. 8.22).

Direct and consensual light reflexes should be tested.

Direct light reflex is elicited preferably in a dark room and by asking the patient to look at a distance (in order to avoid accommodation reflex). A bright light is then

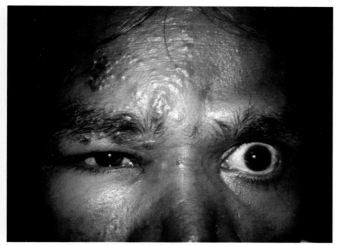

Fig. 8.31: Herpes zoster ophthalmicus

4. Postganglionic Nerve Lesions

Causes

A. Cavernous sinus lesion (associated with III, IV and VI cranial nerve palsies)
   Mandibular branch of V nerve is characteristically spared.
B. *Gradenigo's syndrome:* This is due to osteitis of the apex of the petrous temporal bone, associated with otitis media and results in
   a. Ipsilateral Vth nerve palsy (ophthalmic and maxillary divisions)
   b. Ipsilateral VIth nerve palsy
   c. Retro-orbital pain.
C. Superior orbital fissure syndrome (associated with III, IV, VI cranial nerve palsies, maxillary and mandibular branches being spared).

Seventh Cranial Nerve (Facial Nerve)

Anatomical Peculiarity

The upper half of the face has a bilateral representation by the facial nerve, whereas the lower half of the face has a unilateral representation.

Inspection

1. Observe the face for any asymmetry which may be related to paresis of facial muscles
2. Observe the symmetry of blinking and eye closure and the presence of any tics or spasms of the facial musculature
3. Observe spontaneous movements of the face, particularly the upper and lower facial musculatures during actions such as smiling.

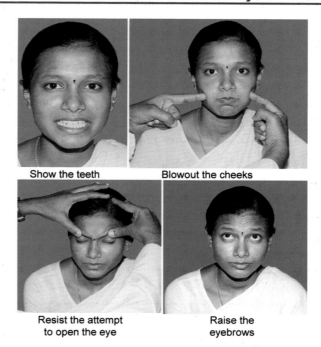

Show the teeth   Blowout the cheeks

Resist the attempt   Raise the
to open the eye   eyebrows

Fig. 8.32: Testing the motor functions of facial nerve

Examination of Motor Function

The motor function of the facial nerve is tested by asking the patient (Fig. 8.32).
1. To raise the eyebrows
2. Wrinkle the fore head by asking the patient to look upwards at the examiner's hand, held above
3. Close the eyes as tightly as possible
4. To show the teeth; the angle of the mouth is drawn to the healthy side
5. To blow out the cheeks against the closed mouth; air can be made to escape from the mouth more easily on the weak or paralysed side by tapping the inflated cheek with the finger
6. To purse the mouth
7. To whistle.

Voluntary and emotional responses of all muscles are compared.

The tone of the muscles of facial expression is noted.

Examination of Sensory Functions

Taste

- The tongue must be kept protruded during the entire test and the patient should not be allowed to speak during the examination.
- Examine the anterior two-third portion of each half of the tongue separately.

Localisation of Level of Facial Nerve Lesion (Figs 8.33 and 8.34)

Site	Lesion	Clinical features
Cortex (supranuclear)	Cerebral infarction Haemorrhage Tumour	Contralateral facial weakness mainly of lower face (UMN palsy) often associated with hemiparesis on the same side
Pons (nuclear)	Infarction Demyelination Haemorrhage Tumour	LMN type of ipsilateral face weakness; often VI nerve also affected; contralateral hemiparesis
Cerebellopontine angle	Acoustic neuroma Meningioma	LMN type of ipsilateral face weakness; deafness and tinnitus; ophthalmic division of V nerve affected
Facial canal (petrous bone)	Bell's palsy Mastoiditis Herpes-zoster (Ramsay Hunt Syndrome)	LMN type of ipsilateral face weakness ± loss of taste, salivation and lacrimation, if lesion is proximal to chorda tympani ± hyperacusis if lesion is proximal to nerve to stapedius
Parotid gland	Tumour Sarcoidosis	Selective weakness of parts of face due to branch involvement
Neuromuscular junction	Myasthenia gravis	Associated ptosis and external ophthalmoplegia, dysphagia, dysarthria, ± limb weakness
Muscles	Muscular dystrophy Myositis	Limb muscles also weak; tenderness of muscles involved

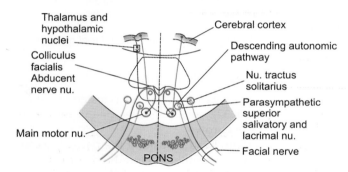

Fig. 8.33: Central connections of facial nerve nuclei

- Gently hold the protruded tongue with a swab, and wipe off the saliva.
- Use strong solutions of sugar and common salt and weak solutions of citric acid and quinine to test for 'sweet', 'salty', 'sour' and 'bitter' taste respectively. Quinine should be applied last.
- Ask the patient to identify the substance by pointing to the appropriate word written on a card.

Examination of the Secretory Functions

Lacrimation

Increased lacrimation is usually apparent and decreased lacrimation may be determined from the history.

Schirmer's Test

Keep a piece of special blotting paper under the lower eyelid and remove it after 5 minutes. Normally at least

10 mm of the blotting paper will be dampened by the evoked tear secretion.

Nasolacrimal Reflex

Reflex secretion of tears usually produced by stimulation of nasal mucosa by irritating substances such as dilute solutions of ammonia or formaldehyde.

Afferent	Trigeminal nerve
Efferent	Greater superficial petrosal nerve (a branch of facial nerve).

Salivation

- Increased or decreased salivation is also apparent from the history
- Place highly flavoured substance upon the tongue
- Ask the patient to elevate the tongue
- A copious supply of saliva is seen to flow from the submandibular duct if there is no interference with the secretary functions.

Examination of the Reflexes

Corneal Reflex

Afferent Trigeminal nerve (descending or bulbospinal tract)
Efferent Facial nerve.

Stapedial Reflex

When the stapes is stimulated by a loud noise, normally the reflex contraction of stapedius leads to reduction in transmission of the sound.

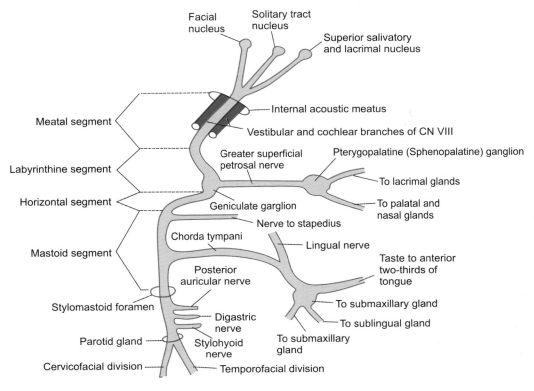

Fig. 8.34: The course of facial nerve

Weakness of the stapedius muscle is not apparent objectively, but the patient may complain of hyperacusis especially for low tones.

Afferent Vestibulocochlear nerve
Efferent Facial nerve.

Common Causes of VII Nerve Palsies

Unilateral	Bilateral
UMN	
Usually vascular	Often vascular (multi-infarct dementia)
Cerebral tumour	Motor neuron disease
Multiple sclerosis	
LMN	
Bell's palsy	Guillain-Barre' syndrome
Parotid tumour	Sarcoidosis-Uveoparotid fever
Head injuries	Leprosy
Skull base tumours	Leukaemia/Lymphoma
Diabetes	
Hypertension	

Facial Nerve Involvement in Leprosy

- Branches are affected
- Upper fibres are more affected
- Patchy involvement
- Asymmetrical involvement.

Bilateral UMN Palsy	Bilateral LMN palsy
Bell's phenomenon—absent	Bell's phenomenon—present
Emotional fibres—spared	Emotional fibres—affected
Associated with long tract signs	Long tract signs absent
Jaw jerk—exaggerated	Jaw jerk—normal
Corneal reflex—present	Corneal reflex—absent

Bell's Palsy

It is due to an acute onset of non-suppurative inflammation of the facial nerve within the facial canal above the stylomastoid foramen, producing a unilateral lower motor neuron type of facial palsy.

- Aetiology of Bell's palsy is not known. At times, Bell's palsy can be bilateral.
- Diabetes mellitus and hypertension have been seen to be associated with Bell's palsy in 10 to 14% of patients, especially after the age of 40 years. These are other causes of LMN type of facial palsy.
- Bell's palsy is associated with the presence of herpes simplex virus 1 DNA in endoneurial fluid and posterior auricular muscle suggesting the possibility that a reactivation of this virus in the geniculate ganglion may be responsible. However, the causal role of this virus is unproven.

Clinical Features

The onset is often sudden. Paralysis is partial in 30% and complete in 70% of cases.

The voluntary, emotional, and associated movements of the upper and lower facial muscles are usually involved.

Frowning and raising the eyebrows are impossible. Bell's phenomenon is noted.

Bell's Phenomenon

- Normally, on closing the eye, the eyeball moves upwards and inwards. This movement is well appreciated in patients with Bell's palsy, when they attempt to close the eye on the affected side.
- The nasolabial furrow is less prominent on the affected side, and the mouth is drawn to the normal side.
- The patient cannot retract the angle of the mouth on the affected side.
- The patient cannot hold air in the mouth on the affected side.
- If lesion extends upwards to involve the nerve above the point at which the chorda tympani leaves it (6 mm above stylomastoid foramen), there is loss of taste on the anterior two-thirds of the tongue, on the affected side.
- In about a third of cases, the branch to the stapedius is involved leading to hyperacusis on the affected side.

Poor Prognostic Factors

1. Age above 60 years
2. Presence of hyperacusis
3. Diminished lacrimation
4. Associated hypertension or diabetes mellitus
5. No return of voluntary power or total inexcitability of the nerve by needle electrode.

Complications

In those cases in which recovery is incomplete, contracture often develops in the paralysed muscles and may give a normal appearance to that side. However, the paralysis becomes evident when the patient smiles.

Clonic facial spasm is an occasional sequel.

Syndrome of crocodile tears: It is characterised by unilateral lacrimation on eating and is due to an aberrant regeneration of facial nerve fibres. Degeneration of the greater superficial petrosal nerve that innervates the lacrimal gland, causes sprouting of nerve fibres from the lesser superficial petrosal nerve (innervates the parotid gland), at the point where they meet. These sprouts from the lesser superficial petrosal nerve innervate the lacrimal gland, thereby causing a flow of tears and not saliva while eating.

Treatment

About 70 to 80% of patients with Bell's palsy recover spontaneously within 2–12 weeks, especially when there is a partial involvement of the facial muscles in the first week.

A short course of steroids, after excluding the concomitant presence of hypertension and diabetes mellitus, (dexamethasone 2 mg tid or prednisone, 60–80 mg/day for five days and gradually tapering over the next five days) may be helpful if the patient is seen within 48 hours of the onset of symptoms.

In one study, Patients treated within 3 days of onset with both prednisone and acyclovir 400 mg 5 times/day for 10 days has a better outcome than with prednisone alone.

Physiotherapy of the affected facial muscles.

Care of the eye, by using eye pads, when there is incomplete closure of the eye on the affected side.

Ramsay-Hunt syndrome: This is due to affection of the geniculate ganglion by Herpes zoster.

Patients present with vesicular lesions over the external auditory meatus and pharynx, lower motor neuron type of facial nerve palsy, loss of taste, salivation and lacrimation and hyperacusis if stapedius is weak. Often the eight cranial nerve may also be affected.

Mimic paralysis: It is due to frontal or thalamic lesions, which abolish the contralateral emotional movements of the face, leaving the voluntary movements unimpaired.

Mobius' syndrome: This is due to a congenital absence of facial nerve nucleus, presenting with lower motor neuron type of facial nerve palsy.

It is usually associated with absence of the sixth nerve nucleus, resulting in associated horizontal gaze palsy.

Melkersson Rosenthal syndrome: There is a recurrent unilateral lower motor neuron type of facial nerve palsy, with facial oedema and a fissured tongue.

The Eighth Cranial Nerve (Vestibulocochlear Nerve)

Examination of Auditory Function

A. By the Use of the Human Voice

- Patient should not face the examiner.

- Non-test ear must be adequately blocked or masked by the use of Barany's apparatus or by producing a noise in the non-test ear by friction of hair over that ear. This test must preferentially be done in a sound-proof room.
- Examiner should use unfamiliar words or spondee (i.e. words which will not give a clue to the patient as to the context of the question asked)
  Example: If the patient is asked 'what is your age?' the patient may only hear the word 'age' and guess the question asked.

Normal conversational voice should be heard at 20 ft.

Whispering voice should be heard at 10 ft.

B. Watch Test

Quartz watch should be avoided.

The watch test may be used at the bedside if early aminoglycoside toxicity is suspected.

C. Tuning Fork Tests
(A 512 Hz Tuning Fork is Used)

(i) *Rinne's Test:* It compares air conduction with bone conduction. Strike a tuning fork gently and hold it near one external auditory meatus. Mask the other ear and ask the patient if he can hear it. Place the vibrating tuning fork on the mastoid process and ask the patient if he can hear it and tell him to say the moment the sound ceases. When he does so, at once place the parallel blades of the fork near the external auditory meatus. Normally, the vibrating note continues to be heard.

In a normal person, air conduction is better than bone conduction. This is called positive Rinne test.

If bone conduction is better than air conduction, it is known as negative Rinne test (Fig. 8.35).

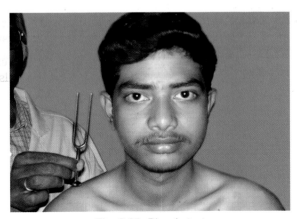

Fig. 8.35: Rinne's test

Interpretation
Rinne Positive
  (i) normal ear
  (ii) nerve deafness (sensorineural deafness)*
Note: *In sensorineural deafness, both air and bone conduction are decreased. However, air conduction is still better than bone conduction. Presence of sensori-neural deafness can be definitely ascertained by doing the absolute bone conduction test or by audiometry.

Rinne Negative = Bone better than air
  (i) middle ear deafness (conductive deafness)

(ii) *Weber's Test:* The vibrating tuning fork is placed on the centre of the forehead, or vertex of the head. The patient is asked if he can hear the vibrating sound at the point of application of tuning fork, or in both ears equally or in any one ear predominantly (Fig. 8.36).

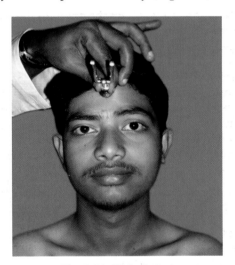

Fig. 8.36: Weber's test

Interpretation

(i) The vibrating sound is heard at the point of application of the tuning fork (no lateralisation)	Normal ears
(ii) The vibrating sound is better heard in the normal ear (lateralised to the normal ear)	Nerve deafness (sensorineural deafness on the opposite side)
(iii) The vibrating sound is better heard in the affected ear (lateralised to the affected ear)	Conductive deafness on the same side

(iii) *Absolute Bone Conduction Test (Schwabach test):* It is the most simple and reliable test, provided the examiner has normal auditory function. The essence of the test is to compare the bone conduction of the patient with that of the examiner. The bone conduction is made absolute for clinical purpose by occluding the external auditory meatus. The vibrating tuning fork is placed on the mastoid bone of the patient first, and when the patient ceases to hear the vibrations, it is placed on the examiner's mastoid bone.

Interpretation

(i) ABC equal for patient and examiner (the patient ceases to hear the vibration of the tuning fork at the same time as the examiner). This test is recorded as *ABC normal.*

(ii) ABC increased for patient (the patient continues to hear the vibration of the tuning fork, while the examiner ceases to hear it). This test indicates that the patient has *conductive deafness.*

(iii) ABC decreased for patient (the patient ceases to hear the vibration of the tuning fork, while the examiner continues to hear it). This test indicates that the patient has *sensorineural deafness.*

Audiometric Tests

1. Subjective Hearing Tests

(i) *Pure tone audiometry:* Quantitative measurement of hearing—particularly important in detecting early nerve deafness.
*   High tone loss is characteristic of nerve deafness.
*   Low tone loss is characteristic of middle ear deafness.

(ii) *Speech discrimination audiometry:* Discrimination of speech is affected, in about 75% of VIII nerve tumours.

(iii) *Loudness recruitment (alternate biaural loudness balance test):* Phenomenon of recruitment is due to lesions of cochlear end organ. To ears showing recruitment, a puretone will be just audible when the intensity is slightly greater than the hearing threshold, but intense sounds (80–100 dB) create a sensation of loudness atleast as great as that experienced by a normal ear at that intensity.

(iv) *Decruitment*

Tone Decay Tests: Measure the decay of an auditory stimulus presented to the test ear.

Decay of less than 15 dB	-	Normal
Decay in excess of 20 dB	-	Neural lesion.

2. Objective Hearing Tests

(i) *Impedence measurements:* Impedence of the tympanic membrane is estimated by measuring the amount of sound reflected from the membrane under various external pressures.

(ii) *Evoked response audiometry.*

Test of Vestibular Function

Fistula Sign

Increase the pressure in external acoustic meatus by otoscopy or by the use of a Siegel's pneumatic speculum or by repeatedly pressing the tragus of the ear against the external auditory meatus. If jerk nystagmus results, then a 'fistula sign' is said to be present, suggesting that the entire bony labyrinthine wall has been breached so that pressure changes are transmitted directly to the membranous labyrinth.

Oculocephalic Reflex or Doll's Eye Movement

1. Stand behind the patient at the head end of the bed.
2. Slightly flex and support the patient's head.
3. Briskly rotate the head from one side to the other and note lateral movements of the eyes.

The normal response is for the patient's eyes to deviate to the left as the patient's head is turned to the right and vice versa. It is a definite sign of normal midbrain function. Its absence suggests brain death.

Positional Vertigo

Vertigo is induced by certain head postures or by sudden changes in head position.

Provocative Test for Positional Vertigo

*   Support the patient's head, with eyes open, and lower it briskly below the horizontal plane of the couch, turning the head to one side.
*   Repeat the test, turning the head to the other side.
*   Note the response of the eyes to head movement, and look for presence of nystagmus.
*   A person with positional vertigo will develop vertigo with the above test and nystagmus will also be seen.
*   Nystagmus will not be seen in normal people and patient is asymptomatic (no vertigo).

	Labyrinthine lesion	*Central lesion*
1.	Nystagmus develops after an interval of 5–15 sec	Nystagmus develops immediately
2.	Adaptation rapidly occurs	Adaptation does not occur
3.	Nystagmus directed towards the side of lesion	Direction of nystagmus altered by varying the head posture
4.	Cannot usually be elicited again on repeated testing	Can be readily reproduced within 10–15 minutes
5.	Visual fixation inhibits nystagmus	Visual fixation does not inhibit nystagmus

Causes of Multiple Cranial Nerve Palsies

Site	Cranial nerves involved	Usual cause
Sphenoid fissure (superior orbital)	III, IV, first division of V and VI	Invasive tumours of sphenoid bone
Lateral wall of cavernous sinus	III, IV, first division of V and VI often with proptosis	Aneurysms or thrombosis of cavernous sinus; invasive tumours from paranasal sinuses and sella turcica; benign granulomas
Retrosphenoid space	II, III, IV, V and VI	Large tumours of middle cranial fossa
Apex of petrous bone	V, VI	Petrositis; tumours of petrous bone
Internal auditory meatus	VII, VIII	Tumours of petrous bone (dermoid etc.); infectious processes; acoustic neuroma
Pontocerebellar angle	V, VII, VIII and sometimes IX	Acoustic neuroma, meningioma
Jugular foramen	IX, X and XI	Tumours and aneurysms
Posterior laterocondylar space	IX, X, XI and XII	Tumours of parotid gland, carotid body and metastatic tumour deposits
Posterior retro parotid space	IX, X, XI, XII and Horner's syndrome	Tumours of parotid gland, carotid body; metastatic tumour deposits; tuberculous adenitis

Pure motor cranial nerves are III, IV, VI, XI and XII cranial nerves.

Pure sensory cranial nerves are I, II and VIII cranial nerves.

Mixed motor and sensory cranial nerves are V, VII, IX and X cranial nerves.

Spinomotor System

The spino motor system is primarily concerned with the execution of smooth and coordinated voluntary movements.

The components of the motor system:
1. The corticobulbar and corticospinal (upper motor neuron).
2. The basal ganglia and cerebellum.
3. The neuromuscular system (lower motor neuron).

A particular movement is initiated when the idea of the movement is first invoked in the association areas of the cortex in which recall of acquired motor skills (praxis) is stored. The appropriate motor cells of the precentral cortex are then activated and impulses travel down the pyramidal tracts, and activate the appropriate anterior horn cells and the motor units. Simultaneously the movement is influenced and controlled by the activity of the cerebellum and of the components of the extrapyramidal motor system.

Lesions of the motor system might result in total weakness (paralysis), or partial weakness (paresis) or involuntary movements or ataxia.

The Corticobulbar and Corticospinal (Pyramidal) System

The upper motor neurons, which constitute this pathway, arise in part from nerve cells in the precentral motor cortex of the cerebrum. Some of these neurons arise from the giant Betz cells which are common in this area. Pyramidal fibres originate from primary motor cortex, premotor cortex, supplementary motor cortex, somatosensory cortex (areas 1, 2, 3, 5, 7).

One-third of the fibres arise from area 4, one-third from area 6 and the rest from parietal lobe (Fig. 8.41).

The somatic body representation in the precentral motor cortex is such that the face, hands, fingers, upper limb and trunk occupy the lateral surface of the cortical hemisphere and the leg and foot area lies partly on the medial surface of the hemisphere and partly on its

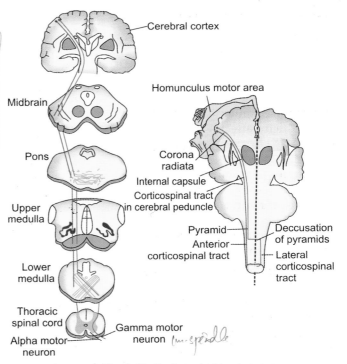

Fig. 8.41: Corticospinal tract

superior aspect. The maximal representation in the cortex is for the lip, thumb and other fingers. Each cortical hemisphere controls movement of the body on the opposite side.

In man, the pyramidal tract contains about 10,00,000 fibres. Nerve fibres arising from these cortical cells (including Betz cells) then come together in the corona radiata and converge upon the internal capsule. In the internal capsule, the fibres lie in the middle third of the posterior limb. From the internal capsule the tract passes down in the middle three-fifths of the cerebral peduncle to enter the midbrain. In the pons it is broken into bundles by transverse pontine fibres. In the medulla it again becomes a compact tract. Throughout the brainstem, the tract gives off corticobulbar fibres which travel to the contralateral motor nuclei of the cranial nerves. In the lower part of the medulla, most fibres of the pyramidal tract decussate to form the crossed pyramidal tract which descends in the lateral column of the spinal cord on the opposite side. A small proportion do not do so and continue downwards in the anterior column, forming the direct or uncrossed pyramidal tract which extends downwards only as far as the dorsal spinal cord and they supply the axial muscles.

Fibres of the pyramidal tract do not synapse directly with the anterior horn cells, but end in the posterior horn cells and from there through internuncial neurons in the grey matter of the spinal cord, the fibres synapse in the anterior horn cells. From the anterior horn cells, the lower motor neuron arise.

Signs of Pyramidal Tract (Upper Motor Neuron) Lesion

1. No muscle wasting (however, muscle wasting can occur in the late stages due to disuse atrophy)
2. Increased muscle tone (in the form of clasp knife spasticity affecting mainly the antigravity muscles, flexor group of muscles in the upper limb and extensor group of muscles in the lower limb)
3. Paralysis of voluntary movement
   a. Early distal weakness involving fine movements of the hand
   b. Other muscles that are involved early are
      i) Shoulder abductors
      ii) Muscles of hand grip
      iii) Hip flexors
      iv) Foot dorsiflexors
   c. The weakness is more in extensors of the upper limbs and flexors of the lower limbs (opposite to that of tone distribution)
   d. The group of muscles first affected are the last to recover (fine distal movements of the hand are the last to recover)

4. Absent abdominal reflex
5. Positive Babinski's sign (extensor plantar response)
6. Brisk or exaggerated deep tendon reflexes and sustained clonus.

The Extrapyramidal System

This consists of basal ganglia and their connections.

It is a complex system of neurons and fibres which have reciprocal connections with the cerebral cortex, thalamus, cerebellum, brainstem nuclei and spinal cord. This system refers to all the descending tracts other than the corticospinal tract (rubrospinal tract, tectospinal tract, reticulospinal tract and vestibulospinal tract).

The Basal Ganglia

The basal ganglia are group of nuclei situated deep within the substance of the cerebral hemispheres and brainstem, and include the caudate nucleus, putamen, globus pallidus (or pallidum), the claustrum, subthalamic nucleus, and substantia nigra (Fig. 8.42).

The putamen and pallidum together form the lentiform nucleus.

The caudate, putamen, and pallidum nuclei are collectively referred to as corpus striatum. The corpus striatum plays an important role in the regulation of posture.

Phylogenetically, the pallidum (paleostriatum) is older than the caudate nucleus and putamen (neostriatum).

The globus pallidus (pallidum) is the final efferent-cell station of the basal ganglia, its activity being

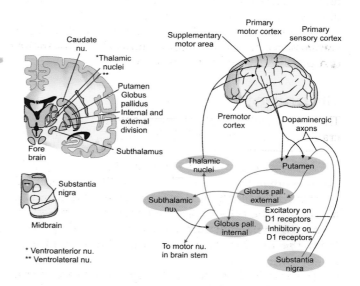

Fig. 8.42: Basal ganglia and its connections

Contd...

Muscle	Main segmental nerve supply	Peripheral nerve	Test
Flexor digitorum sublimis	C_8	Median	The patient flexes the fingers at the proximal interphalangeal joint against resistance from the examiner's fingers placed on the middle phalanx
Flexor digitorum profundus	C_8	Median and ulnar	The patient flexes the terminal phalanx of the fingers against resistance, the middle phalanx being supported
Abdominal muscles	T_6–T_{12}	Ilioinguinal, iliohypogastric	The patient lies on his back and attempts to raise the head against resistance. Note is made of the movement of the umbilicus. In case of lower abdominal muscle weakness, the umbilicus is pulled upwards by the healthy upper abdominal muscles. It is pulled downwards in presence of upper abdominal muscle weakness. In case of lesion at the level of T_{10} spinal segment, the umbilicus moves up by atleast 3 cm on contracting the abdominal muscles
Erector spinae muscle	All segments	Posterior rami of spinal nerves	The patient lies prone and then attempts to raise his shoulders off the bed
Ilio-psoas	$L_{1,2,3}$	Femoral	The patient lies on his back and attempts to flex his thigh against resistance
Adductor longus	$L_{2,3}$	Obturator	The patient attempts to adduct the leg against resistance
Gluteus medius and minimus	L_4–S_1	Superior gluteal	The patient, lying prone, flexes the knee and then forces the foot outwards against resistence. These muscles also abduct the extended leg
Gluteus maximus	L_5, S_1	Inferior gluteal	The patient lying prone, should tighten the buttocks so that each can be palpated and compared; then he is instructed to try to raise the thigh against resistance
Hamstrings (biceps, semitendinosus, semimembranosus)	$L_{4,5} S_{1,2}$	Sciatic	The patient lying prone, attempts to flex the knee against resistance
Quadriceps femoris	$L_{3,4}$	Femoral	The patient, lying on his back, attempts to extend the knee against resistance
Tibialis anterior	$L_{4,5}$	Anterior tibial	The patient dorsiflexes his foot against the resistance of the examiner's hand placed across the dorsum of the foot
Tibialis posterior	L_4	Medial popliteal	The patient plantar-flexes the foot slightly and then tries to invert it against resistance
Peronei	$L_5 S_1$	Musculocutaneous	The patient everts the foot against resistance. Isolated weakness may be the earliest sign of peroneal muscular atrophy
Gastrocnemius	S_1	Medial popliteal	The patient plantar flexes the foot against resistance
Extensor digitorum longus	L_5	Anterior tibial	The patient dorsiflexes the toes against resistance
Extensor hallucis longus	L_5	Anterior tibial	The patient attempts to dorsiflex the great toe against resistance
Flexor digitorum longus	$S_{1,2}$	Medial popliteal	The patient flexes the terminal phalanges of the toes against resistance

Muscle power is tested in the different muscle groups, from head to foot.

Any weakness detected is noted and analysed by comparing with the power of the similar group of muscles on the normal side.

Note is made as to the predominant groups of muscles involved (proximal, distal or both proximal and distal). The causes of predominant proximal muscle weakness, predominant distal muscle weakness or both proximal and distal muscle weakness are the same as listed for muscle wasting.

The quantitative assessment of power can be done by grading the muscle power as suggested by the Medical Research Council.

Grade 5 Normal power.
Grade 4 Movement against resistance.
Grade 3 Movement against gravity.
Grade 2 Gravity eliminated movement (lateral movements in bed).
Grade 1 There is a visible or palpable flicker of contraction, but no resultant movement of joint.

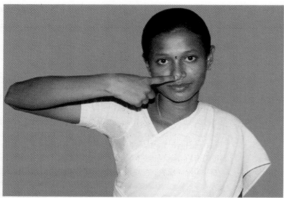
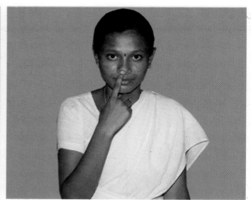

Correct method-Testing with arm in abducted position

Incorrect method

Fig. 8.47: Finger nose test

Grade 0   Total paralysis.
Grade 4 power covers a broad range – (4 –, 4, and 4+) denoting movement against slight, moderate and stronger resistance.

Normally, the larger the muscle group, the greater is the power exhibited by that muscle group. Exceptions to this rule are seen in the following:

a. The power of the muscles of mastication (small muscles) is greater than the power of the pectoral muscles (large muscles).
b. The power in muscular dystrophies is weak, in spite of their larger size (pseudohypertrophy).
c. Some amount of muscle power is retained inspite of the muscle wasting seen in motor neuron disease.

Coordination

Coordination of the limbs can be tested effectively only when the power of the muscle is greater than grade 3.

It is always better to explain the procedure properly to the patient so that the patient can perform the act smoothly.

The limbs are examined on both sides and the results compared.

All tests for coordination are done initially with eyes open and then with eyes closed (to detect posterior column lesions).

Coordinated action of the muscles is under cerebellar control, and influenced by the extrapyramidal system. Intact proprioceptive sense, combined with an accurate image of one's own body and its relationship to the environment are equally essential for the movement to be completed satisfactorily. Lesions in these sites may therefore produce incoordination.

Methods of Testing Coordination

1) Testing Coordination in the Upper Limbs

a) *The finger-nose test:* In this test, the patient is asked to keep his upper limb outstretched and then to touch the tip of his nose with his forefinger. This act is repeated and the ability to carry out this action smoothly is noted and compared with the opposite limb (Fig. 8.47).
b) *The finger-finger-nose test:* This test is performed in a similar manner as the finger-nose test, except that the patient is asked to touch the examiner's finger before touching his nose. This test helps to detect mild degrees of incoordination (Fig. 8.48).

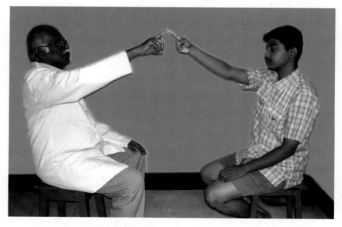

Fig. 8.48: Finger finger nose test

c) *Tapping in a circle test:* A circle l cm in diameter is drawn and the patient is given a pencil and asked to tap out a series of dots, all within the circle. In any ataxia the patient will spread the dots irregularly over a wide area, outside as well as inside the circle.

d) *Dysdiadochokinesis:* This is a failure to efficiently perform rapidly alternating movements. This test may be carried out by asking the patient to alternatively and rapidly pronate and supinate the forearm and hand while clapping the other hand. In presence of incoordination, this alternating rapid movement cannot be carried out smoothly.

2) Testing Coordination in the Lower Limbs

a) *The heel-knee test:* The patient is asked to place the heel of one foot over the knee of the other foot and then to move the heel down over the tibia. This test is repeated with the other foot and presence or absence of incoordination is noted (Fig. 8.49).

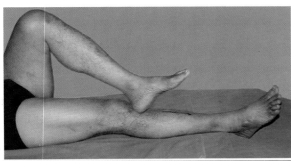
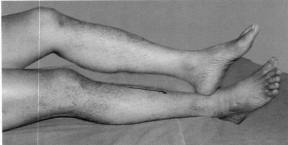

Fig. 8.49: Heel-knee test

b) *Foot pat test:* The patient is asked to pat the ground with the heels of both feet alternatively in the sitting

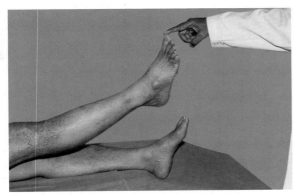

Fig. 8.50: Testing coordination in lower limbs (method 2)

position. In presence of incoordination this test cannot be carried out smoothly (Fig. 8.50).

Involuntary Movements

A note is made as to the presence of involuntary movements.

They may be grossly visible (dystonias) or may require careful examination to detect their presence (e.g. muscle fasciculation).

They may be seen at rest or may become manifest when the patient assumes certain postures or when he walks.

They are mainly due to lesions affecting the extra-pyramidal system.

Common Involuntary Movements

Chorea (Caudate Nucleus)

This is described as a semi-purposive, irregular, non-repetitive and brief, jerky movements arising in the proximal joints and appearing to flit from one part of the body to another randomly. The movements are absent during sleep, and increased on attempting voluntary movement. Emotional disturbance exacerbates this involuntary movement. It is due to lesion in the caudate nucleus.

Causes of Chorea

Sydenham's chorea
Chorea gravidarum
Huntington's chorea
Hereditary chorea
Hemichorea
    Stroke
    Tumour
    Trauma
    Post-thalamotomy
Drug induced chorea
    Neuroleptic drugs
    Phenytoin
    Alcohol
    Contraceptive pill
Symptomatic chorea
    Encephalitis lethargica
    Subdural haematoma
    Cerebrovascular disease
    Neuroacanthocytosis
    Dentato-rubro-pallido-luysian degeneration
    Hypoparathyroidism
    Hypernatraemia
    Polycythaemia rubra vera
    SLE

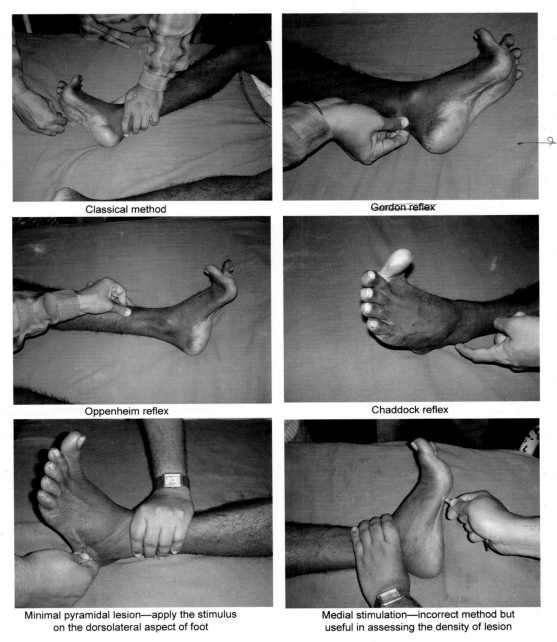

Classical method

Gordon reflex

Oppenheim reflex

Chaddock reflex

Minimal pyramidal lesion—apply the stimulus
on the dorsolateral aspect of foot

Medial stimulation—incorrect method but
useful in assessing the density of lesion

Fig. 8.53: The plantar reflex

This sign indicates pyramidal tract lesion and may be taken as an equivalent of Babinski sign in case of amputation of both lower limbs.

Abnormalities of Tendon Reflexes

Diminished or Absent Tendon Reflexes

These are seen in lower motor neuron lesions involving any part of the reflex arc
a. Lesion of the sensory nerve (polyneuritis)
b. Lesion of the sensory root (tabes dorsalis)
c. Lesion of the anterior horn cell (poliomyelitis)
d. Lesion of the anterior root (compression)
e. Lesion of the peripheral motor nerve (trauma, poly-neuritis).

Exaggerated Tendon Reflexes

Reflexes may be brisk if the patient is agitated, frightened, or anxious. Exaggerated tendon reflexes suggest the presence of pyramidal tract lesion.

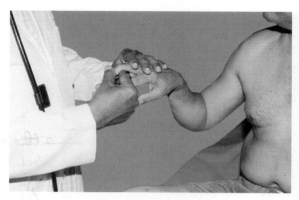

Fig. 8.54: Hoffman reflex

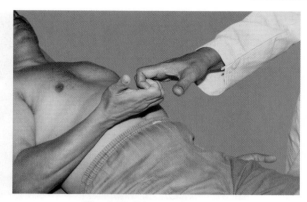

Fig. 8.55: Wartenberg's reflex

Reflex	Technique	Segmental Innervation and Peripheral Nerve	Normal Response
Jaw jerk	The patient is asked to keep his mouth partly open with his mandible hanging loosely. A finger is placed over the chin and a downward stroke is delivered with the knee hammer	Pons (trigeminal nerve)	Slight elevation of the mandible
Trapezius jerk	The finger is placed over the trapezius muscle on the shoulder and the finger is stroked with the knee hammer	Spinal accessory nerve and $C_{1,2}$	Slight elevation of the shoulder
Biceps jerk	The upper limb is partially flexed at the elbow. Press the forefinger gently on the biceps tendon in the antecubital fossa and then strike the finger with the knee hammer (Fig. 8.56)	C_5 (musculocutaneous nerve)	Flexion of the elbow and visible contraction of the biceps muscle
Supinator jerk	The upper limb is partially flexed at the elbow in a midprone position. Strike the lower end of the radius about 5 cm above the wrist (Fig. 8.57)	$C_{5,6}$ (radial nerve)	Contraction of the brachioradialis and flexion of the elbow
Triceps jerk	The upper limb is flexed at the elbow. Keep the patient's hand across the trunk and strike the triceps tendon 5 cm above the elbow (Fig. 8.57)	$C_{6,7}$ (radial nerve)	Extension of the elbow and contraction of the triceps
Finger flexion	Allow the patient's hand to rest with palm upwards, the fingers slightly flexed. The examiner gently interlocks his fingers with the patient's and strikes them with knee hammer (Fig. 8.57)	C_8 (median nerve)	Slight flexion of all fingers
Knee jerk	The knees are partially flexed and rested on the examiner's forearm. The quadriceps tendon is then struck with knee hammer (Fig. 8.58)	$L_{2,3,4}$ (femoral nerve)	Extension of the knee and visible contraction of the quadriceps
Ankle jerk	The patient's leg is externally rotated and flexed at the knee. The patient's forefoot is gently dorsiflexed and the achilles tendon is then struck with the knee hammer (Fig. 8.58)	S_1 (medial popliteal nerve)	Plantar flexion of the foot and visible contraction of the gastrocnemius

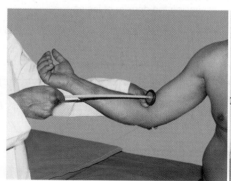

Sitting position

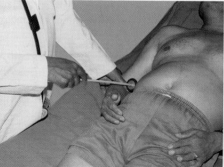

Supine position

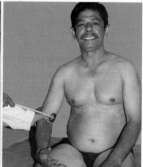

Reinforcing the reflex

Fig. 8.56: Methods of eliciting biceps reflex

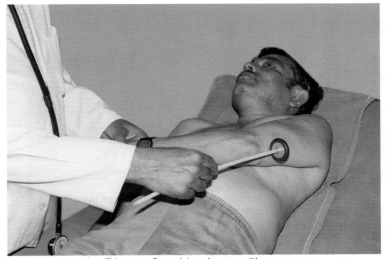

Triceps reflex—lying down position

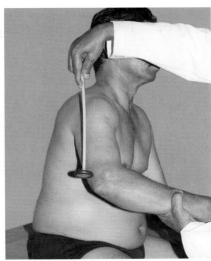

Triceps reflex—sitting position

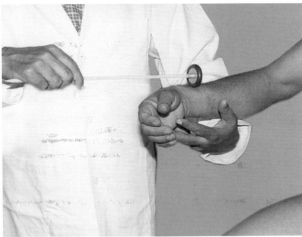

Supinator reflex—sitting position

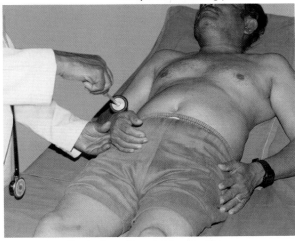

Supinator reflex—supine position

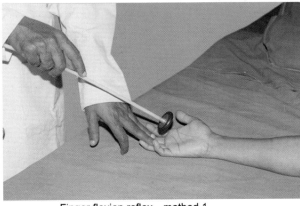

Finger flexion reflex—method 1

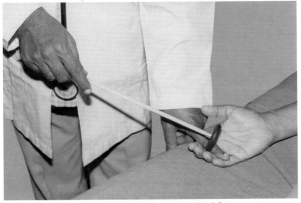

Finger flexion reflex—method 2

Fig. 8.57: Deep tendon reflexes

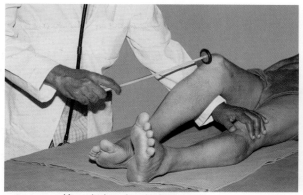

Knee jerk—classical method

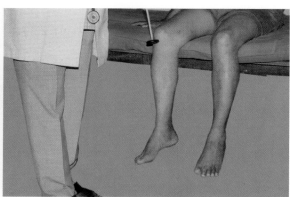

Method of eliciting pendular knee jerk

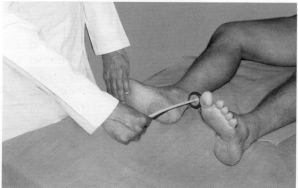

Ankle jerk—classical method

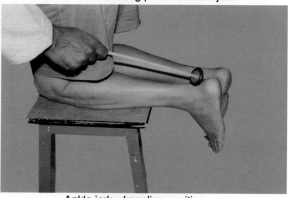

Ankle jerk—kneeling position

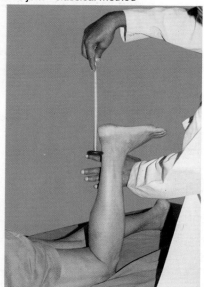

Ankle jerk—prone position
slow relaxation is best observed

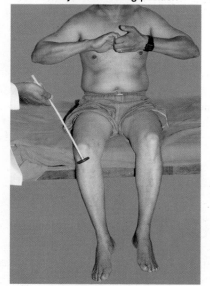

Knee jerk—jendrassik's manoeuvre

Fig. 8.58: Deep tendon reflexes

The Sensory System

Perception of normal sensation demands moment to moment nervous system activity.

Abnormalities of sensory phenomena are described under two categories.

1. Positive Phenomena

These include tingling, pins and needles, pricking, band like sensations, electric shock like or lightning like sensations. These are produced as a result of ectopic generation of volleys of impulses at some site of lowered neural threshold either in central or in peripheral nervous system. Positive phenomena represent heightened activity in sensory pathways and are not necessarily associated with any demonstrable sensory deficit.

2. Negative Phenomena

These result from loss of sensory function and are characterized by numbness or diminution or absence of sensation in a particular distribution. These are accompanied by definite sensory loss on examination. Atleast 50% of the fibres innervating a particular site should be lost before sensory deficit could be demonstrated.

If the rate of loss is slow, patient may not appreciate the sensory loss and it is very difficult to demonstrate them clinically.

In case of posterior column sensory loss, the patient cannot walk or stand unaided and sometimes show continuous worm like involuntary movements called 'pseudoathetosis' in the arms and hands especially when the eyes are closed.

Similarly, patients have imbalance, with clumsiness of precision movements and unsteadiness of gait which is termed as sensory ataxia. This again gets worsened with the eyes closed or in the dark.

Cutaneous Afferent Innervation

It is subserved by
1. Nociceptors (naked nerve endings) and
2. Mechanoceptors (encapsulated terminals)
   a. Pacinian corpuscles (vibration or tickle sense)
   b. Meissner's corpuscles and hair follicle receptors (tapping)
   c. Krause's end bulb
   d. Merkel's cells (pressure) and Ruffini's endings (touch and pressure).

Small Fibres Subserve *pain & temp*
- Pain (cutaneous nociceptors)
- Temperature (cutaneous thermoreceptors for hot and cold). *crude touch*

Large Fibres Subserve *Position & vibration*
- Vibration (mechanoreceptors—Pacinian corpuscles)
- Joint position (joint capsule, tendon endings and muscle spindles)
- Touch is appreciated by cutaneous mechanoreceptors and naked nerve endings (large and small fibres). *light touch   2 point discrimination*

Sensory Pathways

From the peripheral nerves sensations reach dorsal roots and dorsal horn of spinal cord.

Spinothalamic System

Small fibres subserving pain and temperature (small myelinated and unmyelinated fibres) ascend for 2–3 segments and cross and ascend in lateral spinothalamic tract through spinal cord, brainstem to ventroposterolateral nucleus (VPL) of thalamus and from there to postcentral gyrus of parietal cortex (area 3, 1, 2) (Fig. 8.65).

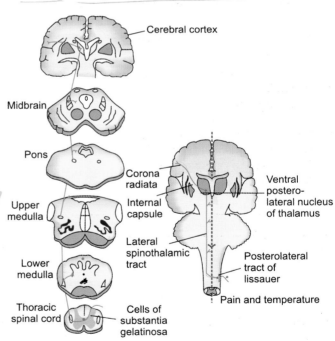

Cerebral cortex

Midbrain

Pons

Corona radiata

Internal capsule

Ventral postero-lateral nucleus of thalamus

Upper medulla

Lower medulla

Lateral spinothalamic tract

Posterolateral tract of lissauer

Pain and temperature

Thoracic spinal cord

Cells of substantia gelatinosa

Fig. 8.65: Pain and temperature pathways

Lemniscal System

Large fibres subserving tactile, postition sense and kinesthesia project rostrally in the ipsilateral posterior

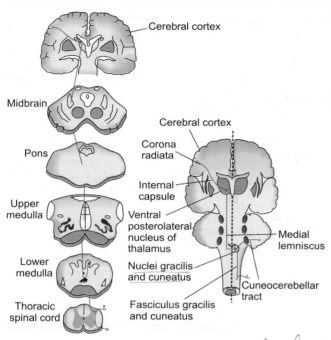

Fig. 8.66: Posterior column Medial lemniscus

post column and make their 1st synapse in the gracile and cuneate nuclei of lower medulla. The 2nd order neuron decussates and ascends in medial lemniscus located medially in medulla and in the tegmentum of pons and midbrain and synapses in VPL. The 3rd order neurons project to parietal cortex (Fig. 8.66).

Definitions

Paraesthesia: Abnormal sensation perceived without an apparent stimulus.

Dysesthesia: Perverted interpretation of sensation such as burning or tingling feeling in response to tactile or painful stimulation.

Hypesthesia or hypoesthesia: Reduction of cutaneous sensation to a specific type of testing such as pressure, light touch, warm or cold stimuli.

Anaesthesia: Complete absence of skin sensation to the above stimuli and to pin prick.

Hyperesthesia: Exaggerated perception of sensations in response to mild stimuli (light touch/stroking of skin).

Allesthesia or synesthesia: When sensation of touch is experienced at a site remote from point of stimulation.

Allochiria: Referring of a sensation to the opposite side of the body.

Hypalgesia: Diminished perception of pain (nociception).

Hyperalgesia: Exaggerated perception of pain

Allodynia: Ordinarily nonpainful stimulus is experienced as painful and excruciating.

Hyperpathia: Excessive reaction to pain, usually with a raised threshold to stimulation. It includes hyperesthesia, hyperalgesia, allodynia.

Phantom or spectral sensations: Spontaneous sensations referred to insensitive areas (in lesions of cord/cauda equina).

Phantom limb: It is the sensation of continued presence of an absent portion of body or of pain, paraesthesia or movement in the absent limb.

Causalgia: It is a neuritis characterised by disagreeable, burning type of pain often accompanied by trophic changes and is seen in lesions of median and sciatic nerves.

Meralgia paraesthetica: Painful paresthesia in the area of distribution of lateral femoral cutaneous nerve, seen in diabetes mellitus.

Digitalgia paraesthetica: An isolated neuritis of dorsal digital nerve of one of the fingers.

Acro-paraesthesia: A disease characterised by tingling, numbness, burning and painful extremities, chiefly of tips of fingers and toes often accompanied by cyanosis.

Modalities of Sensation to be Tested

Exteroceptive sensations: Pain, light touch and temperature (derived from sources outside the body).

Proprioceptive sensations: Sense of position, passive movement, vibration and deep pain (impulses from body itself).

Cortical sensations: Tactile localization, two point discrimination, stereognosis, graphesthesia.

Visceral or interoceptive sensations: These sensations are rarely examined as a clinical bedside routine.

Arrangement of Sensory Fibres

Posterior column: Fibres from lower part of the body are displaced medially as more fibres enter since they do not cross at the spinal segmental level.

Spinothalamic tract: Fibres from lower part of the body are displaced more laterally to those from upper part since they cross at the spinal segmental level.

Thalamus: Fibres from lower part of body lie laterally to those from trunk and arms and fibres from face lie most medially of all.

Sensory cortex: Fibres from lower limb terminate near the superior longitudinal fissure and from the face, in lower part of post-rolandic gyrus (post-central gyrus). Hand and mouth occupy larger areas than other parts of body.

Sensory Dermatomes

Clues (Fig. 8.67)

1. Patient is considered to be standing with the palm of the hands facing forwards
2. C_1—no cutaneous supply; supplies meninges C_2—occiput, earlobe, angle of jaw
3. C_4—above clavicle
4. C_5—deltoid; outer aspect of shoulder tip
5. C_6—radial half of forearm including thenar eminence and thumb
6. C_7—(longest spinous process—longest finger) middle finger
7. C_8—little finger, hypothenar eminence, and ulnar aspect of hand
8. T_1—ulnar aspect of forearm
9. T_2—ulnar aspect of arm
10. T_3—lies in axilla
11. T_4—nipple
12. T_8, T_{10}, T_{12}—supply rib margin, umbilicus and pubis respectively
13. L_1—inguinal ligament.
14. L_3—lies at knee
15. L_4—medial aspect of leg
16. L_5—lateral aspect of leg (runs diagonally from outer aspect of tibia to the inner aspect of foot)
17. S_1—includes little toe, tendo-Achilles, strip of skin above it and sole
18. S_2—calf muscle and hamstring
19. $S_{3, 4, 5}$—perianal region.

Rule of 3

C_3—nape of neck
T_3—axilla
L_3—knee
S_3—perianal.

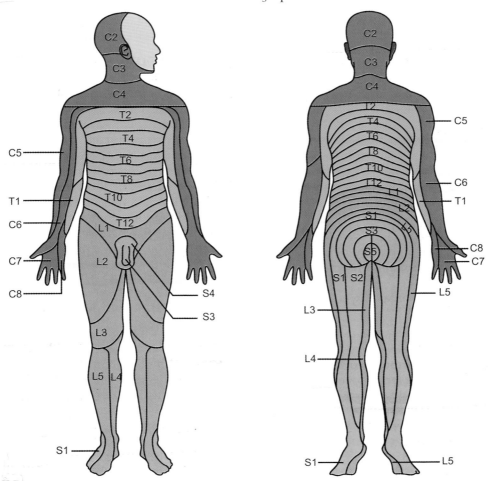

Fig. 8.67: Dermatome pattern

Method of Examination

Preliminary Screening

After instructing the patient, choose a part of patient's body which is expected to be normal (from history) and touch him precisely.

Ask him a. if he can feel anything
 b. what is that he can feel
 c. if it is sharp or blunt

Later do detailed analysis always moving from impaired to normal sensation.

Touch

A small piece of cotton wool is used. After similar preliminary screening, tell the patient to shut his eyes and to say 'yes' if he feels anything.

 Cotton wool is shaped to a point and the skin is touched lightly, testing again in dermatome areas and mapping out abnormalities. Fine camel's hair brush can also be used to test. Do not stroke hairy areas.

Pain

Tested using a sharp pin with a rounded head. Same preliminary screening is adopted.

 Note: Pulp is insensitive to pain but very sensitive to light touch.

Deep Pain

Tested by firm squeezing over muscles (usually calf muscle) and tendons. Patient is asked to indicate when the pressure becomes painful and the examiner gauges whether the force applied is painful in normal people.

Temperature

Preliminary Screening
Patient can compare the temperature of a cold object such as a tuning fork in the main sensory areas of the body.

 After this, use test tubes containing hot water (44°C) and cold water (30°C).

Sensory Levels

Spinal segments do not correspond to vertebral levels owing to the disparity in their lengths, i.e. spinal cord is shorter than vertebral canal and ends at L_1. To find out the segmental level do the following.
- For lower cervical vertebrae, add 1
- For thoracic 1–6,   add 2
- For thoracic 7–9,   add 3
- 10th thoracic arch overlies lumbar 1 and 2 segments

- 11th thoracic arch overlies lumbar 3 and 4 segments
- 12th thoracic arch overlies lumbar 5
- First lumbar arch overlies the sacral and coccygeal segments
- In the lower dorsal region the tip of a spinous process marks the level of the body of vertebra below.

 In cord lesions, there may be a clear cut upper level of sensory abnormality defined by a zone of hyperaesthesia.

 Remember to test for sacral sparing.

 While testing for a sensory level by moving the pin from lower to higher spinal segments, there is a danger of error, i.e. a sudden increase in intensity of stimulus, e.g. between C_4 and T_4 due to *summation of sensory stimuli*. To overcome the error, careful examination of upper limb including axilla should be carried out.

Examination over the Trunk

Earliest sensory deficit in the trunk may be detected anteriorly closer to midline supplied by distal terminal segments of the nerves. However, because of overlapping, exact level or site of sensory loss can be made out clearly only by examining paraspinal region.

Proprioceptive Sensations

Position Sense

1. Patient's eye should remain closed while testing.
2. Place the patient's arm in a particular position, then move it away and ask him to replace it himself and then to place the opposite limb in a similar position.
3. Ask him to touch the forefinger of one hand with the forefinger of the other and make it harder by changing different positions.
4. Let him adopt similar positions with legs and ask him to raise one leg so as to touch his own outstretched hand with his big toe.
5. Ask him to place his forefinger accurately on tip of nose and his heel accurately on his knee.

Sense of Passive Movement (Joint Sense)

1. Eyes remain closed
2. After fixing the joint, the digit or toe at the terminal interphalangeal joint is moved up or down (15°–30°) by holding the sides of digits between the finger and the thumb not touching the adjacent toe or finger. Pulp of the finger not to be touched (Fig. 8.68).

 The patient is asked to say in which direction the movement occured after clearly explaining which movement is up or down.

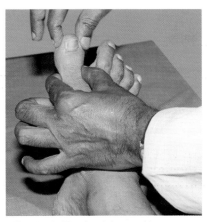

Fig. 8.68: Testing joint position sense

3. Repeat it several times avoiding alternate movements and if any error is made the test should be continued until atleast 6 successive correct responses are given.
4. If digit movement could not be detected in the first place, same test is carried out at the wrist, elbow and knee.
5. It is common in posterior column deficit to have numbness in the affected limb which cannot be demonstrated objectively.

Romberg's Test for Position Sense

Patient stands upright with the feet together and eyes closed (Fig. 8.69). Where there is a proprioceptive or

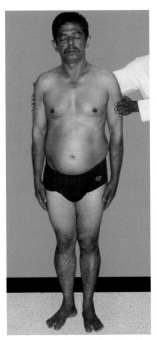

Fig. 8.69: Romberg's test

vestibular deficit, balance is impaired only when the eyes are closed, and the patient may fall if not caught.

Minimal lesions can be demonstrated by asking the patient to stand on his toes with the eyes closed.

Vibration Sense

This is also first impaired at the periphery of limbs. Ideally tested with the vibrating tuning fork with a frequency of 128 cycles per second with the eyes closed. 128 Hz tuning fork decays later (15–20 seconds) compared to 512 Hz and hence is preferred. Only the stem of the tuning fork should be touched and not the prongs (Fig. 8.70).

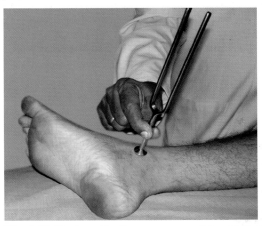

Fig. 8.70: Testing vibration sense—medial malleolus

Tuning fork is struck and placed on bony points starting peripherally at the terminal phalanx, then successively over medial or lateral malleoli, tibial tuberosity, anterior superior iliac spine, ribs or costal margin, lower end of radius, elbow and clavicle (Tables 8.71 and 8.72).

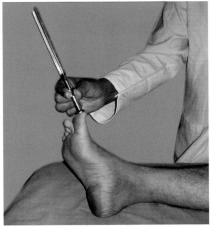

Fig. 8.71: Testing vibration sense over great toe

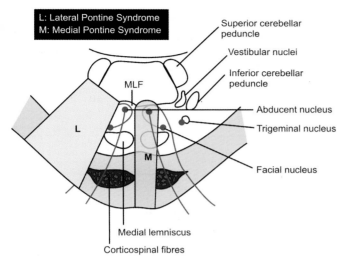

L: Lateral Pontine Syndrome
M: Medial Pontine Syndrome

Fig. 8.83: Pontine syndromes

A. Medial

Symptoms	Structures Involved
Internuclear ophthalmoplegia	Medial longitudinal fasciculus
Myoclonic syndrome	Inferior olivary nucleus
Contralateral loss of position sense and vibration sense	Medial lemniscus

B. Lateral (Syndrome of Superior Cerebellar Artery)

Symptoms	Structures Involved
Cerebellar ataxia	Superior surface of cerebellum, superior and middle cerebellar peduncles
Horizontal gaze palsy	Parapontine reticular formation (PPRF)
Horner's syndrome	Descending sympathetic fibres
Dizziness, nausea, vomiting, horizontal nystagmus	Vestibular nucleus

Pontine Syndromes

Superior pontine syndrome (paramedian branches of upper basilar artery) (Fig. 8.83).

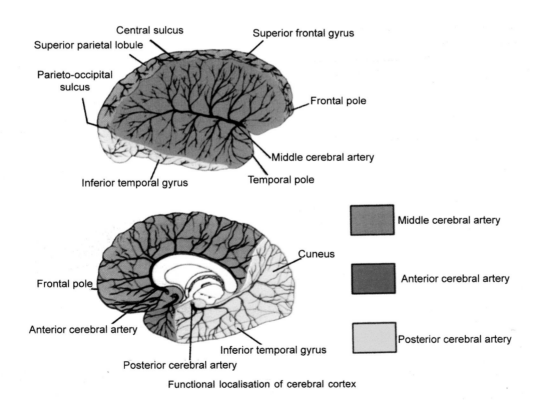

Functional localisation of cerebral cortex

Fig. 8.84: Functional localisation of cerebral cortex

Localisation of Site of Lesion

Site of Lesion	Localising Clinical Features
Cortex	Aphasia Bladder involvement Cortical sensory loss Denial Epilepsy (focal fits) Flaccid mono or hemiplegia
Internal capsule (most common site)	Hemiplegia, hemianaesthesia hemianopia Spasticity marked
Thalamus	Fleeting hemiparesis or hemiplegia in the side opposite to the lesion. Impairment of superficial and loss of deep sensation on opposite side. Elevation of threshold to cutaneous tactile, thermal and painful stimuli, intolerable, spontaneous pains and hyperpathia
Midbrain	Upper level—Weber's syndrome (III nerve palsy + contralateral hemiplegia)—cerebral penducle Lower level—Benedikt's syndrome (III nerve palsy + contralateral cerebellar or rubral tremor + contralateral hemiplegia)
Pons	Millard-Gubler syndrome (ipsilateral facial and gaze palsy + contralateral hemiplegia), Foville's syndrome (lpsilateral VI, VII nerves + contralateral hemiplegia)
Medulla	Medial medullary syndrome Lateral medullary syndrome
Spinal cord (rare)	Same side hemiplegia; No cranial nerve lesion

Ataxia is present in all lesions due to involvement of middle cerebellar peduncles. In superior pontine involvement, superior peduncle may also be involved.

Vestibular nucleus is involved in superior pontine (lateral) and inferior pontine (medial and lateral) syndromes.

V, VII, and VIIIth nerves are affected in the inferior lateral pontine syndromes.

VI nerve is affected in medial inferior pontine syndrome.

V nerve nucleus (motor and sensory) is affected in lateral mid pontine syndrome.

Young Stroke

Young stroke refers to stroke occurring in persons below 40 yr of age.

Causes

I. *Infants and Children*
Congenital heart disease
Arteriovenous malformation
Thrombosis of veins.

II. *Children and Young Adults*
a. *Cardiovascular*
Rheumatic heart disease
Infective endocarditis
Embolism
Prosthetic valve
Mitral valve prolapse
Left atrial myxoma.
b. *Specific arteritis*
TB
Syphilis
Nonspecific arteritis
Aorto-arteritis
Moya moya disease
Takayasu's arteritis
Trauma
Drugs.
c. *Collagen vascular disorders*
Systemic lupus erythematosus
Antiphospholipid syndrome
Spontaneous dissection of cartoid.
d. *Inborn errors of metabolism*
Homocystinuria
Fabry's angiokeratosis.
e. *Haematological*
Sickle cell disease
Idiopathic thrombocytopaenic purpura.
f. *Thrombophilia*
Congenital
1. Activated protein C resistance syndrome (Factor V Leiden)
2. Protein C, S deficiency
3. Antithrombin III deficiency
4. Hyperhomocystenaemia (MTHFR mutation)
5. Tissue plasminogen activator deficiency
6. Hyperfibrinogenaemia
7. Factor XII deficiency
8. High concentration of factor VIII
9. Heparin cofactor II deficiency
10. Prothrombin gene mutation.
Acquired
1. Increasing age
2. Cancer
3. Pregnancy
4. OCP and HRT
5. Antiphospholipid syndrome

6. Nephrotic syndrome
7. Myeloproliferative disorders
8. Paroxysmal nocturnal haemoglobinuria
9. Hyperhomocystenemia
10. High level factor VIII
11. Heparin induced thrombocytopaenia
12. Hyperviscosity.

Investigations (Figs 8.86 to 8.89)

I. *Baseline investigations*
   1. Full blood count, ESR
   2. Serological tests for syphilis
   3. Blood glucose and urea
   4. Serum electrolytes and proteins
   5. X-ray chest
   6. ECG and ECHO
   7. Carotid Doppler.
II. Special investigations (especially young patients)
   1. Antinuclear antibodies (ANA) for SLE, rheumatoid arthritis
   2. Antibodies to double stranded DNA (SLE)
   3. Anticardiolipin antibodies (SLE)
   4. Lupus anticoagulant (antiphospholipid antibodies)—SLE
   5. Serum cholesterol (familial hyperlipidaemia).

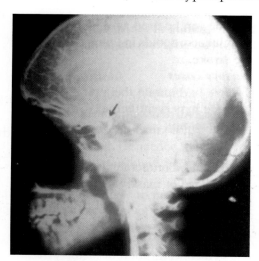

Fig. 8.86: Carotid angiogram—MCA occlusion

III. CT Scan—Indications
CT scan is mandatory for proper initial evaluation in all cases of stroke to categorise them into either ischemic or haemorrhagic origin.
1. To confirm diagnosis (haemorrhage can be detected immediately whereas it may take 48 hours for infarcts to be detected).

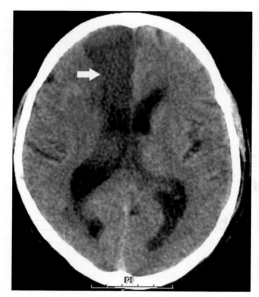

Fig. 8.87: Infarct in anterior cerebral artery territory

2. To decide the line of management (to decide on therapy with anticoagulants or antiplatelet drugs).
3. To identify the presence of underlying tumour, haematoma or vascular malformation which can simulate stroke.

IV. *MRI:* It is the preferred modality of investigation in cases of posterior fossa infarcts and for patients having TIA.

V. *Angiography:* It is not usually indicated but indicated only to rule out specific causes such as arterial dissection.

VI. *Cardiac Evaluation* (for sources of thromboembolism).

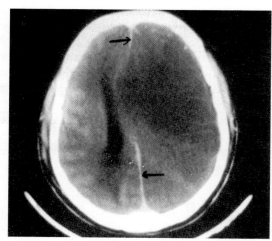

Fig. 8.88: CT brain—large right cerebral infarct with hyperdense SAH in the interhemispheric fissure

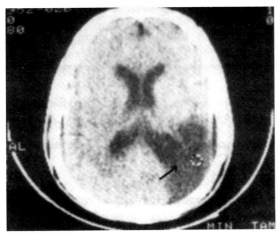

Fig. 8.89: CT brain—watershed zone infarct

CT Findings in Cerebral Infarction

Stage of infarct	CT findings
Hyperacute (< 12 hours)	Normal (50 to 60%), hyperdense artery (25 to 50%), obscuration of lentiform nuclei
Acute (12 to 24 hours)	Low density basal ganglia, loss of grey-white matter interface (insular ribon sign), sulcal effacement
1 to 7 days	Mass effect, wedge shaped low density area involving white and grey matter, haemorrhagic transformation, gyral enhancement
1 to 8 weeks	Contrast enhancement persists, mass effect resolves
Months to years	Encephalomalacic change, volume loss, rarely calcification

Management

I. Specific Management

1. *Medical Management*

a. *Blood pressure:* There is likely to be a stress induced hypertensive state in acute stroke. So, all cases may not need antihypertensive drugs. However, oral anti-hypertensive drugs are indicated in persistent or accelerated hypertension or when there are signs of end organ damage. Sudden lowering of blood pressure can exacerbate infarction.

A patients blood pressure at presentation should not be lowered unless it is more than 185/ 110 mmHg, as the ischemic penumbral tissue will infarct with even minor drop in systemic blood pressure, because cerebral autoregulation in this zone is impaired.

MRI Findings in Cerebral Infarction

Stage of Infarction	MRI findings
Immediate	Intravascular contrast enhancement; Alteration of perfusion/diffusion coefficient
< 12 hours	Anatomic changes of T_1 images (gyral thickening, sulcal effacement loss of grey-white interface)
12 to 24 hours	Hyperintensity, mass effect, leptomeningeal enhancement
1 to 3 days	Obvious abnormality in T_1 and T_2 images (early parenchymal contrast enhancement, haemorrhagic transformation)
4 to 7 days	Parenchymal enhancement, Haemorrhage (in 25%)
1 to 8 weeks	Mass effect resolves, decreased signal on T_2 images, enhancement persists, haemorrhage signal evolves
Months to years	Encephalomalacic changes, volume loss in affected area, haemosiderin staining (in significant haemorrhage)

b. *Anticoagulants*—Indications
   1. When there is a definite source of emboli (AF, dissection of carotid artery)
   2. Stroke evolving over hours or days especially in posterior circulation stroke
   3. Repeated TIAs (embolic)
   4. Cortical venous thrombosis

c. *Treatment of cerebral oedema*

Cerebral oedema represents an excess accumulation of water within the brain tissues.

Pathophysiology
   i. Vasogenic oedema refers to the influx of fluids and solutes into the brain, due to incompetent blood-brain barrier.
   ii. Cytotoxic oedema refers to cellular swelling in response to exogenous toxins, brain ischaemia and trauma.

Management
   1. Head end elevation to 30°.
   2. Osmotherapy by oral glycerol (30 ml TDS), and mannitol (25-100 gm 4th hrly).
      Mannitol is contraindicated in cardiac failure and renal failure.
   3. Pressor therapy to maintain adequate mean arterial pressure to ensure cerebral perfusion pressure of more than 70 mmHg.
   4. Hyperventilation to reduce $PaCO_2$ to 30–35 mmHg.

5. Frusemide can be used as an adjuvant with Mannitol.
6. Avoid glucocorticoids in trauma, ischaemia and haemorrhagic stroke.
   In refractory cases
7. High dose barbiturate therapy.
8. Aggressive hyperventilation.
9. Hemicraniectomy.
10. Hypothermia.

Relief of the increased intracranial tension in CVA is needed only in haemorrhage or massive infarction, causing midline shift.

d. *Thrombolysis*
Indications
   i. Clinical diagnosis of stroke.
   ii. Onset of symptom to time of drug administration < 3 hr.
   iii. CT scan showing no haemorrhage or significant edema.
   iv. Age > 18 yrs.
   v. Consent by patient or surrogate.

Contraindications
   i. Sustained BP > 185/110.
   ii. Platelets < 1 lakh, PCV < 25%, Glucose < 50 or > 400 mg%.
   iii. Use of heparin within 48 hr or prolonged PTT or INR.
   iv. Rapidly improving symptoms.
   v. Prior stroke or head injury in 3 months.
   vi. Major surgery in preceeding 14 days.
   vii. Minor stroke symptoms.
   viii. GI bleeding in preceeding 21 days.
   ix. Recent MI.
   x. Coma or stupor.

Dose of rtPA (recombinant tissue plasminogen activator): 0.9 mg/kg IV (max 90 mg). 10% of the total dose bolus, followed by remainder of total dose over 1hr.

e. *Antiplatelet drugs*
These are used in the primary as well as secondary prevention of stroke
   i. *Aspirin:* It is given in a dose of about 150 mg/day so as to suppress the production of TXA$_2$.
   ii. *Ticlopidine:* This is recommended at present in a dose of 250 mg PO bid for patients who cannot tolerate aspirin and for those who develop recurrent stroke while on aspirin. The side effects are skin rash, diarrhoea, reversible neutropenia, and therefore patients need more careful monitoring.
   iii. *Glycoprotein IIb IIIa inhibitors:*
       Abciximab 0.25 mg/kg IV bolus
       Clopidogrel 75 mg PO QID.

2. *Surgical Management*
Carotid endarterectomy is useful in patients with TIA with haemodynamically significant (> 70%) carotid stenosis.

II. General Management
a. Attend to bladder, bowel, back, base of lungs and eyes
b. Patients should be ideally placed in the semiprone position if unconscious to prevent aspiration
c. Proper nursing, feeding, (if needed, through Ryle's tube)
d. Intake and output chart should be maintained
e. Physiotherapy
   i. It is started immediately to prevent joint contractures and to promote recovery of strength and coordination
   ii. Physiotherapy of the chest is done to prevent lung infection.

Subclavian Steal Syndrome

This occurs due to stenosis or occlusion of the subclavian artery proximal to the origin of the vertebral artery. The increased metabolic demand of the left or right arm musculature during exercise is met by retrograde blood flow down the vertebral artery and this results in symptoms of brainstem ischaemia.

Clinical Features

Unequal pulse and BP between two upper limbs and bruit over supraclavicular fossa over the affected subclavian artery.

Lacunar Infarction

Lacunar infarcts are small deep infarcts (usually < 1.5 cm in diameter) secondary to disease of the small perforating branches within the brain substance.
   The major risk factor is hypertension, which produces microatheroma, lipohyalinosis and dissection of the tiny penetrating vessel.

Clinical Features

1. *Pure Motor Stroke:* There is complete or incomplete weakness of one side of body involving the whole or two out of three body areas (face, upper limb, leg). Lesion is in the internal capsule or basis pontis.
   Pure motor hemiparesis with motor aphasia may occur due to a lesion in genu and anterior limb of internal capsule and adjacent corona radiata (white matter) as a result of involvement of lenticulo striate artery.

Heubner's recurrent artery can also be involved resulting in faciobrachial monoplegia.

2. *Pure Sensory Stroke:* Lesion is in the ventrolateral thalamus.
3. *Sensory and Motor Stroke.*
4. *Ataxic Hemiparesis:* This is a combination of hemiparesis and ipsilateral cerebellar ataxia often marked with dysarthria, clumsiness of hand and unsteadiness. Lesion is in the base of pons or genu of internal capsule.

Diagnosis

It can be diagnosed by CT (for supratentorial lesions) or MRI for both (supra and infratentorial lesions).

Treatment

1. Control of hypertension should be done only after the progression of the disease ceases, i.e. when the patient stabilizes. Immediate reduction in BP worsens the condition and hence gradual reduction of BP is advised
2. Aspirin in a dose of 60 to 150 mg per day
3. Physiotherapy
4. Use of heparin is controversial.

Cortical Venous Thrombosis (Dural Sinus Thrombosis)

Cortical venous thrombosis (CVT) is a less common cause of cerebral infarction than arterial disease.

Patient usually presents with headache, drowsiness, seizures and a rapidly evolving focal neurological deficit.

Causes

Local

1 Head injury (with or without fracture)
2. Intracranial surgery
3. Local sepsis (sinuses, ear, scalp, mastoids and nasopharynx)
4. Bacterial meningitis
5. Tumour invasion of dural sinuses
6. Dural or cerebral AVM.

Systemic

1. Pregnancy, puerperium, oral contraceptive pills
2. Septicaemia
3. Dehydration
4. Haematological disorders (sickle cell anaemia and polycythaemia)

5. Antifibrinolytic drugs
6. Nephrotic syndrome.

Clinical Features

General

- Seizures with focal neurological deficit with or without altered sensorium
- Raised intracranial pressure with headache and vomiting
- Features simulating intracranial space occupying lesion.

Sites of Involvement

a. *Cavernous sinus:* Proptosis, ptosis, headache, external and internal ophthalmoplegia, papilloedema, reduced sensation in ophthalmic division of trigeminal nerve.
b. *Superior sagittal sinus:* Headache, papilloedema, seizures. May involve veins of both hemispheres causing advancing motor (paraplegia) and sensory (cortical sensory) deficits.
c. *Transverse sinus:* Hemiparesis, seizures, papilloedema, involvement of cranial nerves IX, X and XI.

Investigations

1. Blood culture
2. CSF examination (increased pressure, protein may be raised, leucocytosis)
3. CT scan can show the presence of clot in the affected sinuses/adjacent area of infarction.
   a. *Direct signs*
      i. *Cord sign:* In plain CT scan, hyperdensity of the straight sinus and cortical vein which is due to fresh blood clot within the vein or sinus.
      ii. *Empty delta sign:* This is seen in contrast CT, contrast enhancement of the walls of the superior sagittal sinus with hypodense area within it (Fig. 8.90).
   b. *Indirect signs*
      Diffuse brain oedema: It is characterised by hypodensity of the white matter; compression of lateral ventricle and effacement of cortical sulci. It may be unilateral or bilateral.

      CT may be normal at first and then at one week delta sign develops.
4. Carotid angiography (sinus with thrombus fails to fill).

Parkinson's Disease

It is a movement disorder of unknown aetiology due to degeneration of the neurons in the nigrostriatal dopaminergic system.

There is an imbalance between dopamine and acetylcholine neurotransmitters (either an increase in acetylcholine or a decrease in dopamine level).

Clinical Features

1. General

- Expressionless face with staring look with infrequent blinking
- Greasy skin
- Soft, rapid, indistinct monotonous speech
- Flexed posture (universal flexion).

2. Gait

- Patients walk with short steps, with a tendency to run (as though they catch their own centre of gravity)
- Slow to start walking
- Shortened stride
- Rapid small steps, tendency to run (festination)
- Reduced arm swinging
- Impaired balance on turning
- Propulsion and retropulsion and lateropulsion
- Kinesia paradox (patients can run fast during emergency).

3. Tremor

Resting tremor (4–6 Hertz)

- Usually first in fingers/thumb
- Coarse, complex movements, flexion/extension of fingers (pill rolling and drum beating movements)
- Abduction/adduction of thumb
- Supination/pronation of forearm
- May affect arms, legs, feet, jaw, tongue
- Intermittent, present at rest and when distracted
- Diminishes on action and disappears during sleep.

4. Rigidity = Unused door = diff flexion extension.

- It is seen predominantly in the limbs
- Cogwheel type, mostly appreciated in upper limbs especially in wrist joints (there is a phasic element to stiffness in all directions of movement)
- Plastic (lead pipe) type, mostly appreciated in the legs and trunk
- In the trunk, rigidity manifests itself by the presence of a flexed, and stooped posture.

5. Hypokinesis

- Slowness in initiating movements
- Impaired fine movements, especially of fingers
- Poor precision of repetitive movements
- Handwriting–micrographia.

Staging

Grading	Clinical features
Grade I	Unilateral involvement
Grade II	Bilateral involvement
Grade III	Bilateral with mild postural imbalance
Grade IV	Bilateral with moderate postural imbalance and requires assistance
Grade V	Bedridden

Eye Signs in Parkinsonism

Decreased blink rate
Hypometric saccades   Involuntary spasmodic
Impaired smooth pursuit   → contraction of orbicularis oculi.
Reflex blepharospasm (glabellar, Myerson's sign)
Blepharoclonus
Spontaneous blepharospasm
Oculogyric crises (postencephalitic parkinsonism)
Reversed Argyll Robertson pupil (postencephalitic parkinsonism). = can't accommodate but reactive to light

Investigations

1. Serological tests for syphilis (all patients)
2. CT brain (Fig. 8.102)

   Indications
   a. Patients under age 50

Causes of Parkinsonism

Mechanism	Example
Impaired release of dopamine	Idiopathic Parkinson's disease
Drugs depleting dopamine stores	Reserpine, tetrabenazine
Toxins damaging dopaminergic neurones	Methyl-phenyl-tetrahydropyridine (MPTP), manganese
Viral infection	Encephalitis lethargica Japanese 'B' encephalitis
Trauma	Repeated head injury (punch drunk syndrome)
Blockade of striatal dopamine receptors	Phenothiazines Butyrophenones
Damage to striatal neurones	Viral infection Multisystem atrophy
Miscellaneous	Wilson's disease Huntington's disease Cerebral tumour Neurosyphilis

b. Signs entirely unilateral
c. Atypical signs (e.g. pyramidal).

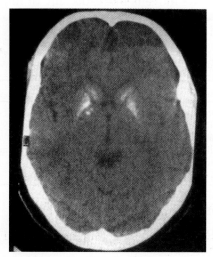

Fig. 8.102: CT brain—basal ganglia calcification in hypoparathyroidism—causing Parkinsonism

3. Tests to exclude Wilson's disease (in young patients (2nd to 4th decade)
   a. Serum ceruloplasmin
   b. Serum copper
   c. Urine copper
   d. Liver function tests.

Treatment

1. Treat the underlying disease
2. Withdraw the drugs in drug induced parkinsonism
3. Drug therapy.

Principles of Drug Therapy
a. Avoid anticholinergics in old age (to avoid urinary retention and glaucoma)
b. Selegiline and bromocriptine can be used in all ages
c. Avoid early use of L-dopa
d. Avoid intake of vitamin B_6 along with L-dopa
e. *Neuroprotective therapies.*
Neuroprotectives halt or delay the nigrostriatal degeneration. Neurorestorative therapies not only halt , but restore normal or near normal function in surviving neurons.
a. Monoamine oxidase inhibitors: Selegiline blocks oxidative enzyme MAO-B, it induces secretion of neurotropic factors, increase formation of oxidative enzyme superoxidases dismutase, alter glutamate receptor activity, and blocks apoptosis. Rasageline is a newer selective MAO-B inhibitor.

b. Free radical scavengers: Vitamin E is a free radical scavenger which is tried.
c. Neurotropic factor: Glial derived neurotropic factor can protect and rescue nigral neurons.
d. Neuroimmunophilin: Immunophilins are proteins that serve as receptors to immuno-suppressant drugs. Immunophilin ligands has been found to stimulate neurite growth
e. Glutamate antagonist: Remacimide .
4. Surgery—stereotactic thalamotomy and palidotomy.
5. Supportive therapy (physiotherapy and speech therapy).

Parkinsonism Plus Syndromes

It refers to disorders in which the classical signs of parkinsonism are combined with other signs of neurological dysfunction, particularly autonomic, cerebellar, oculomotor or cortical.
• Progressive supranuclear palsy
• Multiple system atrophy
   1. Shy-Drager syndrome
   2. Olivopontocerebellar degeneration
   3. Striatonigral degeneration
• Corticobasal degeneration

Treatment of Parkinsonism

Stage	Features	Drugs
Early (stage I and II)	Tremor Rigidity	*Under age 65* Anticholinergics Amantidine *Over age 65* Avoid anticholinergics Amantidine *All ages* Deprenyl 5 mg bd (selegiline) (MAO–B inhibitor)
Moderate (Stage III)	Tremor Rigidity Hypokinesias	a.*L–DOPA combinations b. Anticholinergics c. In younger patients consider low dose bromocriptine + L–DOPA combinations. Frequent small doses of L–DOPA combination are preferred.
Severe (Stage IV)	Tremor Rigidity Hypokinesias Dyskinesias Fluctuations	Frequent small doses of L–DOPA combination (1.5–3 hourly) ± selegiline 10 mg/d ± low dose bromocriptine 15–30 mg/d

* Carbidopa can be combined to prevent peripheral degradation of L-Dopa in the ratio of 1 : 4 or 1 : 10.

- ALS/PD/dementia complex of Guam
- Alzheimer's disease
- Pick's disease
- Diffuse Lewy body disease.

Parkinsonism plus sydromes may be suspected if there is

1. Prominent akinesia and rigidity without tremor at onset
2. Rapid progression
3. Development of neurologic signs indicating disease outside the basal ganglia.

Multisystem Atrophy

Common name	Clinical features	
	Early	Late
Shy–Drager syndrome	Dysautonomia	Parkinsonism Cerebellar signs Motor neuron disease signs with amyotrophy and corticospinal signs Ocular palsies Dementia
Olivopontocerebellar atrophy (ADCA)	Cerebellar dysfunction plus Parkinsonism	Dysautonomia Corticospinal signs
Striatonigral degeneration	Parkinsonism	Dysautonomia Cerebellar signs

Motor Neuron Disease

Motor neuron disease is a disease of motor neurons and refers to progressive involvement of upper or lower motor neurons, without sensory system involvement. It is a disease of unknown origin which leads to degeneration of Betz cells, pyramidal fibres, cranial motor nerve nuclei and anterior horn cells.

Genetic Classification

I. Upper and lower motor neurons (familial ALS)
   A. Autosomal dominant
   B. Autosomal recessive (juvenile)
   C. Mitochondrial
II. Upper motor neurons
   A. Familial spastic paraplegia (FSP)
      1. Autosomal dominant
      2. Autosomal recessive
      3. X-linked
   B. Adrenomyeloneuropathy
III. Lower motor neurons
   A. Spinal muscular atrophies
      1. Infantile: Werdnig-Hoffman disease
      2. Childhood
      3. Adolescent: Kugelberg-Welander disease
   B. X-linked spinobulbar muscular atrophy
   C. G_{M2} gangliosidosis
      1. Adult Tay-Sach's disease
      2. Sandhoff disease
      3. AB variant
IV. ALS-plus syndromes
   A. ALS with frontotemporal dementia
   B. Amyotrophy with behavioral disorder and parkinsonian features.

Amyotrophic Lateral Sclerosis

It is the most common form of motor neuron disease. It occurs mostly as a sporadic form (90–95%) and rarely familial (autosomal dominant 5–10%).

Pathogenesis of ALS-MND

Genetic	Familial ALS mapped to chromosome 21(positive in 20% of families) Positive only in 1% of sporadic cases
Glutamate	Excitatory neurotransmitter that facilitates calcium entry into the neuronal cells inducing cell death. Glutamate antagonist Riluzole has only shown doubtful benefit.
Autoimmune	i. Possible higher instance of monoclonal paraprotein and lympho-proliferative disease ii. Association with anti-GM1 antibodies iii. Possible anti-calcium channel antibodies
Free radical accumulation	Trial with free radical scavenger, N-acetylcysteine, showed no significant benefit
Neurotrophic growth factors	No evidence of depletion of growth factors in ALS. Administration of neurotrophic factors may rescue nerve cells. BDNF and ILGF studies nearing completion.
Environmental factors	Cycas circinalis(Guamanian ALS phenotype) High iron levels

Clinical Classifications

Disease	Features	Incidence	Prognosis
1. Amyotrophic lateral sclerosis (ALS)	UMN & LMN signs (pyramidal tracts and anterior horn cells)	50%	5 years
2. Progressive muscular atrophy (PMA)	LMN signs (anterior horn cells)	10%	10 years
3. Primary lateral sclerosis (PLS)	UMN signs (pyramidal tract)	5%	3 years
4. Progressive bulbar palsy (PBP)	LMN signs (cranial nerve nuclei)	25%	2 years
5. Pseudobulbar palsy	UMN signs (corticobulbar fibres)	10%	2 years

Clinical Features

1. It often starts unilaterally, later involves contralateral side, often symmetrically in a matter of a few weeks to months.
2. There is progressive muscle wasting which usually begins in the small muscles of hand (first thenar group of muscles and then forearm muscles).
3. It usually presents with UMN signs (spasticity, ↑ DTR and Babinski in the lower limbs) and LMN signs (fasciculation, wasting, weakness) in the upper limbs.
4. Foot and wrist drop may occur.
5. The characteristic feature is the recent onset of cramping with volitional movement in the early morning (during stretching in bed).
6. Ultimum moriens (serratus anterior, lower fibers of latissimus dorsi, upper fibers of trapezius and triceps are spared or involved very late).
7. The ocular muscles and sphincters of the bowel and bladder are characteristically spared.
8. The cause of death in motor neuron disease is respiratory paralysis.

[margin note: ∴ LMN dominant in LL & UMN in UL   ∴ LL will show UMN & vice versa]

Differential Diagnosis

1. Compressive myelopathy at cervicomedullary junction or spinal cord especially at cervical region (root pains, segmental sensory loss are against the diagnosis of MND)
2. Syringomyelia (dissociated sensory loss is against the diagnosis of MND)
3. Subacute combined degeneration (posterior column and lateral column involvement)
4. Chronic lead poisoning (only LMN signs)
5. Poliomyelitis (flaccidity; no UMN signs).

Poor Prognostic Factors

1. Respiratory muscle involvement
2. Increased CSF proteins
3. Autonomic dysfunction.

Progressive Muscular Atrophy (Predominant LMN Involvement)

1. It contributes to 10% of the cases of motor neuron disease.
2. The male : female ratio is 5 : 1.
3. It presents with diffuse wasting and weakness of hand muscles and gradually progresses to involve proximal part of limbs.
4. Deep tendon reflex is diminished or absent.
5. This has best prognosis of all motor neuron diseases.

Progressive Bulbar Palsy

It comprises 20–30% of ALS, and may have initial bulbar symptoms (unilaterally or bilaterally).

Other Causes of Bulbar Palsy

Disease	Test
Motor neurone disease	ENMG
Thyrotoxicosis	FT4 and TSH
Polymyositis	CK and biopsy
Myasthenia gravis	Anti Ach AB, Tensilon, ENMG
Exclude pseudobulbar palsy by MRI and Local obstruction by ENT exam and endoscopy	

Clinical Features

1. Orbicularis oris muscle is the first muscle to be affected.
2. Other muscles affected are muscles of the jaw, other facial muscles, tongue, pharyngeal and laryngeal muscles.
3. Wasting and fibrillations of tongue, dysarthria and dysphagia and loss of palatal and gag reflexes are seen.
4. Patient dies within 6 months to 2 1/2 years due to respiratory infections, general weakness and debility.

Primary Lateral Sclerosis (Predominant UMN Involvement)

1. This is usually insidious in onset beginning with spastic paraparesis of the lower limbs.
2. The age of onset is > 5th decade and there is no family history.
3. It has a gradually progressive course.
4. It is symmetrical in distribution.
5. Clinical features are limited to those with cortico-spinal dysfunction.

Pseudobulbar Palsy (UMN Fibres Corticobulbar Tracts) of Cranial Nerves

Clinical Features

1. Brisk DTR including jaw jerk and snout reflex and gag reflex
2. Emotional instability
3. Dysarthria and dysphagia
4. Small spastic tongue.

The dysarthria may ultimately lead on to mutism.

Other Causes of Pseudobulbar Palsy

1. Multiple sclerosis
2. Double hemiplegia at or above the internal capsule
3. Multiple cerebral embolism (multiple infarctions)
4. Diffuse atherosclerosis (cerebral atrophy).

Variants of Motor Neuron Disease

1. Madras Motor Neuron Disease

The salient features are:
a. The age of onset is between 10–30 years.
b. It has male preponderance (2 : 1).

c. It accounts for 10% of motor neuron disease in South India.
d. There is gradual asymmetric involvement of limbs in > 50% cases, with the slowly progressive involvement of all four limbs over many years finally manifesting as a classical amyotrophic lateral sclerosis.
e. There is a weakness of facial and bulbar muscles (in 60–70%).
f. Sensorineural deafness is frequent (30%).
g. There is decreased serum citrate and increased serum pyruvate levels.
h. The patient may present with an abnormal glucose tolerance test.
i. Longevity is prolonged.

2. Monomelic Amyotrophy (MMA)

The clinical features are
a. Slow/nonprogressive wasting and weakness confined to one limb, usually in the upper limb.
b. It is seen all over India and age of onset is between 15 and 25 years.
c. It has male preponderance.
d. The characteristic pattern of muscle wasting is seen in the upper limb muscles (commonest forearm flexors, followed by small hand muscles, arm muscles biceps/triceps).
e. The brachioradialis muscle is spared.

3. The Wasted Leg Syndrome (WLS) (LMN signs in lower limb)

a. It is a nonprogressive unilateral wasting disease of leg muscles.
b. The characteristic features are gross wasting of lower limb muscles mainly posterior crural (calf muscle) followed by anterior crural and quadriceps.
c. DTR are preserved.

Differentiation between Bulbar and Pseudo-bulbar palsy

	Bulbar palsy	Pseudo-bulbar palsy
Type of lesion	LMN- from motor brain stem nuclei (V to XII)	UMN- bilateral cortico-bulbar lesions
Speech	Monotonous, nasal	Spastic dysarthria
Facial muscles	Lip and facial muscles are weak	Stiff spastic facial muscles
Chewing	Saliva pools and dribbles, occasionally nasal regurgitation	Chewing trouble, food may stay in mouth or spill over and may choke
Gag reflex	Depressed	Brisk
Tongue	Atrophy with fasciculations	Small and spastic
Emotion	No emotional incontinence	Emotional incontinence

4. Juvenile MND of North India

a. It is a nonfamilial disorder and the age of onset is between 10 and 30 years.
b. Types
  i. Group I involves distal muscles of extremities
   • Slow progression
   • No cranial nerve involvement
  ii. Group II resembles classical ALS
   • More rapid progression.

5. Guamin ALS (locally called 'Lytico')

a. The age of onset is between 10 and 30 years
b. It has a more marked UMN signs
c. Positive family history is present in 50% cases.
d. It has a high incidence of associated Parkinsonism dementia (PD) complex.

6. Crural ALS (UMN and LMN in lower limb)

It predominantly involves lower limbs.

7. Hemiplegic Type (Mills variant)

It predominantly involves upper and lower limbs on the same side of the body.

8. MND with Dementia

The dementia is found in 5–10% of sporadic cases and 10–15% of familial cases.

9. MND with Parkinsonism

a. It usually follows post encephalitic Parkinsonism. Parkinsonism can precede MND by months to decades.
b. It runs a more benign course.

Secondary Causes of Motor Neuron Disease (Differential Diagnosis for MND)

1. Structural lesions
  a. Parasagittal or foramen magnum tumours
  b. Cervical spondylosis
  c. Syringomyelia
  d. Spinal cord AVM
2. Infections
  a. Bacteria—tetanus, Lyme's disease
  b. Viral—poliomyelitis, herpes-zoster
3. Physical agents
  a. Toxins (lead, aluminium and other metals)
  b. Drugs (strychnine, phenytoin)
  c. Electric shock
  d. Irradiation
4. Immunologic
  a. Autoimmune
  b. Polyradiculoneuropathy
5. Paraneoplastic syndrome
6. Metabolic
  a. Hypoglycaemia
  b. Hyperparathyroidism
  c. Hyperthyroidism
  d. Deficiency of folate, vitamin B_{12} and vitamin E
7. Hereditary biochemical disorders
  a. Hexosaminidase deficiency
  b. Superoxide dismutase deficiency
  c. Hyperlipidaemia.

Investigations

1. Electrophysiological studies
  a. Fibrillation potentials
  b. Positive sharp waves
  c. Increased amplitude
  d. Increased duration of motor unit action potentials (in addition to fibrillations and fasciculations—polyphasic potentials)
  e. The electrophysiological dysfunction present in > 2 extremities is diagnostic of amyotrophic lateral sclerosis
2. CSF in MND
  a. Cytology is normal
  b. Protein is increased in 20–30 % of patients with ALS
3. *Serum CK levels:* There is a mild to moderate rise occurring in 35–100% cases, secondary to muscle wasting.
4. *Cranial MRI in MND:* Gyral atrophy, decrease in precentral gyrus width and increase in central sulcus width are seen in ALS.

Treatment

There is no specific treatment
1. Symptomatic treatment (supportive care and speech therapy).
2. Treatment of secondary causes of motor neuron disease.
3. However, insulin like growth factors, ciliary neurotrophic factors, thyroid releasing hormone are used to improve the muscle strength (they are under trial).
4. Riluzole.

Cerebellar Signs

These are common in established case of multiple sclerosis.

Ocular

1. Optic neuritis is common at the onset of disease but uncommon during the later course of the disease
2. The other ocular signs are central scotoma, diplopia, nystagmus, retrobulbar neuritis and exaggerated pallor of the optic disc in the temporal region
3. Cranial nerve involvement (III nerve palsy, internuclear ophthalmoplegia or VI nerve palsy).

Paroxysmal Symptoms

1. Trigeminal neuralgia
2. Facial weakness
3. Deafness and vertigo
4. Brainstem lesions (dysarthria)
5. Epilepsy
6. Mental symptoms (emotional change, euphoria, delusion and terminal dementia).

Events Influencing the Course

1. *Pregnancy*: There is regression of symptoms and signs during pregnancy.
2. *Infections*: There is an increase in symptoms and signs either preceding or following or during infections.
3. *Inoculation*: The symptoms manifest or relapse immediately after the inoculation against a variety of infections.
4. Trauma increases the relapse rate.
5. *Uhthoff's phenomenon*: The worsening of symptoms (increased weakness and decreased vision) on exposure to heat (hot bath) or after exercise (fatigue).
6. *Emotional stress*: The symptoms may exacerbate immediately after the emotional stress.

Criteria for Diagnosis

a. Age of onset is between 10 and 50 years
b. Lesions are dissociated in time and place
c. Predominant involvement of white matter
d. The interval between episodes should be about one month; when it progresses over 6 months the disease is said to be chronic.

Investigations

No test is pathognomonic and diagnostic.
1. *CSF analysis*: Pleocytosis, raised protein (0.5 to 1 gm/dl) and - IgG (70%)
2. *CSF electrophoresis*: It reveals oligoclonal bands

3. The visual, auditory and somatosensory evoked potentials are prolonged.
4. *MRI*: It is very sensitive for detecting lesions produced by multiple sclerosis (presence of periventricular plaque) (Figs 8.104 and 8.105).

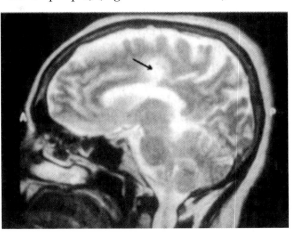

Fig. 8.104: MRI brain—periventricular plaque in multiple sclerosis

Treatment

Treatment may be divided into three categories.
1. Disease modifying drugs.
   a. RRMS.
      1. Interferon beta 1b (8 MIU S/C alternate day)
      2. Interferon beta 1a (6 MIU IM once weekly)
      3. Glatiramer acetate (20 mg S/C daily)
   Treatment duration for 6 months
   b. SPMS.
      1. Interferon beta 1b (8 MIU S/C alternate day)
      2. Mitoxantrone (12 mg/m^2 IV every 3rd month)
   c. PPMS. No approved therapy currently.

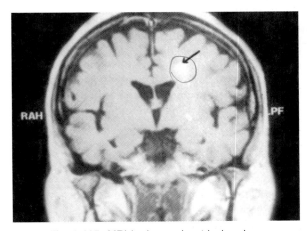

Fig. 8.105: MRI brain—periventricular plaque in multiple sclerosis

2. Acute exacerbation—Methyl prednisolone 1 gm IV OD × 3 days followed by oral Prednisolone 60 mg OD × 5 days tapering doses.
3. Symptomatic treatment .
   a. Spasticity with
      Baclofen 15-18 mg/day divided doses
      Tisanidine 2-8 mg/d TDS
      Diazepam 1-2 mg TDS
   b. Pain—   Carbamazepine 100-1200 mg/day
      Gabapentine 300-3600 mg/day
      Phenytoin 300-400 mg/day
      Amitriptyline 25-150 mg/day
   c. Paroxysmal symptoms—Carbamazepine, Gabapentine or Acetazolamide may be given.
   d. Bladder hyperreflexia—treated with anti-cholinergics like Oxybutinin 5 mg TDS, Tolterodine 1-2 mg BD or Propantheline 7.5-15 mg QID.

Clinical Variants

1. Neuromyelitis Optica (Devics syndrome).
   Acute optic neuritis with myelitis.
2. Acute MS (Marburg's variant)
   It is a fulminant acute disease, usually fatal within one year.

Prognosis

1. Thirty-five per cent relapse in 5 years
2. Sixty-five per cent relapse in 20 years
3. Twenty per cent die of complications.

Meningitis

Meningitis is an infection of the pia-arachnoid and the CSF of the arachnoid space.

Causes

1. *Neonates: E.coli*
2. *Children*: (1 month to 15 years)
   a. *Haemophilus influenzae*
   b. *Streptococcus pneumoniae*
   c. *Neisseria meningitidis.*
3. *Adults*
   a. Young—*Meningococcus*
   b. Older—*Streptococcus pneumoniae.*
4. *Elderly and Immuno compromised persons*
   a. *Pneumococcus*
   b. *Listeria*
   c. TB
   d. Gram-negative organisms
   e. *Cryptococcus.*

5. *Viral*
   a. Enteroviruses
   b. Herpes simplex viruses
   c. Mumps virus
   d. Influenza virus
   e. Japanese encephalitis virus
   f. Arbo viruses
   g. Rabies virus
   h. HIV.
6. *Nosocomial and post-traumatic meningitis:*
   a. *Klebsiella pneumoniae*
   b. *E. coli*
   c. *Pseudomonas aeruginosa*
   d. *Staph. aureus*
7. Meningitis in special situations:
   a. CSF shunts – Staphylococcal
   b. Spinal procedures—Pseudomonas.

TB Meningitis is common in extremes of age, in children and elderly.

Clinical Features (Figs 8.106 to 8.108)

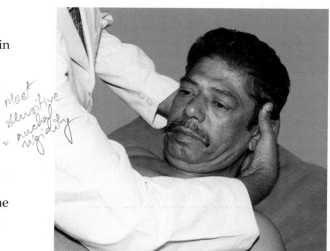

Fig. 8.106: Method of examination for neck stiffness

1. Meningeal signs (positive Kernig's sign, Brudzinski's sign and opisthotonus) (Figs 8.107 and 8.108).
2. Raised intracranial pressure signs.
3. Septic signs (fever, arthritis, odd behaviour, rashes, petechiae (meningococcus), shock, DIC, tachycardia, tachypnoea).

The meningeal signs are invariably present in 50 per cent of patients and their absence does not rule out bacterial meningitis. In 10–20% of cases cranial nerve palsy occurs (IV, VI and VII). Occasionally focal neurological deficits such as visual field defects, dysphasia and hemiparesis can occur.

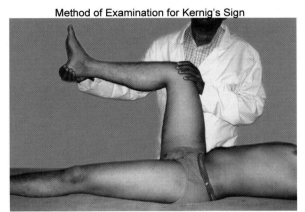

Fig. 8.107: Stage 1—flex the hip to 90 degrees with the knee flexed

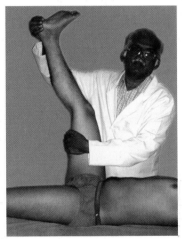

Fig. 8.108: Stage 2—extend the knee. Palpate for hamstring spasm

Predisposing Factors

1. Head injury (fractures of base of the skull)
2. Sinusitis, mastoiditis and otitis media

3. Immunosuppressed states (carcinoma, HIV, splenectomy for sickle cell disease)
4. Diabetes mellitus
5. Pneumonia
6. Alcoholism
7. CSF shunts.
8. Iatrogenic (after LP).

Investigations

CSF Analysis

- The only investigation that will confirm the diagnosis is lumbar puncture and CSF analysis.
- Lumbar puncture is contraindicated in the presence of gross papilloedema with or without neurological deficit or meningococcemia (risk of bleed). However LP has to be planned after a preliminary CT scan.
- Early CSF analysis may be normal and the lumbar puncture should be repeated if the meningeal signs persist.
- Send 3 bottles of CSF (8 drops or ½ CC in each bottle) for urgent gram stain and culture, virology study and biochemical study (especially glucose).

CSF Glucose Decreased

1. Bacterial meningitis (markedly low in pyogenic meningitis than in TB meningitis)
2. Carcinomatous meningitis
3. Haematomyelia
4. Epidural haemorrhage.

Encephalitis

Encephalitis is an infection of the brain. The viruses causing encephalitis are herpes simplex (most common); measles, mumps, varicella, poliomyelitis, Japanese B encephalitis and arboviruses.

Empirical Treatment of Meningitis

Age and likely micro-organisms	Choice of antimicrobials
Neonates: *E.coli*—β haemolytic streptococci—Listeria monocytogenes	Ampicillin + Cefotaxime
Children < 14 years: *H.influenzae* – Meningococci –*S. pneumoniae*	Cefotaxime or Ceftriaxone + Vancomycin
Adults: Pneumococci - Meningococci	Cefotaxime 2 g IV q4h or Ceftriaxone 2 g IV q12h +Vancomycin
Elderly and immunocompromised: Pneumococci – *Listeria monocytogenes* – Gram-negative organisms	Ampicillin 2 g IV q4h +Cefotaxime 2 g IV q4h or Ceftriaxone +Vancomycin 500-750 mg IV q6h
Nosocomial and post-traumatic:*K.pneumoniae* – *E.coli* – *S.aureus* –*Pseudomonos aeruginosa*	Ampicillin 2 g IV q4h +Ceftazidime 2 g IV q8h + Vancomycin 500-750 mg IV q6h

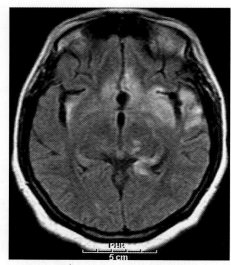

Fig. 8.109: Herpes-simplex encephalitis

No Organisms seen in CSF

Ceftriaxone 2 g IV q12h or Cefotaxime 2 g IV q4h along with Vancomycin 500-750 mg IV q6h can be given. Add additionally ampicillin 2 g IV q4h for immunocompromised and aged (>50 years).

Vancomycin should not be used alone.

Adjuvant Therapy – Dexamethasone

Dexamethasone exerts its beneficial effect by inhibiting the synthesis of IL-1 and TNF from inflammatory cells at the level of m-RNA, decreasing CSF outflow resistance and stabilizing the blood brain barrier. Dexamethasone 10 mg IV should be given 20 minutes before the first dose of an antibiotic and continued 6th hourly for 4 days.

The rationale for giving dexamethasone 20 minutes before the administration of antibiotic is that it inhibits the production of TNF by macrophages and microglia only if it is given before these cells are activated by endotoxin. Do not use dexamethasone when the patient is in shock.

Symptoms and Signs

They are headache, fever, fits, altered sensorium with or without neurological deficit, signs of increased intracranial pressure, and meningeal signs.

Investigations

1. *CT scan*: It is useful to differentiate encephalitis from cerebral abscess and CNS tumours (Fig. 8.109).
2. *Lumbar puncture*: The CSF pressure is increased with increased protein and lymphocytic pleocytosis.

3. *EEG*: It shows diffuse slowing with epileptiform discharge in herpetic encephalitis.
4. *Isotope scan*: The increased temporal lobe isotope uptake on a brain scan is a feature of herpetic encephalitis.
5. *Brain biopsy*: It is useful in potentially treatable herpetic encephalitis.
6. The serology and immunological tests are useful in confirming the diagnosis.

Management

1. Skilled nursing care
2. Maintenance of fluid balance and nutritional status
3. The raised ICP is reduced by dexamethasone 4 mg 6th hourly
4. The herpes simplex virus encephalitis is treated with acyclovir 10 mg/kg IV 3 times daily for 10 days.

Prognosis

The highest mortality is seen in herpes-simplex (mortality rate of 15–20%).

Slow Virus Disease

Slow virus diseases involving central nervous system mainly occur many months or even years after the infection with transmissable agents which have properties different from conventional viruses.

Subacute Sclerosing Pan Encephalitis (SSPE)

It has a chronic progressive and eventually fatal course. It is caused by measles virus. It occurs in children and adolescents.

Clinical Features

1. Intellectual deterioration, apathy and clumsiness.
2. Myoclonic jerks, rigidity and dementia.

Investigations

1. CSF analysis:
   Lymphocytic pleocytosis or acellular, markedly elevated gamma globulin (antimeasles antibodies)
2. EEG:
   Periodic burst of triphasic waves.
3. Brain tissue—culture positive for measles virus (immunocytochemical methods)

Kuru

- The cardinal features are severe cerebellar ataxia with associated involuntary movements (choreo-athetosis, myoclonus and tremor) (Fig. 8.110).

Conditions	Appearance	Cells	Glucose	Protein	Organism
Normal	Clear	Lymphocyte < 4/mm³	2/3rd of plasma glucose level	20–40 mg%	Nil
Pyogenic	Turbid	Polymorphs 1000/mm³	< 2/3rd of plasma glucose (40 mg%)	1–5 gm%	Present
Tuberculosis	Clear or yellow Fibrin web	PMN/LYM/mixed	< 2/3rd plasma glucose	1–5 gm%	AFB present in cob-web
Aseptic (viral)	Clear	Mononuclear 50–1500/mm³	Normal	Normal or raised	Nil
Malignancy	Clear	Lymphocytes 0–100	Low	Normal or elevated	Nil

Treatment			
Organism	Choice of antibiotic	Dose	Duration
Pneumococcus	Benzyl penicillin or ceftriaxone	20 lakhs 2 hourly or 40 lakhs 4 hourly 2 gm IV 12 hourly	10 to 14 days
Meningococcus	Benzyl penicillin or cefotaxime	20 lakhs 2 hourly or 40 lakhs 4 hourly 2 gm IV 4 hourly	10 to 14 days
Haemophilus influenzae	Chloramphenicol or cefotaxime or ceftriaxone	1 to 1.5 gm IV 6 hourly 2 gm IV 4 hourly 2 gm IV 12 hourly	10 days
Listeria monocytogenes	Ampicillin + Gentamicin	2 gm IV 4 hourly 3 to 5 mg per kg/day 8 hourly	3 to 4 weeks
Gram-negative organisms	Cefotaxime or Ceftriaxone	2 gm IV 4 hourly 2 gm IV 12 hourly	2 weeks

- Mental impairment and frontal release signs.
- The source of transmission is due to ingestion of infected human brain material (cannibalistic practices).

Creutzfeldt-Jakob Disease

It mostly occurs as sporadic, although 5–15% are familial with an autosomal dominant inheritance

Clinical Features

The clinical manifestations are severe and progressive dementia, pyramidal and extrapyramidal motor disturbances and signs and symptoms of cerebellar dysfunction.

Investigations

1. *EEG*: The typical pattern of periodic sharp wave complexes consists of a generalized slow, background interrupted by bilaterally synchronous sharp wave complexes occurring at intervals of 0.5–2.5 sec and lasting for 200–600 milli seconds
2. *CT and MRI*: This shows generalised cortical atrophy (The degree of clinical dementia is disproportionate to the amount of tissue lost)
3. *Brain biopsy*: It is the gold standard for diagnosis of Creutzfeldt-Jakob disease. The pathologic hallmarks are spongiform changes (small round vacuoles) within the neuropia, neuronal loss, hypertrophy and proliferation of glial cells and absence of significant inflammation or white matter involvement. The above changes are predominantly seen in the basal ganglia, cerebellum and thalamus. The brain stem and spinalcord are usually spared.

Autonomic Nervous System

Autonomic nervous system is composed of sympathetic and parasympathetic pathways. They function below the conscious level and respond rapidly to the changes that threaten to disturb the constancy of the internal environment.

Sympathetic outflow is from the lateral grey column of the spinal cord from T_1–L_2 (thoraco-lumbar outflow). This outflow communicates with the ganglionic fibres that innervate the blood vessels, heart, lungs, hair follicle, sweat glands and abdomino-pelvic viscerae.

The parasympathetic system spreads from the brainstem through IIIrd, VIIth, IXth and Xth cranial nerves and sacral segments of the spinal cord ($S_2S_3S_4$) (craniosacral outflow). They synapse in the parasympathetic ganglia and the postganglionic fibres innervate the end organs.

The sympathetic ganglia are situated in the paraspinal region, close to the cord whereas parasympathetic ganglia are situated close to the respective end organs.

Both sympathetic and parasympathetic systems are under the control of hypothalamus (anterior hypothalamus-parasympathetic, posterior hypothalamus-sympathetic) (Fig. 8.110).

Neurological Diseases in Patients with HIV

1. Myopathy
2. Peripheral neuropathy
   a. GBS Guillian Barre
   b. CIDP
   c. Mononeuritis multiplex
   d. Distal symmetric polyneuropathy
3. Myelopathy
   a. Vacuolar myelopathy
   b. Pure sensory ataxia
   c. Paraesthesia/Dysaesthesias
4. Aseptic meningitis
5. HIV encephalopathy
6. Neoplasms
   a. Primary CNS lymphoma
   b. Kaposi's sarcoma
7. Opportunistic infection
   a. Toxoplasmosis
   b. Cryptococcosis
   c. Progressive multifocal leucoencephalopathy
   d. CMV
   e. Syphilis
   f. Tuberculosis
   g. HTLV 1.

Treatment is mainly symptomatic.

Cervical Spondylosis

It is a degenerative disorder involving the discs, cervical spines and joints of the cervical region. It affects men more than women.

Mechanism of Degeneration

1. Narrowing of the intervertebral disc space (due to nucleus pulposus herniation or annulus bulging)
2. Osteophytic spur formation (dorsal surface of vertebral bodies)
3. Partial subluxation of vertebrae
4. Hypertrophy of the dorsal spinal ligament and dorsolateral facet articulations.

5. Hypertrophied ligamentum flavum with fibrosis and calcification
6. C5-C6 intervertebral disc has strong attachment to the vertebral column and this predisposes to degenerative changes.

The most common intervertebral joint to undergo degenerations is between C_5–C_6. It is due to maximal movements occuring at this cervical spine. However C_6–C_7 and at times C_4–C_5 can also be involved.

Symptoms and Signs

Radiculopathy

1. Neck pain (local and referred pain)
2. Sensory loss and paraesthesiae in the corresponding dermatomes (due to sensory root involvement)
3. Weakness and wasting of the muscles supplied (due to motor root involvement) and inverted biceps reflex (C_5 lesion)
4. The wasting of the small muscles of the hand is uncommon.

Spurling's Sign

In cervical spondylosis, cervical extension results in narrowing of the vertebral canal thereby producing severe pain in neck.

Shoulder Abduction Relief Sign

Abduction of shoulder relieves pain in cervical spondylosis.

Cervical Angina Syndrome

C6 – C7 disc prolapse can cause pain over the chest simulating angina.

Myelopathy

The most common presentation is spondylotic myelopathy. It presents with insidious onset of spastic weakness of the legs, dragging of the toes and stiffness of the legs. An accompanying radiculopathy is reported in

Differential Diagnosis of Leg Pain

Features	Neurological	Arterial	Venous	Rheological
Site of pain	Along a dermatome	Usually calf region	Always calf	Usually whole leg
Method of relief	Lying down for atleast 30 minutes	Standing still for few minutes	Elevation of legs	Standing still
Confirmatory signs	Abnormal neurological signs after exercise	Absent distal pulse	Oedema and other signs of chronic venous congestion	Bounding pulse
Confirmatory test	Myelogram	Ankle: arm systolic ratio < 0.8	Venogram	CBC and ESR

40–80% of cases. The features of root involvement are asymmetric, asymptomatic or present with focal weakness or wasting or loss of a reflex.

The sensory signs (loss of VS, PS, Rombergism +) in myelopathy is due to posterior column involvement.

Differential Diagnosis for Cervical Spondylosis

1. Compression of cord or root (TB, secondaries or *NF)
2. Carcinomatous infiltration or radiotherapy.
3. Peripheral nerve lesions (distal ulnar or median nerve)
4. Motor neuron disease
5. Syringomyelia
6. Multiple sclerosis
* Neurofibromas

Lumbar Canal Stenosis

It is a congenital disorder causing narrowing of the lumbar canal. Symptoms are exacerbated by degenerative changes. The narrowest part of the lumbar canal is present between L_4 and L_5 vertebrae. It is the most common condition causing cauda equina lesion.

Predisposing Factors

Achondroplasia
Spondylolisthesis
Acromegaly.

Mechanism

1. The compression by the disc causes further narrowing of the canal during erect posture
2. The physiological hyperemia occurring during exercise.

Clinical Features

1. It is three times more common in men than women
2. The age of onset is 40–50 years
3. There is history of postural low backache (the pain is provoked by sitting, standing, bending or lifting)
4. There are symptoms of neurogenic claudication (appearance of pain, numbness in the legs during walking).

The signs are
a. Stiffness of the lumbar spine
b. Reversal of normal lordosis
c. Stooped posture
d. Absence of ankle reflex.

Differentiation between Intervertebral Disc Prolapse and Lumbar Canal Stenosis

Features	Intervertebral disc prolapse	Lumbar canal stenosis
Age	3–4 decade	4–6 decade
Onset	Acute	Gradual
Pain	Back and lower limb	Back and lower limb
Neurogenic claudication	May be positive	Rapid onset
SLR	Restricted	Normal
Sitting posture	Aggravation of pain	Pain not aggravated
*Pain relief on stooping	—	Present

* Stoop test

Procedure

1. Ask the patient to walk
2. Ask the patient to continue to walk even after the development of neurogenic claudication.
3. Patient continues his walk with a stooped posture.

Characteristics of Neurogenic Claudication

- Pain is not in the exercising muscle but along the dermatome
- Patient cannot walk but may be able to cycle long distance
- During the episode reflexes are usually absent
- In early stages pain is relieved by sitting and stooping position
- Elevation of the limb does not relieve pain.

Investigations

1. Measurement of Movement of the Spine

Procedure
a. Mark 2 points over skin about 10 cm above and 5 cm below L_5 vertebra in the midline with the patient erect. (total 15 cm)
b. Ask the patient to bend forward as far as possible. Normally interpoint distance increases by more than 5 cm. (i.e. more than 20 cm) (Fig. 8.116).

Interpretation: In disc prolapse, the interpoint distance is less than 20 cm due to restricted movement on bending forwards.

2. Plain X-ray Neck

Anteroposterior
Lateral-Neutral
    Flexion
    Extension
Oblique (for delineating intervertebral foramina)

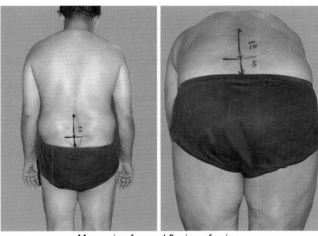

Measuring forward flexion of spine

Fig. 8.116: Schober's test

Features
1. Loss of normal cervical lordosis
2. Spondylotic bars
3. IV disc narrowing and subluxation
4. Reduction of sagittal diameter is less than11 mm or 7 mm (in neck extension).

3. Plain X-ray Lumbar Spine AP and Lateral View
- Inter pedicular distance decreased
- AP diameter < 15 mm

$$\frac{\text{AP diameter of canal} \times \text{inter pedicular distance}}{\text{AP diameter of body} \times \text{Transverse diameter of the body}}$$
$$= > 1.4 \text{ indicates lumbar canal stenosis}$$

4. Myelography
It provides evidence of nature of cord, nerve roots and dimension of the vertebral canal and the root outlets.

5. CT Scan and MRI
They are extremely valuable after myelography.

It provides evidence of overall transverse axial dimensions of the canal and the foramina and helps in the better assessment of cord compression.

MRI is the first choice when investigating suspected lesions of the spinal cord.

6. EMG Study
It provides differentiation of root lesions from other plexopathies and thoracic outlet problems.

Management
Medical
1. Rest
2. Analgesics
3. Cervical immobilisation with soft cervical collar (cervical spondylosis)
4. Spinal braces (lumbar canal stenosis)
   Cervical collar/spinal braces should be worn for a maximum of two to three weeks. Prolonged passive cervical/lumbar support may lead to muscle weakness and interfere with rehabilitation.

Surgical
Indications
1. Failure of medical treatment
2. Objective signs of root lesion or cord lesion.

Procedure: Decompression by laminectomy

Lumbar Disc Prolapse
The patient is usually an adult between 20 and 40 years of age. The commonest site of lumbar disc prolapse is L4- L5.

Symptoms
Low back ache
Acute back ache is severe with the spine held rigid by muscle spasm and any movement at the spine is painful.

Chronic back ache is dull and diffuse usually made worse by exertion, forward bending, sitting or standing in one position for a long time.

Sciatic pain
- The pain radiates to the gluteal region, back of the thigh and leg.
- In S1 root compression pain radiates to the posterolateral calf and heel.
- In L5 root compression pain radiates to anterolateral aspect of the leg and ankle.

Femoral root pain:
- In a disc prolapse at a higher level L2-L3 pain radiates to the front of thigh.

Tests for Nerve Root Compression
Tests for Sciatic Nerve Root (L5-S1) (Fig. 8.117)
Straight leg raising Test: (SLR)
Raise the affected leg with the knee in extended position (while preventing knee flexion on the normal side), pain

Neurological Deficit in Disc Prolapse

Level	Nerve root	Motor weakness	Sensory loss	Reflexes
L5-S1	S1 root	Weakness of plantar flexors of the foot	Over lateral side of the foot	Ankle jerk absent
L4-L5	L5 root	Weakness of EHL and dorsiflexors of the foot	Over dorsum of the foot and lateral side of the leg	Ankle jerk normal
L3-L4	L4 root	Weakness of extension of the knee	Over the great toe and medial side of the leg	Knee jerk absent

at 40° or less denotes positivity and it is suggestive of root compression.

Bragaard Test

Gentle dorsiflexion of the ankle precipitates further tension to the nerve root on reaching the limit in straight leg raising test.

Lasegue Test

First the thigh is lifted to 90° with the knee bent. The knee is then gradually extended. If the nerve sheath is pressed, patient will experience pain in the back of the thigh or leg and the pain radiates to the back.

Bowstring Sign

After performing the Lasegue's test, apply firm pressure with the thumb over the posterior tibial nerve in the middle of the popliteal fossa and over the hamstring tendon. Now, the posterior tibial nerve is strtched like a bowstring across the popliteal fossa causing pain locally and radiation to the back.

Flip Test

The patient is seated on the edge of the couch with the hips and knees flexed to 90 degrees. Gently extend the knee. When there is root irritation, the patient will 'flip' backwards to relieve the tension on the nerve root. In the absence of root compression, full extension of the knee is possible.

Test for Femoral Nerve Root (L2-L3-L4) (Fig. 8.118)

Femoral Nerve Stretch Test

In prone position femoral roots are slack and there is no pain. Tighten the femoral roots by flexion of the knee which causes pain in the back. If there is no pain femoral roots are further stretched by extension of the hip. This test is positive when the femoral roots are compressed.

Management

Conservative Treatment

1. Absolute rest
2. Drugs—Analgesics and muscle relaxants
3. Physiotherapy
4. Lumbar traction
5. Trans-cutaneous electrical nerve stimulation.

Surgical Treatment

Indications:
* Failure of conservative treatment
* Central disc prolapse with neurological deficit
* Recurrent disc prolapse
* Bladder/bowel involvement
* Acute disc prolapse with excruciating pain – not relieved by drugs.

Operative procedures:
1. *Fenestration:* The ligamentum flavum bridging the two adjacent laminae is excised and the spinal cord is exposed.
2. *Laminotomy:* In addition to fenestration, a hole is made in the lamina.
3. *Hemilaminectomy:* The whole of the lamina one side is removed.
4. *Laminectomy:* The laminae on both sides are removed.

Paraplegia

Paraplegia means weakness or paralysis of the lower limbs, sparing the upper limbs. It can occur in disorders of the cerebrum, spinal cord, spinal roots, peripheral nerves or muscles.

I. Intracranial Causes

1. Trauma : Parasagittal region
2. Tumour : Parasagittal meningioma
3. Thrombosis

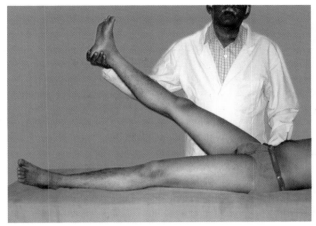

Stage 1- Straight leg raising test

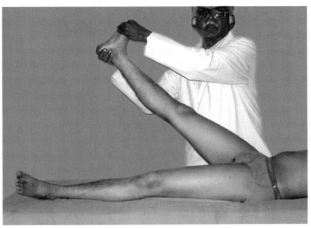

Stage 2- Dorsiflexion of ankle (Bragaard test)

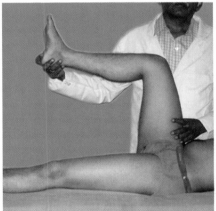

Lasegue test   Stage 1- Flex the hip with knee flexed

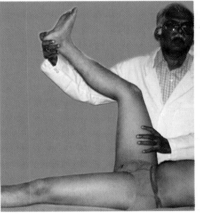

Stage 2- Extend knee, look for Lasegue sign

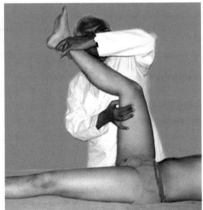

Stage 3- Press with thumb (Bowstring's sign)

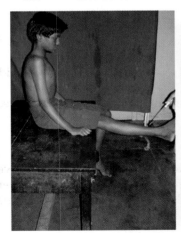

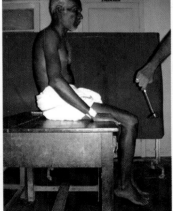

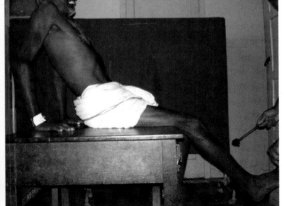

Negative response ➡ Flip test ◄ Positive response - on extending the knee the patient flips backwards due to tension on the nerve root

Fig. 8.117: Stretch test—sciatic nerve roots

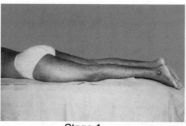
Stage 1

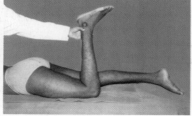
Stage 2

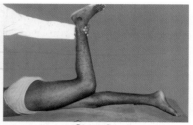
Stage 3

Fig. 8.118: Stretch test—femoral nerve roots

a. Arterial
   i. Unpaired anterior cerebral artery
   ii. Bilateral anterior cerebral artery
b. Venous
   i. Sagittal sinus thrombosis

True cortical lesion may cause flaccid paraplegia with bladder involvement and there may be difficulty in differentiating it from LMN type of paraplegia.

The following features help in differentiating from LMN lesions
1. Cortical sensory loss
2. Jacksonian fits

However spastic weakness can occur due to involvement of descending pyramidal fibres in subcortical regions.

Cerebral Palsy (Cerebral Diplegia)

Cerebral palsy may result in tetraplegia where the degree of involvement is more in the lower limbs than the upper limbs.

Causes

1. Birth injuries
2. Cerebral anoxia
3. Faulty myelination
4. Maternal infection.

Clinical Features

1. It is present from childhood
2. Lower limbs are affected more than upper limbs
3. The limbs are clumsy
4. UMN signs (stiffness of muscle, - DTR, scissor gait, Babinski's sign)
5. Early bladder involvement is present
6. It presents with delayed motor development with or without cognitive dysfunction
7. Other features are
   a. Cerebellar ataxia
   b. Speech disturbance
   c. Convulsions.

II. Spinal Causes

It may be acute or chronic.

Acute Causes

1. Fracture dislocation
2. Vascular
   a. Endarteritis (TB, syphilis)
   b. Thrombosis of anterior spinal artery
3. Haematomyelia (AVM, angioma)
4. Epidural abscess
5. Necrotizing myelitis.

Acute Transverse Myelitis

Clinical Features (Fig. 8.119)

It is of acute onset with total transection of cord. At times it may evolve over a period of several days to weeks.
1. Back pain or root pain may or may not be present

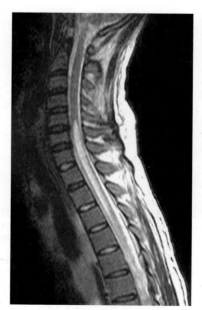

Fig. 8.119: Transverse myelitis

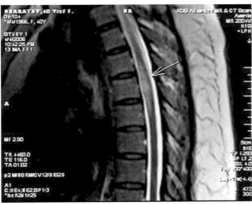

Demyelination in spinal cord

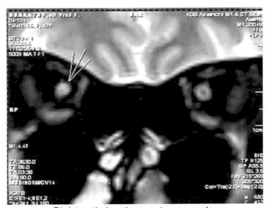

Right optic involvement seen as loss
of central low intensity signal

Fig. 8.120: Devic's disease

2. Motor loss (total) ⎫ below the level
3. Sensory loss (all modalities) ⎬ of lesion
4. Bladder involvement
5. The most common site is mid thoracic region
6. 70% of patient recover within 3 months

Devic's Disease (Neuromyelitis Optica)

A form of transverse myelitis with demyelination of both optic nerve and optic chiasma. The optic nerve involvement may precede or follow the transverse myelitis (Fig. 8.120).

Causes of Pure Spastic Paraplegia

1. Motor neuron disease
2. Erb's paraplegia
3. Hereditary spastic paraplegia
4. Lathyrism
5. Fluorosis.

Compressive Myelopathy

Mechanism of Cord Involvement

1. Pressure effect
2. Ischaemia (arterial)
3. Congestion (veins)
4. Interruption of CSF flow (Froin's syndrome).

Mode of Compression

In general, slow spinal compression affects the pyramidal tract first, the posterior column next, and the spinothalamic tract last. In compression at cervical region, the order of involvement is first ipsilateral upper limb, and ipsilateral lower limb and then lower limb of contralateral side and finally contralateral side of upper limb. This is known as Elseberg phenomenon.

Effects of the lesion

1. Anterior horn cell: LMN signs (wasting, weakness and fasciculations)
2. Posterior root: root pain or girdle pain (trunk)
3. Posterior column: Lhermitte's sign (unpleasant sensation) Constriction band around the trunk
4. Pyramidal system: UMN signs (stiffness and spasticity).

In compressive lesions, the involvement of diaphragm is rare due to partial involvement and in traumatic conditions it is common.

However these fine differentiating features do not hold true at all times in all cases of compressive myelopathy.

Localisation of Spinal Cord Lesions at Different Segmental Levels

Foramen Magnum

The clinical features depend upon the position and size of the tumour.
a. Atrophy of sternomastoid muscle
b. Downbeat nystagmus
c. C_2 sensory loss and cerebellar signs
d. Horner's syndrome
e. Lower cranial nerve palsy

Cervicomedullary Junction

Hemiplegia Cruciata

The paresis or paralysis of ipsilateral lower limb and contralateral upper limb. This is due to arm fibres crossing before the leg fibres at the lower part of the medulla and this is the reason for hemiplegia cruciata.

Differentiation between Intramedullary and Exrtamedullary Lesions of the Cord

Features	Extramedullary	Intramedullary
Motor system		
1. Upper motor neuron sign	Common and persist	Less common
i. Spasticity		
ii. Muscle spasm		
2. Lower motor neuron signs		
i. Muscle atrophy	One or two segments at the site of root compression	Wide due to anterior horn involvement
ii. Trophic changes of the skin	Not common	Present
iii. Fasciculation	Rare	Common
Sensory system		
1. Root pain	Common	Rare
2. *Funicular pain	Not present	Present
3. Dysesthesias and paresthesias	Rare	Common
4. Dissociated sensory loss	Absent	Present
5. Sacral sensation	Lost	Sacral sparing for pain and temperature
6. Joint position sense	Lost	Spared
7. Lhermitte's sign	Present	Absent
Autonomic nervous system		
Bowel and bladder disturbances	Late	Early
Investigations		
1. X-ray of the spine	Bony changes may be seen	Not seen
2. Effect of lumbar puncture	Signs and symptoms are precipitated or increased	No such effect
3. Alteration in CSF	Frequently present	Absent
4. Manometry changes (Quecken stedt's)	Early change	Late change

*Funicular pain—Diffuse, burning pain

Differentiation between Intradural and Extradural Lesions of the Cord

Features	Intradural	Extradural
Mode of onset	Asymmetrical	Symmetrical
Vertebral pain (Local tenderness)	Not common	Common

C₂ Segment Level

Suboccipital pain or sensory loss; descending tract of V nerve (pain and temperature loss over the face) exaggerated trapezius reflex.

C₃ Segment Level

Loss of trapezius reflex.

C₅ Segment Level

1. Inverted biceps jerk
2. Inverted brachioradialis jerk (supinator jerk)
3. Sensory loss over deltoid.

C₆ Segment Level

The loss or diminished biceps and supinator reflexes with exaggerated finger flexor reflex.

C₇ Segment Level

1. Paresis of flexors and extensors of the wrist and fingers
2. Preservation of biceps and supinator reflexes
3. Exaggerated finger flexor reflexes
4. Inverted triceps reflex.

C₈ and T₁ Segment Level

1. Weakness and wasting of the small muscles of the hand
2. UMN signs in the lower limb
3. Uni or bilateral Horner's syndrome.

Thoracic Segments

1. Girdle pain or paraesthesia
2. Segmental LMN involvement (very difficult to make out clinically)
3. Autonomic nervous system dysfunction.

T₃ Segment Level

Sensory impairment in axilla.

T₄ Segment Level

Sensory impairment below the level of nipple.

T₆ Segment Level

The abdominal reflex is impaired or lost (in all quadrants).

T₁₀ Segment Level

Positive Beevor's sign (intact upper abdominal reflexes and absent lower abdominal reflexes with pull of umbilicus more than 3 cm on raising the head).

T₁₂ Segment Level

Abdominal reflex preserved.

L₁ Segment Level

1. The sensory loss in the lower limbs starts from the level of groin.
2. Brisk ankle and knee jerks
3. Absence of cremasteric reflex.

Features	Conus medullaris (S₃ S₄ S₅ and coccygeal)	Cauda equina
1. Onset	Symmetrical	Asymmetrical
2. Dissociated sensory loss	Present	Not present
3. Root pain	Rare	Common
4. Fasciculation	Rare	Common
5. Decubitus ulcer	Rare	Common
6. Bladder and bowel	Early	Early or late depending on root involvement

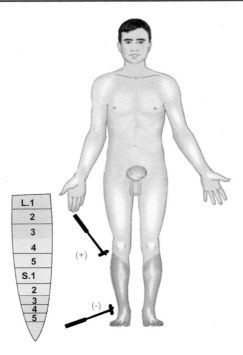

Fig. 8.122: Epiconus lesion (L₄-S₂)

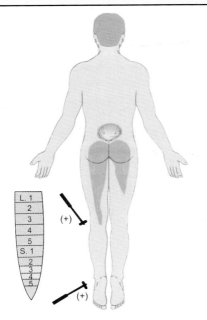

Fig. 8.121: Conus lesion (S3, S4)

Features	Conus medullaris (S₃ S₄ S₅ and coccygeal) Pure conus	Epiconus (L₄L₅S₁S₂)
Bladder involvement	distension	–
Faecal incontinence	present	not present
Saddle anaesthesia	present	not present
Motor symptoms	absent	paralysis of muscles of lower limb

However, it may be difficult to clinically distingush lesions confined to each of these fine anatomical divisions, and there may be an overlap of signs of conus and epiconus producing extensor plantar reponse (Figs 8.121 and 8.122).

Most Common Causes of Paraplegia

1. Trauma
2. Tumour
3. Tuberculosis
4. Thrombosis
5. Transverse myelitis.

Paraplegia in Flexion and Paraplegia in Extension

Muscle tone is maintained by spinal reflex arc, extrapyramidal system, corticospinal tract and cerebellum. The final modulation is controlled by intact corticospinal tract. When corticospinal tract alone is affected, the extrapyramidal system (especially reticulospinal tract) takes the upper hand, resulting in increased tone of antigravity muscles (paraplegia in extension). When the influence of the extrapyramidal system is cut off, the spinal arc takes over and there is a relative increase in tone of the flexors (hamstring and ilio-psoas) more than the extensors (paraplegia in flexion).

Features	Paraplegia in extension	Paraplegia in flexion
1. Mode of transection	Incomplete transection (only corticospinal tract involved)	Complete transection (affects both corticospinal and extra-pyramidal)
2. Evolution	Early	Late
3. Flexor withdrawal reflex	Not present	Present
4. Mass reflex	Not present	Present Any stimulus below the level of lesion produces a. Flexor spasm b. Emptying of the bladder and bowel c. Seminal emission

Persistent Flaccid Paraplegia in UMN Lesions

1. Urinary tract infection
2. Malnutrition
3. Bed sore
4. Stress and strain.

Bladder Innervation

Pattern of Innervation (Fig. 8.123)

1. Parasympathetic—S_2 S_3 S_4 segments
2. Sympathetic—thoraco-lumbar outflow (T_{11} T_{12} L_1 L_2 segments)
3. Somatic—pudendal nerve from S_2 S_3 S_4.

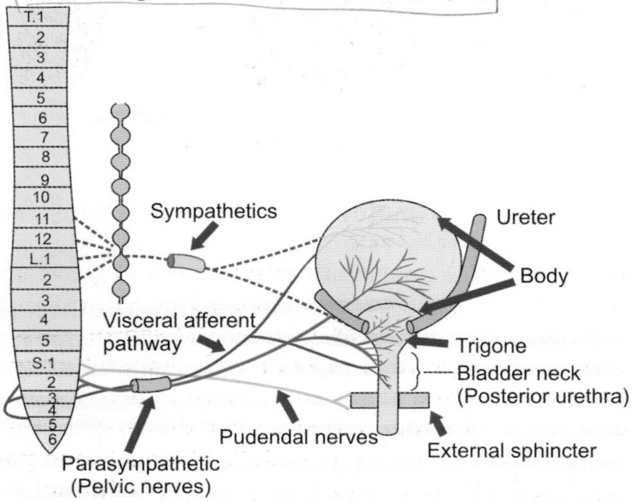

Fig. 8.123: Urinary bladder and its innervation

Motor

1. Detrusor muscle—parasympathetic S_2-S_4 through pelvic nerve.
2. Trigone muscle—sympathetic T_{11}-L_2 segments through presacral and hypogastric nerves.
3. External sphincter and perineal muscle—pudendal nerve.

Sympathetic system involvement results in retrograde ejaculation of semen into bladder (infertility). Bladder function is predominantly maintained by para-sympathetic system. The parasympathetic system dysfunction leads to the following types of bladder.

1. Incomplete Spastic or Uninhibited Bladder (Cortical Bladder)

Cortical lesions
a. Post-central—Loss of awareness of bladder fullness, incontinence
b. Precentral—Difficulty in initiating micturition
c. Frontal—Inappropriate micturition, loss of social control (It is akin to infant's bladder—frequent voiding at every 100 cc and no residual urine).

2. Complete Spastic or Reflex Bladder or Automatic Bladder or Hypertonic Bladder

Lesions in the spinal segments above S_2 S_3 S_4.

3. Autonomous Bladder or Hypotonic

Lesions at S_2 S_3 S_4 and cauda equina.

4. Sensory Paralytic Bladder (Afferent pathway)

- Impairment of afferent pathways innervating the bladder
- Common causes
  Diabetes mellitus
  Syringomyelia
  Tabes dorsalis
- Intact voluntary initiation of micturition
- Urinary retention-Overflow incontinence
- Frequent urinary tract infection

5. Motor Paralytic Bladder (Efferent pathway)

- Lesions involving efferent motor fibers innervating detrusor
- Lumbar canal stenosis
- Lumbo-sacral meningo- myelocele
- Complication following-Radical hysterectomy, Abdomino-perineal resection
- Painful urinary retention

Drug Therapy in Bladder Dysfunction

Drugs	Indications	Mechanism of action
Bethanechol 25-50 mg QID	Retention without obstruction as in neurogenic bladder or postoperative -Facilitates emptying	Stimulation of parasympathetic nervous system → detrusor contraction
Prazosin 1-2 mg BID/TID Terazosin 1-4 mg Doxazosin 1-4 mg	Outlet obstruction as in benign prostatic hypertrophy or bladder neck obstruction/dysfunction	α_1 blockade of external sphincter *= relaxation (symp) pudendal n)*
Hyoscyamine 0.125mg HS or 0.25 mg TID Imipramine 25-100 mg HS	Urge incontinence	Relaxes detrusor and increases internal sphincter tone
Oxybutynin 5 mg TID/QID Tolterodine tartarate (Detrol/Detrositol) 2 mg TID/QID	Urinary incontinence Increased frequency and urgency as a result of neurogenic or overactive bladder	Anticholinergics and direct antispasmodics cause relaxation of detrusor, Muscarinic receptor antagonist -relaxes detrusor and increases internal sphincter tone

In cauda equina lesion and in tabes dorsalis, the bladder is more atonic and accepts a very large volume of urine (atonic bladder).

In compressive myelopathy, paraplegia in flexion denotes dense lesion. In transverse myelitis, paraplegia in flexion is an early sign of recovery.

Myelogram Appearance (Figs 8.124 and 8.125)

1. Extramedullary
   a. Extradural—Brush border appearance
   b. Intradural—Meniscus sign
2. Intramedullary
   a. Obliteration of subarachnoid space
   b. Enlargement of cord.

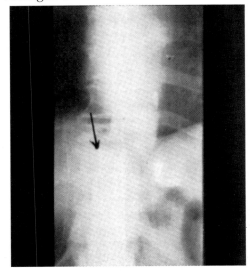

Fig. 8.124: Myelogram—extradural obstruction at D_{10} level

3. Arachnoiditis
   Candle guttering appearance (multiple areas of patchy deposits).

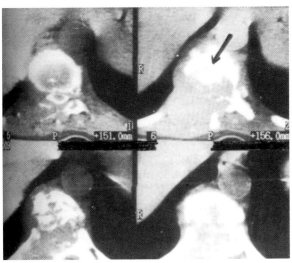

Fig. 8.125: CT dorsal spine—destruction of vertebra due to secondaries

Syringomyelia

It is defined as a chronic progressive degenerative disorder of spinal cord characterised clinically by brachial amyotrophy and segmental sensory loss of dissociated type (loss of pain and temperature with retained touch) and pathologically by cavitation of central part of spinal cord usually in the cervical region but extends upwards into medulla oblongata and pons (syringobulbia) or downwards into thoracic or lumbosacral segments.

Classification

Group I   Idiopathic polymyositis
Group II Idiopathic dermatomyositis
Group III Dermatomyositis (polymyositis) associated
          with neoplasia
Group IV Childhood dermatomyositis associated with
          vasculitis
Group V   Polymyositis with collagen vascular disease

Clinical Features

I. Idiopathic Polymyositis

1. It is insidiously progressive over weeks or months
2. The female and male ratio is 2 : 1
3. The ocular muscles are spared
4. The reflexes are disproportionately reduced (carcinoma with polymyositis and polyneuropathy or Eaton-Lambert syndrome should be considered)
5. The other features are dysphagia (25%) and cardiac abnormalities (ECG changes, arrthythmias, CCF secondary to myocarditis)
6. The respiratory symptom is dyspnoea (due to lympho-cytic pneumonitis, pulmonary edema and pulmonary fibrosis).

II. Idiopathic Dermatomyositis

1. The skin changes may precede or follow the muscle syndrome
2. The localized or diffuse erythema; maculopapular eruption
3. Scaling eczematoid dermatitis, exfoliative dermatitis
4. "Heliotrope rash"—butterfly distribution
5. Itching and periorbital edema
6. Subcutaneous calcification
7. Erythematous rash over the anterior chest—V sign
8. Erythematous rash over the back and shoulders—Shawl sign.

III. Dermatomyositis (Polymyositis) Associated with Neoplasia

1. The malignancy may antedate or postdate the onset of the myositis by up to 2 years.
2. The most common malignancies (ca lung, breast, ovary, GIT and myeloproliferative disorders).

IV. Childhood Dermatomyositis Associated with Vasculitis

It is associated with vasculitis in skin and GIT.

V. Polymyositis with Collagen Vascular Disease

Dysphagia is a common symptom of this group (due to the involvement of the smooth muscle of the distal 1/3 of esophagus in systemic sclerosis).

It is associated with connective tissue disorder (rheumatoid arthritis, systemic lupus erythematosus, systemic sclerosis, malignancy, sarcoidosis).

Extramuscular Manifestations

1. Systemic symptoms—fever, malaise, weight loss, arthralgia and Raynaud's phenomenon.
2. GI symptoms—Dysphagia, GI ulcerations.
3. Cardiac symptoms—AV conduction defects, tachyarryhthmias, dilated cardiomyopathy, congestive cardiac failure and myocarditis.
4. Pulmonary symptoms—may result from interstitial lung disease and thoracic myopathy.

Investigations

1. *Serum enzymes* (CK, aldolase, AST, LDH and ALT) are increased
2. *ESR* is raised
3. *EMG:* It reveals a markedly increased insertional activity (muscle irritability) together with the typical myopathic triad of motor unit action potentials which are of low amplitude, polyphasic and have an abnormally early recruitment.
4. *Muscle biopsy:* The muscle biopsy reveals inflammatory cell infiltrates, destruction of muscle fibres with a phagocytic reaction, and perivascular (perivenular) inflammatory cell infiltration (hallmark of polymyositis).

Treatment

Step 1: Oral prednisolone 1 mg/kg/day for 3-4 weeks followed by tapering slowly over a period of 10 weeks to 1 mg/kg every alternate day.

Step 2: Immunosuppressive drugs—usually started when the patient fails to respond to glucocorticoids after 3 months of treatment, glucocorticoid resistance, glucocorticoid related side effects, rapidly progressive disease with respiratory failure.
   A. Azathioprine 3 mg/kg/day.
   B. Methotrexate 7.5 mg weekly for 3 weeks followed by gradual increase up to 25 mg/week.

Step 3: IV 1 g 2 gm/kg divided over 2-5 days per course repeated every 6-8 weeks.

Step 4: Other drugs—Cyclophosphamide, chlorambucil, mycophenolate mofetil.

Muscular Dystrophies

They are a group of hereditary disorders characterised by progressive degeneration of selective group of muscles without involvement of nervous system.

Classification

The 'pure' muscular dystrophies:
1. *X-Linked muscular dystrophy*
   a. Severe (Duchenne)
   b. Benign (Becker)
   c. Benign with acanthocytes (Mcleod syndrome)
   d. Benign with early contractures (Emery-Dreifuss)
   e. Scapuloperoneal (rare)
2. *Autosomal recessive muscular dystrophy*
   a. Limb-girdle (usually scapulohumeral, rarely pelvifemoral)
   b. Distal type
   c. Childhood type, resembling Duchenne
   d. Congenital muscular dystrophy
3. *Autosomal dominant muscular dystrophy*
   a. Facioscapulohumeral
   b. Scapuloperoneal
   c. Late-onset proximal (limb-girdle)
   d. Benign early onset with contractures
   e. Distal
   f. Ocular
   g. Oculopharyngeal.

Duchenne Dystrophy

1. *Inheritance:* X-linked recessive
2. *Age of onset:* Between 3 and 10 years
3. Proximal muscles of upper limbs and lower limbs are predominantly affected, later involving the diaphragm, neck muscles, extraocular muscles, and facial muscles. Patients may become bed bound within 1st decade of life.
4. Pseudohypertrophy of the muscle is present (enlargement of calf muscle, quadriceps and deltoids)
5. The associated features are macroglossia, absence of incisor teeth, low (less than 10% of normal) I.Q., skeletal atrophy and deformity (long bones become pencil thin and fracture), and cardiac involvement (persistent tachycardia, tall R-waves in the right precordial leads and deep Q-waves in limb leads and left precordial leads).

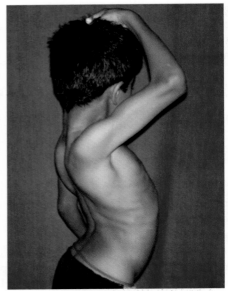

Fig. 8.129: Lumbar lordosis in Duchenne dystrophy

Investigations

1. The serum CK value is 20 to 100 times the normal
2. EMG—myopathic pattern
3. Muscle biopsy—The dystrophin deficiency is seen (Western blot analysis).

Treatment

Prednisolone 0.75 mg/kg/day significantly slows the progression of disease up to 3 yr.

Becker's Dystrophy

1. *Inheritance:* X-linked recessive
2. *Age of onset:* Between 5 and 25 years
3. The pelvic and pectoral muscles are predominantly affected
4. The patients are unable to walk after about 25 years of onset (benign course)
5. The associated features are cardiac involvement, contractures, skeletal deformity and hypertrophy of the muscles.

Investigations

Same as in Duchenne dystrophy.

Prognosis

The longevity is better than Duchenne dystrophy.

Limb Girdle Muscular Dystrophy

1. *Inheritance:* Autosomal recessive and equally affects both sexes.

2. *The age of onset:* Between 10 and 30 years.
3. Pelvic and shoulder girdle muscles are predominantly affected.
4. Patients notice disability only after 10 to 20 years of onset.
5. The proximal tendon reflexes are absent except ankle jerk.
6. The pseudomuscular hypertrophy is an associated feature (calves and deltoids).
7. The cardiac involvement and mental deficiency are rare.

Investigations

The serum enzymes are raised.

Prognosis

Normal lifespan.

Facio-scapulo-humoral Dystrophy

1. *Inheritance:* Autosomal dominant and equally affects both sexes.
2. The muscles predominantly affected are facial muscles, shoulder girdle muscles and serratus anterior.
3. The biceps and triceps jerks are diminished.
4. Patients may have absent pectoralis and biceps muscles.
5. The progression is slow and disability is less (pseudohypertrophy is rare).

Investigation

The serum enzymes (CK) are raised.

Prognosis

Normal lifespan.

Oculopharyngeal Dystrophy

Clinical Features

1. *Inheritance:* Autosomal dominant.
2. Patients have external ophthalmoplegia. Ptosis and/or dysphagia occur in the 4th to 6th decades.
3. Mild neck and limb weakness can occur.

Investigations

a. The serum CK may be 2–3 times normal.
b. *Biopsy:* The distinct feature is the presence of tubular filaments, of 8.5 nm in diameter within muscle nuclei.

Treatment

a. Cricopharyngeal myotomy may improve swallowing (does not prevent aspiration)

b. Eyelid crutches improve vision in patients with ptosis.

Congenital Muscular Dystrophy

It is mostly sporadic (without CNS involvement) and sometimes of autosomal recessive inheritance.

Clinical Features

1. It is present at birth or within a few months of life.
2. The signs and symptoms are hypotonia, proximal limb weakness, and joint contractures at the elbows, hips, knees and the ankles (contractures at birth is known as arthrogryposis).

Types

1. *Fukuyama congenital muscular dystrophy:* The features are generalised tonic-clonic seizures and delayed development of both mental and verbal status, microcephaly and enlarged ventricles.
2. *Cerebro-ocular-dysplasia muscular dystrophy:* The features are cataract, retinal dysplasia and hypoplasia of the optic nerve.

Investigation

Serum CK level ranges from normal to 20 times normal.

Treatment

Supportive care.

Congenital Myopathies

1. Central Core Disease

The features are
1. Inheritance: Autosomal dominant and may be sporadic also
2. Decreased fetal movements and breech presentation
3. Skeletal abnormalities (congenital hip dislocation, scoliosis, pes cavus, and clubbed feet)
4. Hypotonia and delayed motor milestones.

Investigations

1. Serum CK is normal
2. EMG: Myopathic pattern
3. Muscle biopsy shows single or multiple central or eccentric discrete zones (cores) devoid of oxidative enzymes and diminished PAS staining.

Treatment

It is essential because it predisposes to malignant hyperthermia during general anaesthesia.

2. Nemaline Myopathy
Clinical Features

1. *Inheritance:* Autosomal dominant and may be sporadic
2. Severe neonatal hypotonia with respiratory distress are present
3. Patients may have delayed milestones and they have long, narrow facies or head, high arched palate and open mouth appearance due to prognathous jaw
4. The other skeletal abnormalities are pectus excavatum, kyphoscoliosis, pes cavus, and clubbed foot
5. Myocardial involvement is an unusual presentation.

Investigations

1. Serum CK is normal
2. *EMG:* Myopathic pattern
3. *Muscle biopsy:* The diagnostic features are clusters of small rods or nemaline bodies.

3. Centronuclear Myopathy
It is of X-linked recessive inheritance.

Types

1. Neonatal Form
The clinical features are
a. Severe hypotonia and weakness at birth
b. Respiratory distress
c. Poor prognosis.

2. Late Infantile-childhood Form
The clinical features are
a. Delayed milestones (especially walking)
b. Ptosis
c. Ophthalmoplegia
d. Marfanoid features.

3. Childhood-adult Type
The clinical features are
a. Onset: Second or third decade
b. Sparing of ocular movements
c. Mild nonprogressive limb weakness
d. No skeletal abnormalities.

Investigations

1. Normal or slightly elevated CK level
2. EMG features are
   a. Positive sharp waves
   b. Fibrillation potentials
   c. Complex and repetitive discharges.

3. *Muscle biopsy:* The features are rows of central nuclei often surrounded by a halo.

Treatment
Supportive care.

Dystrophia Myotonica

1. Inheritance: Autosomal dominant
2. Age of onset: Between 20 and 60 years
3. The predominant muscles affected are temporalis, facial, masseter, sternomastoid ('hatchet face' and swan neck) and distal group of muscles (quadriceps and tibialis anterior). Sternomastoid is absent in some cases. Patients may have a transverse smile (due to delayed relaxation)
4. The tendon reflexes are depressed
5. Difficulty in releasing the hand after making 'fist'
6. The patient is unable to walk within 15 to 20 years of onset of the disease
7. The associated features are early frontal baldness, ptosis, gynaecomastia, cardiac involvement (cardiomyopathy and mitral valve prolapse) bronchiectasis, altered oesophageal, bowel and biliary tree motility, testicular atrophy, bone changes, mental defect (dementia) hypersomnia, and abnormalities of serum immunoglobulin
8. Patients have 'phenomenon of anticipation', i.e., the disease occurs much earlier in successive generations
9. Formation of dimple in thenar muscles or tongue or wrist extensors on percussion.

Investigations

1. Serum CK level—normal or mildly elevated
2. EMG   Myopathic pattern
3. Muscle biopsy

Management

1. Phenytoin for myotonia (Other drugs which can be used for myotonia are quinine and procainamide. They should not be used in patients with heart block).
2. Pace maker for heart blocks.

Prognosis
Poor.

Myotonia Congenita (Thomson's Disease)

1. Inheritance: Autosomal dominant
2. Age of onset: From birth
3. Muscular hypertrophy occurs in the second decade.
4. Athletic ability is poor (due to slowness and stiffness)

5. It is worse in the cold seasons (performance of winter games is not possible)
6. The peculiar features are
    a. Formation of dimple in the thenar muscles of the hand and tongue after percussion
    b. Demonstration of myotonia (difficulty in opening the hand after making 'fist')
7. Patients have normal life expectancy.

Paramyotonia Congenita

1. The myotonia (tonic spasm of muscle) and muscle paralysis occur on exposure to cold
2. It is similar to hyperkalaemic periodic paralysis
3. The responsible gene on chromosome 17q 13.1–13.3 causes a defect of the sodium channel a subunit.

Drugs and Myopathy

1. Drugs causing focal damage or fibrosis
    a. Intramuscular opiates
    b. Antibiotics
    c. Paraldehyde
2. Drugs causing necrosis
    a. Heroin
    b. Clofibrate
    c. Epsilon aminocaproic acid
3. Drugs causing myoglobinuria/rhabdomyolysis
    a. Heroin
    b. Methadone
    c. Amphetamine
    d. Barbiturates
    e. Diazepam
    f. INH
    g. Carbenoxalone
    h. Amphotericin B
4. Drugs causing hypokalaemia
    a. Diuretics
    b. Carbenoxalone
    c. Liquorice
    d. Purgatives
5. Drugs causing inflammation
    a. Procainamide
    b. D-penicillamine
    c. L-dopa
6. Drugs causing subacute or painless proximal myopathy
    a. Corticosteroid
    b. Chloroquine
    c. β-blocker
7. Drugs causing myasthenic syndrome
    a. D-penicillamine
    b. Aminoglycoside antibiotic

8. Drugs causing malignant hyperpyrexia
    a. Suxamethonium
    b. Halothane
    c. Cyclopropane
    d. Enflurane, ketamine.

Inflammatory Muscle Disease

1. Bacterial
    a. *Clostridium welchii* gas gangrene
    b. Diphtheria—extraocular myopathy
2. Viral
    a. Influenza—mimics acute poliomyelitis
    b. Bornholm disease—general myalgia and inter costal tenderness
3. Parasite
    a. *Trichinella spiralis* (trichinosis)—extraocular myopathy
    b. *Taenia solium* (cysticercosis) muscle hypertrophy (thigh and deltoid region).

Myasthenia Gravis

Myasthenia gravis is a neuromuscular disorder characterised by weakness and fatiguability of skeletal muscles due to decrease in number of Ach receptors at neuromuscular junction due to antibody. It occurs at any age and is more common in young adults. This may be associated with other autoimmune disorders (thymic tumours, thyrotoxicosis, rheumatoid arthritis and disseminated lupus erythematosus).

It is more common in females than males. It has a predilection for extraocular muscles and muscles of mastication, facial, pharyngeal and laryngeal muscles. The respiratory and limb muscles (proximal and asymmetric) may also be affected.

Myasthenia Gravis and Thymoma

1. Thymus gland is the primary source of T cells and it undergoes atrophy after the age of 12 years.
2. It is hyperplastic and enlarged in 70% of cases of myasthenia gravis.
3. The cells in the hyperplastic follicles are B cells, plasma cells and T-helper cells.
4. Myoid cells in the thymus sensitize the immune system to the Ach receptor protein.

Clinical Features

1. It is insidious in onset.
2. The exacerbations occur in pregnancy or before menses.

Empty Sella Syndrome

Types

Primary

Empty sella syndrome is due to congenital incomplete diaphragma sella which allows CSF to enter into the sella as an extension of the subarachnoid space. Normal pulsatile CSF pressure then compresses the pituitary and gradually expands the sella turcica. Primary empty sella is most often found in obese, middle-aged women.

This may result in compression of the pituitary stalk and thereby decreased transport of hypothalamic releasing hormones to the anterior pituitary (usual hormone deficiencies are those of gonadotrophic hormone and GH). There is no abnormality in function of the posterior pituitary gland.

Secondary

Empty sella syndrome is found in various pituitary tumours following infarction, ablation, destruction by surgery, radiotherapy, or following shrinkage after medical therapy.

Treatment

1. No treatment other than reassurance (primary)
2. Hormone replacement may be useful in secondary empty sella syndrome of pituitary origin.

Craniopharyngioma

It is a tumour of developmental origin arising from Rathke's pouch. The peak incidence is in the second decade of life.

Craniopharyngiomas are cystic in 60% of cases, solid in 15% of cases and combined cystic and solid in 25% of cases.

The tumour originates above the sella. It causes pressure on the optic chiasma, hypothalamus and pituitary, resulting in increased intracranial pressure, visual defects, endocrine hypofunction (e.g. GH deficiency in children), hyperprolactinemia and mental deficiency.

Investigations

1. X-ray skull—enlargement or erosion of sella with supra- or intrasellar calcification
2. CT and MRI are useful.

Treatment

1. Surgery

2. Radiation therapy
3. Hormone replacement therapy.

Disorder of the Neurohypophysis

Diabetes Insipidus (DI)

Diabetes insipidus is the excretion of a large amount of dilute urine (hypotonic polyuria).

The criteria to be satisfied in order to establish this diagnosis are:
   a. Polyuria of more than 3 lit/day (more than 50 ml/kg/day)
   b. Urine osmolality less than 300 mOsm/kg
   c. Urine specific gravity less than 1.010.

Aetiology

Diabetes insipidus may result from any one of the three defects:
1. Inadequate secretion of arginine vasopressin (AVP) or anti-diuretic hormone (ADH) known as *central*, or *neurogenic DI*.
2. Impaired renal responsiveness to AVP, known as *nephrogenic DI*.
3. Increased water intake of primary polydipsia, known as *dipsogenic DI*.

Central DI

Causes of Central DI

1. Familial (autosomal dominant)
2. Acquired
   a. Idiopathic
   b. Trauma or surgery to the hypothalamus-posterior pituitary region
   c. Tumours (craniopharyngioma, meningioma, metastatic carcinoma, lymphoma, carcinoma of breast and lung)
   d. Infection (encephalitis, meningitis)
   e. Granulomatous disease (sarcoidosis, histiocytosis, Wegener's disease)
   f. Vascular disorders (aneurysm, Sheehan's syndrome, aortocoronary bypass)
   g. Drugs-diphenyl hydantoin and alcohol
   h. Autoimmune-lymphocytic hypophysitis (rare).

Criteria to Diagnose Central DI

a. Inappropriately dilute urine in the presence of strong osmotic or non-osmotic stimuli for AVP secretion.
b. Absence of intrinsic renal disease.

c. A rise in urine osmolality following the administration of AVP.

Clinical Features

Central DI manifests itself clinically when AVP secretory capacity is reduced by more than 75%.

The cardinal symptoms of DI are polyuria, thirst, and polydipsia.

Urine volume varies between a few liters per day in partial DI to 20 liters per day in complete DI, and the onset being abrupt.

The patient has intense thirst and has a preference for cold or iced drinks. If access to water is interrupted, hyperosmolality develops rapidly, and CNS symptoms such as irritability, mental dullness, ataxia, hyperthermia, and coma can develop.

Lab Diagnosis

a. Large urine volume (usually greater than 3 litres per day)
b. Urine osmolality less than 300 mOsm/kg
c. Minimally elevated plasma osmolality of greater than 300 mOsm/kg
d. Inappropriately low serum AVP levels despite slightly elevated plasma osmolality.

Treatment

Treatment is usually with a long acting analogue of vasopressin (desmopressin or DDAVP). The usual dose is 10-20 µg once or twice daily intranasally. A parenteral and oral form of this drug is also available. Other analogues of vasopressin available are lypressin given 2-4 units intranasally or aqueous vasopressin 5-10 units subcutaneously.

Chlorpropamide can be used in patients with partial central DI, as it stimulates AVP secretion. It may be given in a dose of 250-500 mg/day. Hypoglycaemia is a common and sometimes serious side effect.

Clofibrate (500 mg 4 times/day) and carbamazepine (400-600 mg/day) also stimulate AVP release and may be used in partial central DI.

Nephrogenic DI

Nephrogenic DI is a polyuric disorder that results from renal insensitivity to the antidiuretic effect of AVP. This disorder is characterized by
a. Presence of normal rates of renal filtration and solute excretion
b. Persistently hypotonic urine
c. Normal or high levels of AVP

d. Failure of exogenous AVP to raise urine osmolality or to reduce urine volume.

Causes of Nephrogenic DI

1. Hereditary
   a. Autosomal dominant (mutation in aquaporin gene)
   b. Autosomal recessive (mutation in aquaporin gene)
   c. X-linked
2. Acquired
   a. Hypercalcaemia, hypokalemia
   b. Vascular (sickle cell trait or disease)
   c. After treatment for urinary obstruction
   d. Infection (pyelonephritis)
   e. Infiltrative (amyloidosis)
   f. Drugs (lithium, demeclocycline, methoxyflurane)
   g. Low protein diet.

Treatment

The most effective therapy is the combination of thiazide diuretics (5-10 mg/day) and mild salt restriction (increases isotonic proximal tubular fluid absorption and a decrease in the volume of fluids delivered to the collecting duct).

Prostaglandin synthesis inhibitors such as ibuprofen, indomethacin, and aspirin may be used adjunctively to treat this condition (reduce delivery of solutes to the distal tubules, thereby reducing urine volume and increasing urine osmolality).

Chlorpropamide (125-250 mg/day) and carbamazepine (100-200 mg/day) enhance the renal responsiveness to AVP, and may be used to treat this condition.

Dipsogenic DI

Dipsogenic DI is seen when the osmotic threshold for thirst, is paradoxically lower than that for AVP secretion. This reversal of the normal relationship between thirst and AVP secretion results in chronic thirst, polydipsia, and polyuria. The hallmark of primary polydipsia is diluted plasma, diluted urine, and suppressed AVP secretion.

Treatment is focussed on behaviour modification to reduce water intake.

Adipsic Hypernatraemia

This is characterised by chronic or recurrent hypertonic dehydration and deficient AVP response to osmotic stimulation. It is caused by agenesis or destruction of hypothalamic osmoreceptors.

Aetiology

Aquired:
1. Vascular—Occlusion of anterior communicating artery.
2. Tumours—Craniopharyngioma, meningioma, glioma and metastasis.
3. Granulomas—Neurosarcoid and histiocytisis.
4. Trauma
5. Psychogenic
6. Idiopathic
7. Others—Hydrocephalus, AIDS,CMV encephalitis

Congenital:
1. Microcephaly
2. Midline malformations

Genetic: Autosomal recessive.

Clinical Features

Patients have little or no thirst despite their dehydration. There are signs of hypovolumia and muscle weakness, pain, rhabdomyolysis, hyperglycaemia, hyperlipidaemia and ARF may also occur.

Treatment

1. Administration of water by mouth if the patient is alert.
2. If the patient is obtunded, 0.45% saline IV.
3. If diabetes insipidus is present or develops during rehydration, DDAVP should be given.
4. Correct hyperglycaemia and electrolyte imbalance.

Tests to Differentiate Central DI, Nephrogenic DI and Dipsogenic DI

1. *Water deprivation test*: This test is done to distinguish between diabetes insipidus and psychogenic polydipsia. It also helps to determine whether diabetes insipidus is of the central or nephrogenic type.
   The test is carried out as follows:
a. No coffee, tea or smoking on the day of test
b. Free fluids until start of test
c. Light breakfast
d. No fluids for 8 hours after 08.30 a.m
e. Weigh patient at start and after 5 and 8 hours
f. Stop test if patient loses more than 3% of body weight.

After fluid deprivation for 8 hours, urine and plasma osmolality are measured.

In patients with psychogenic polydipsia there is a rise in urine osmolality > 800 mOsm/kg (as urine is concentrated normally), whereas in patients with diabetes insipidus the urine osmolality remains low (due to failure to concentrate urine normally). The plasma osmolality rises in both conditions.

Having detected the presence of DI, it is now possible to differentiate between central and nephrogenic DI. Exogenous desmopressin 2 µg IM or 20 µg intranasally is given and then urine is collected hourly for the next 4 hours.

In patients with central DI the urine osmolality will increase > 800 mOsm/kg. This does not occur in patients with nephrogenic DI, as the exogenous AVP has no action on the renal tubules.

2. *Hypertonic saline infusion test*: A solution of 3% saline is infused to raise serum sodium to 145-150 mEq/liter. Blood samples are obtained for measurements of serum osmolality and plasma AVP levels. Patients with dipsogenic DI and nephrogenic DI exhibit normal stimulation of AVP release in response to the hypertonicity, whereas patients with central DI exhibit little or no rise in plasma AVP levels.

Syndrome of Inappropriate Antidiuretic Hormone Secretion (SIADH)

SIADH is characterised by hyponatremia and submaximal urinary dilution caused by a sustained release of AVP in the absence of osmotic and non-osmotic stimuli. SIADH usually results from a disease or an agent that enhances AVP release or action.

Causes of SIADH

1. Neoplastic diseases
   a. Carcinoma (lung, pancreas, duodenum, bladder, prostate)
   b. Lymphoma, leukaemia
   c. Ewing's sarcoma, mesothelioma
   d. Thymoma (carcinoid).
2. Pulmonary disorders
   a. Pneumonia
   b. Tuberculosis
   c. Asthma, pneumothorax
   d. Cavitation, abscess
   e. Positive pressure breathing
   f. Empyema
   g. Cystic fibrosis.
3. Central nervous system disorders

a. Head injury
b. Meningitis, encephalitis, abscess
c. Guillain-Barré syndrome
d. Cerebrovascular accident
e. Brain tumours
f. Epilepsy
g. Porphyria
h. Peripheral neuropathy
i. Hydrocephalus
j. Shy-Drager syndrome
k. Cavernous sinus thrombosis
l. Multiple sclerosis
m. Psychosis, delirium tremens.

4. Drugs
a. Desmopressin, oxytocin
b. Chlorpropamide
c. Clofibrate
d. Vincristine, vinblastine
e. Cyclophosphamide
f. Carbamazepine
g. Phenothiazines
h. Haloperidol
i. Tricyclic antidepressants
j. Monoamine oxidase inhibitors
k. Nicotine
l. Thiazide diuretics.

In patients with SIADH there is a persistent production of AVP or AVP-like peptide despite body fluid hypotonicity. As a result of the sustained release of AVP, patients retain ingested water and become hyponatremic and mildly volume expanded.

Clinical Features

The signs and symptoms of SIADH are those of water intoxication.

In acute hyponatremia, with serum sodium concentration less than 120 mEq/liter, the syndrome is manifest by somnolence, seizures, coma, and a high mortality rate.

In chronic hyponatremia, even though the serum sodium level may be less than 125 mEq/liter, the patient may remain asymptomatic.

When serum sodium is between 115-120 mEq/liter, the common symptoms are anorexia, nausea, vomiting, headache, and abdominal cramps.

Lab Diagnosis

1. Hyponatremia and low plasma osmolality (hallmark of SIADH).
2. Urine osmolality low but higher than that of plasma.

3. Plasma AVP level elevated in relation to plasma osmolality.
4. Hypouricaemia.

Other causes of hyponatremia should be excluded such as severe congestive heart failure, cirrhosis of liver with ascites, renal failure, or administration of large volume of hypotonic fluids, all of which can cause dilutional hyponatremia.

Salt-losing states such as diarrhoea, adrenal insufficiency or renal disease can also give rise to hyponatremia, but there is associated hypovolaemia.

Pseudo hyponatremia can result from hyperlipidaemia or severe hyperglycaemia. Hyponatremia can also result from hypothyroidism and primary polydipsia.

In hyperlipidaemia and hyperlipidaemic states like hypothyroidism, the osmolality of plasma increases which in turn draws out intracellular fluid causing dilutional hyponatremia.

SIADH can be Differentiated from the Above Conditions as Follows

Diagnosis	Volume status	Urinary sodium concentration (mEq/liter)	Fractional excretion of sodium (%)
SIADH	Normovolaemia	> 20	> 1
Salt wasting			
Renal	Hypovolaemia	> 20	> 1
Extrarenal	Hypovolaemia	< 10	< 1
Dilutional hyponatremia	Hypervolaemia	< 10	< 1

Treatment

Management of acute or symptomatic hyponatremia with a serum sodium concentration less than 120 mEq/liter is a medical emergency. The immediate goal is to raise serum sodium to 125 mEq/liter. The sodium requirement can be calculated according to the following formula:

Sodium requirement = (125 – measured sodium) × 0.6 body weight

Sodium replacement can be accomplished by infusion of hypertonic saline (3%). Rapid rise of serum sodium to levels more than 125 mEq/liter may cause CNS damage such as central pontine myelinolysis. So it is always prudent to correct sodium concentration at the rate of 0.5-1 mEq/hour.

Management of asymptomatic chronic hyponatremia is done by fluid restriction to 800-1000 ml/day or if patient cannot restrict the fluid intake, drugs like demeclocycline (0.62-1.2 g/day) or lithium (these agents interfere with the renal tubular effects of AVP) can be used, and they gradually raise plasma osmolality and serum sodium concentration to normal levels.

Thyroid Disorders

Anatomy and Physiology of Thyroid Gland

Thyroid is an endocrine gland responsible mainly for the maintenance of a normal basal metabolic rate of the body. Anatomically it comprises of two lobes connected together by an isthmus. Histologically it is made up of follicular cells (which secrete thyroid hormones) and parafollicular C-cells (which secrete calcitonin).

The thyroid secretes predominantly thyroxine (T_4) and only a small amount of triiodothyronine (T_3). Production of T_3 and T_4 in the thyroid is stimulated by thyroid-stimulating hormone (TSH) released from the anterior pituitary in response to stimulation by thyrotropin releasing hormone (TRH) released by the hypothalamus. T_3 and T_4 (> 99.9%) circulate in plasma bound to thyroxine binding globulin (TBG). The minute fraction of unbound (free) hormone diffuses into tissues and exerts its metabolic action.

There is a negative feedback of thyroid hormones on the pituitary and so when plasma concentrations of T_3 and T_4 are raised (hyperthyroidism), TSH secretion is suppressed, and conversely when concentration of T_3 and T_4 are decreased (primary hypothyroidism), TSH level is elevated.

Patterns of Thyroid Function Tests in Patients with Thyroid Disease

Type of disease	T_4	T_3	TSH
Conventional hyperthyroidism(95%)	Raised	Raised	Undetectable
T3 hyperthyroidism (5%)	Normal	Raised	Undetectable
Subclinical hyperthyroidism	Normal	Normal	Undetectable
Primary hypothyroidism	Low	Not indicated	Raised
Subclinical hypothyroidism	Normal	Not indicated	Raised
Secondary hypothyroidism	Low	Not indicated	Undetectable

Hyperthyroidism

Hyperthyroidism is the condition resulting from the effect of excessive amounts of thyroid hormones on body tissues.

Causes

Common causes (account for 95% of cases)
1. Graves' disease (autoimmune)   75%
2. Multinodular goitre   15%
3. Solitary thyroid nodule   10%

Rare causes (account for 5% of cases)
1. Thyroiditis (viral, autoimmune, postradiation)
2. Thyrotoxicosis factitia (surreptitious T_4 consumption, especially by female health workers)
3. Exogenous iodine consumption
4. Drugs (amiodarone)
5. TSH secreting tumours (pituitary tumours)
6. HCG producing tumours
7. Struma ovarii (ovarian teratoma).

Clinical Features (Figs 9.8 to 9.11)

1. The skin is warm, moist (due to vasodilatation); the palms are warm, moist and hyperaemic (palmar erythema); Plummer's nails (retraction of nail from its bed) are seen.
2. Dermopathy in the form of peau d' orange (pretibial myxedema) and growth of coarse hair may be seen.
3. Alopecia and vitiligo may be seen (vitiligo may be a marker for autoimmune aetiology for hyperthyroidism).
4. The eyes show retracted upper eyelid (due to increased sympathetic tone) and wide palpebral fissures (the upper limbus is well seen). In severe cases, proptosis may be seen.

Eye Signs in Hyperthyroidism
- Von Graefe's—Lid lag
- Joffroy's—Absence of wrinkling of forehead on looking up
- Stellwag's—Decreased frequency of blinking
- Dalrymple's—Lid retraction exposing the upper sclera
- Möbius—Absence of convergence.

Grading of Eye Signs

NO SPECS
- No eye signs
- Only sign seen in upper eyelid
- Soft tissue involvement
- Proptosis
- Extraocular muscle affected
- Corneal involvement
- Sight loss—due to optic nerve involvement

Grading of Eye Changes

Grading	Features
0	No eye signs
I	Only sign seen is upper eyelid retraction (lid lag sign)
II	Soft tissue involvement with upward gaze palsy and proptosis upto 22 mm
III	Proptosis more than 22 mm with symptoms of epiphora, redness of eye and gritty sensation in the eye
IV	Involvement of extraocular muscles (ophthalmoplegia)
V	Corneal involvement (ulceration)
VI	Optic nerve involvement (complete blindness)

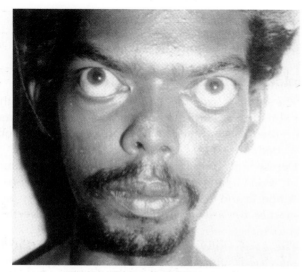

Fig. 9.8: Thyrotoxic ophthalmopathy

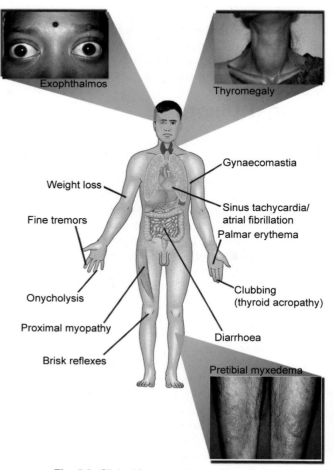

Fig. 9.9: Clinical features of hyperthyroidism

5. Cardiovascular symptoms are palpitations (due to AF, SVT). CCF may be precipitated in long-standing cases. Sleeping pulse rate is greater than 90 per minute. Isolated systolic hypertension can occur.
6. Metabolic symptoms are weight loss despite the increased appetite and intolerance to heat (due to increased BMR).
7. GIT symptoms may be in the form of hyper-defaecation.
8. It may exacerbate bronchial asthma
9. CNS symptoms are nervousness and irritability (very common symptoms). There is fine tremor of outstretched hands, insomnia, inability to relax and proximal muscle weakness. Acute psychosis may occur in about one third of patients with hyper-thyroidism.
10. Women may have amenorrhoea or oligomenor-rhoea and men may have impotence and loss of libido.

On examination, the thyroid gland may be diffusely enlarged and bruit may be heard over the gland due to increased blood flow.

Investigations

1. Serum free T_3 and T_4 levels are elevated
2. Serum TSH level is not detectable
3. Thyroid uptake of radioiodine (^{131}I) is increased
   The test is performed by administering I^{123} orally and measuring the percentage of radionuclide uptake after 4-24 hours. It is most useful for differentiating between high and low uptake types of hyperthyroidism and it should be performed when Graves' disease is not evident.
4. Test for presence of antibodies
   a. Thyroid stimulating immunoglobulin (TSI) is a marker for Graves' disease
   b. TSH-receptor antibody is seen in 75% of patients with Graves' disease.

High RAIU	Low RAIU
Grave's disease	Sub-acute thyroiditis
Toxic multinodular goiter	Painless thyroiditis
Toxic adenoma	Grave's disease with acute iodine load
Hashitoxicosis	Iodine induced hyperthyroidism
Choriocarcinoma	Thyroid hormone therapy
Hydatidiform mole	Metastatic functioning thyroid carcinoma
TSH secreting pituitary tumor	Struma ovarii

c. Antimicrosomal (antiperoxidase) antibody is seen in Graves' disease and also in Hashimoto's thyroiditis.

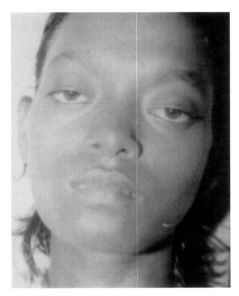

Fig. 9.10: Thyrotoxicosis with myesthenia gravis

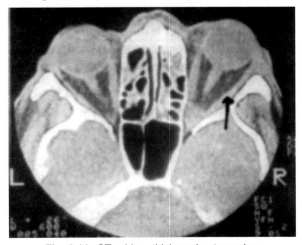

Fig. 9.11: CT orbits—thickened extraocular muscles in thyrotoxicosis

5. Thyroid scan with radioactive iodine is useful in patients with nodular goiter and hyperthyroidism to determine
    a. Whether there is an autonomous hyperfunctioning nodule.
    b. Whether multiple nodules are hyperfunctioning
    c. Whether the nodules are cold and the hyperfunctioning tissue is between the nodules.

Treatment

Management Options for Hyperthyroidism of Graves' Disease

Management	Indications
Antithyroid drugs	First episode in patients less than 40 yrs
Subtotal thyroidectomy	i. Recurrent hyperthyroidism after course of antithyroid drugs in patients less than 40 years ii. Initial treatment in males with large goitres and in those with severe hyperthyroidism (total $T_3 > 9$ nmol/litre) iii. Poor drug compliance
Radioiodine	i. patients > 40 years ii. Recurrence following surgery irrespective of age iii. Other serious illness irrespective of age

1. Immediate control of symptoms can be achieved with propranolol 40 mg/6 hr orally
2. Long-term control of hyperthyroidism can be by use of antithyroid drugs, radioiodine, or surgery
    a. *Antithyroid drugs*: Carbimazole 15 mg tid initially and then reducing to 5 mg tid for 12-18 months, gives symptomatic relief. Relapse may occur in approximately 70% of patients within two years and is commoner with large goitres and severe disease. Adverse reactions such as rashes and neutropenia are relatively common.
    b. Radioiodine ablation of the hyperfunctioning thyroid tissue may be adopted for post-menopausal women and elderly men. Hypothyroidism is common after treatment, and may require replacement therapy. It can also be given in recurrent hyperthyroidism. When given for a fertile female, conception must be postponed for one year.
    c. Surgery should be undertaken only after the thyrotoxic crisis has been controlled. Hypothyroidism is common and relapse of thyrotoxicosis and hypoparathyroidism may occur. Surgery is indicated in presence of large

2. *Adrenal Cushing's Syndrome*
   a. Unilateral adrenal adenoma—surgical removal; since the contralateral adrenal gland is suppressed, glucocorticoid replacement is necessary for several months until adrenal function returns.
   b. Adrenal carcinoma—surgery is the treatment of choice; in inoperable cases mitotane can be used in a dose of 250 mg qid upto 2 to 4 gm/day. MRI can be used for prognostic evaluation.

3. *Ectopic Cushing's Syndrome*
   a. Surgery is the treatment of choice. Adrenalectomy can be considered in cases of indolent yet inoperable tumours such as medullary carcinomas of the thyroid.
   b. Adrenal enzyme inhibitors for reducing hyper-cortisolism in ectopic ACTH syndrome.
   i. Metyrapone *(11-hydroxylase inhibitor) 250-500 mg tid.*
   ii. Aminoglutethimide—*this blocks the conversion of cholesterol to delta-5-pregnenolone, in a dose of 250 mg qid upto 2 g daily.*
   iii. Adrenolytic agents—*mitotane (medical adrenalec-tomy) can be used in addition to the enzyme inhibitors. It is contraindicated in pregnancy. Mitotane has a long half-life and can be detected in adipose tissue even after 2 years and hence it must be avoided in*

fertile females who desire pregnancy later in life. It is a teratogen and induces abortion.
   iv. Ketoconazole—*this blocks steroidogenesis at several levels (esp. 20-22 desmolase catalysing the conversion of cholesterol to pregnenolone). The dose ranges from 400-2000 mg/day. Therapy can be combined with other agents mentioned above.*
   v. Mifepristone is another treatment option.

Adrenal Insufficiency

Adrenal insufficiency can be caused by:
1. A primary disease at the, adrenal level, involving destruction of over 90% of the steroid-secreting cortex (Addison's disease).
2. A destructive process at the hypothalamic-pituitary level, leading to CRH or ACTH deficiency or both.
3. Long-term suppression of the hypothalamo-pituitary-adrenal (HPA) axis by exogenous or endogenus glucocorticoids followed by inappropriate withdrawal.

Causes of Addison's Disease

1. Primary

A. Anatomic Destruction
   a. Idiopathic atrophy—65% (Autoimmune adrenalitis)

Evaluation to Find out if the Patient has Cushing's Syndrome or not

	Test	Abnormality in Cushing's syndrome
1.	Circadian rhythm of plasma cortisol (8.00 and 24.00 samples)	Loss of rhythm
2.	Low dose dexamethasone suppression:	
	a. 1.5 mg at midnight and 9 am plasma cortisol next day	> 180 nmol/l
	b. 0.5 mg 6-hourly for 48 hours and plasma cortisol at 48 hours	> 180 nmol/l
3.	Urinary free cortisol 24-hour excretion or overnight excretion	Elevated (value depends on method used); > 250 µg/day-diagnostic;
4.	Insulin-induced hypoglycaemia	No rise in plasma cortisol

Evaluation to Find out the Cause of Cushing's Syndrome

	Test	Pituitary dependent	Ectopic ACTH	Adrenal tumour
1.	Plasma ACTH 08.00	N (10-80 ng/l) or ↑ (80-300 ng/l)	↑ or ↑↑ (300 ng/l)	Undetectable
2.	Metyrapone 750 mg 4-hourly × 6 doses: measure 11-deoxycortisol at 24.00	↑↑	↑	→↑
3.	High dose dexamethasone 2 mg 6-hourly for 48 hours: Plasma cortisol 48 hours	↓	→	→
4.	Plasma K⁺	N	< 3.5 mmol/l	N
5.	Corticotrophin-releasing factor (1 µg/kg body weight) and measure plasma ACTH and cortisol over 3 hours	↑	→	→

Sporadic
Type I Polyglandular autoimmune syndrome
Type II Polyglandular autoimmune syndrome

b. Surgical ablation
c. Infection
  i. Bacterial   Tuberculosis (20%)
                        Meningococcemia
                        (Waterhouse-Friderichsen
                        syndrome)
  ii. Fungal   Histoplasmosis
                        Cryptococcosis
                        Coccidioidomycosis
  iii. Viral   HIV
                        CMV
d. Inflammation   Sarcoidosis
e. Haemorrhage   Breech delivery
                        Anticoagulant therapy
f. Invasion   Secondaries (breast/lung)

B. *Metabolic*
a. Congenital adrenal
   hyperplasia and hypoplasia
b. Drugs   Enzyme inhibitors
                  (ketoconazole,
                  aminoglutethimide)
                  Metyrapone, Etomidate
                  Cytotoxic (mitotane)
c. Haemochromatosis

C. *ACTH Blocking Antibody (IgG)*

2. Secondary Adrenal Insufficiency

1. Tumours
   Pituitary tumour
   Craniopharyngioma
   Tumour of the third ventricle
2. Pituitary infarction and haemorrhage
   Postpartum necrosis (Sheehan's syndrome)
   Haemorrhage in tumours
3. Granulomatous diseases
   Sarcoidosis
4. Following hypophysectomy
5. Steroid withdrawal
6. Hypopituitarism
7. Suppression of hypothalamo-pituitary axis by exogenous or endogenous steroids.

Clinical Features (Fig. 9.26)

1. *Due to glucocorticoid insufficiency*
   Weight loss   (100%)
   Malaise   (100%)
   Weakness   (100%)

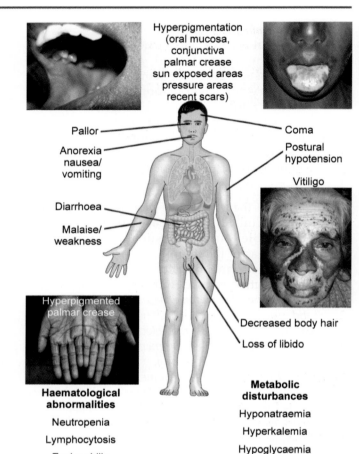

Hyperpigmentation (oral mucosa, conjunctiva palmar crease sun exposed areas pressure areas recent scars)

Pallor — Coma
Anorexia — Postural hypotension
nausea/vomiting
Vitiligo
Diarrhoea
Malaise/weakness
Decreased body hair
Loss of libido
Hyperpigmented palmar crease

Haematological abnormalities
Neutropenia
Lymphocytosis
Eosinophilia

Metabolic disturbances
Hyponatraemia
Hyperkalemia
Hypoglycaemia
Hypercalcemia

Fig. 9.26: Clinical features in Addison's disease

Anorexia   (100%)
Nausea   (50%)
Vomiting   (50%)
Gastrointestinal (diarrhoea or constipation in 50%)
Postural hypotension (this is present in almost all patients and BP should be checked after standing for 1 minute. Systolic pressure should be < 100 mm Hg)
Hypoglycaemia

2. *Due to mineralocorticoid insufficiency*
   Hypotension
3. *Due to increased ACTH secretion*
   Pigmentation is seen in
   • Sun exposed areas
   • Pressure areas, e.g., elbows, knees
   • Palmar creases, knuckles
   • Mucous membranes
   • Conjunctiva
   • Recent scars

4. *Due to loss of adrenal androgen*
Decreased body hair especially in females.

Hyperpigmentation, adrenal calcification and vitiligo are seen only in primary hypoadrenalism. Pigmentation is not seen in secondary hypoadrenalism.

Associated Other Autoimmune Disease

1. Hashimoto's thyroiditis
2. Primary atrophic hypothyroidism
3. Pernicious anaemia
4. Type 1 diabetes mellitus
5. Primary ovarian failure
6. Hypoparathyroidism

Lab Investigations

1. Plasma electrolytes—sodium is low, potassium is high, plasma urea is raised.
2. Blood glucose—may be low in severe adrenal insufficiency
3. Eosinophilia

Special Tests

1. ACTH Stimulation Test (Cosyntropin Test)

Cosyntropin is a potent stimulator of cortisol and mineralo-corticoids.

Procedure

1. Draw blood for baseline serum cortisol, aldosterone and ACTH at 8.00 am.
2. 0.25 mg cosyntropin IV or IM should be given.
3. Obtain blood samples for cortisol and aldosterone 30 min—60 mins following its administration.
   Normal   Plasma cortisol > 550 nmol/lit
   Primary—No change
   Secondary—Subnormal ↑

2. Metyrapone Test

This test is used to confirm diagnosis of adrenal insufficiency and useful especially when secondary causes are suspected.

Metyrapone is an inhibitor of an enzyme required for cortisol synthesis and so its administration leads to a fall in the level of cortisol, rise in ACTH level and rise in 11-deoxycortisol (immediate precursor of cortisol).

Procedure

Metyrapone is given as a single dose of 2-3 g (to be given at midnight with snack). ACTH, serum cortisol and 11-deoxycortisol are measured at 8.00 am the following day.

Interpretation

Type of adrenal insufficiency	ACTH	Serum cortisol	11-deoxy-cortisol
Normal	↑	↓ < 5 µg/dl	↑ > 7 µg/dl
Primary			↑ < 5 µg/dl
Secondary			↑ < 5 µg/dl

*If ACTH test is blunted, then the metyrapone test is unnecessary.

3. Plasma Renin Activity

The values are always high in primary adrenal insufficiency since plasma aldosterone level is low. In secondary adrenal insufficiency plasma renin activity may be normal as serum aldosterone levels are normal.

Management

1. Primary adrenal insufficiency requires replacement with both mineralocorticoids and glucocorticoids.
   a. Glucocorticoid replacement with either
      i. Prednisolone 5 mg in the morning and 2.5 mg in the evening.
         or
      ii. Hydrocortisone (cortisol) 20 mg in the morning and 10 mg in the evening.
         or
      iii. Cortisone acetate 25 mg in the morning and 12.5 mg in the evening.

Increased doses are needed in patients who are obese, and also for patients who are on barbiturates, phenytoin or rifampicin as they enhance metabolism of steroids. Steroid doses should be lowered in patients with liver disease, diabetes mellitus, peptic ulcer or hypertension and also in old age.

Appropriate weight gain and the regression of pigmentation are reliable indices for adequate steroid replacement.

   b. Mineralocorticoid replacement is done with fludrocortisone, a synthetic product, in a dose of 0.05-0.3 mg with adequate salt intake. The dose can be adjusted according to the response.
   c. Patient should be educated regarding:
      i. Adjustment of steroid dose for mild illness (double dose in fever)
      ii. Carrying a card or wearing a bracelet with the name of the disease they are suffering from.
      iii. Administration of 100 mg of hydrocortisone 6th hourly for 24 hours prior and 50 mg IM 6th hourly thereafter.
      iv. In case of gastroenteritis, patients must have parenteral hydrocortisone if oral intake is not possible.

Interpretation of the Test

Cause of adrenal insufficiency	ACTH (Baseline level)	Serum cortisol	Aldosterone
1. Primary	High	Baseline level ↓ and no ↑ after cosyntropin	Baseline aldosterone level ↓ and no ↑ with cosyntropin
2. Secondary	Low or normal	Baseline level ↓ and increases after cosyntropin	Baseline level ↓ or normal and ↑ aldosterone level 30 mins after cosyntropin

d. Sex hormone replacement due to associated primary gonadal insufficiency is required in selected patients.
2. Secondary adrenal insufficiency does not require mineralocorticoid replacement. Other tropic hormones of anterior pituitary should be replaced.
3. HPA suppression can be minimized by giving single morning daily dose of short acting steroids like hydrocortisone and prednisolone or by doubling the total daily dose and giving it on alternate days. This does not hold true for long acting steroids like dexamethasone or betamethasone.
4. Tapering of glucocorticoids: Once prednisolone is reduced to 5 mg/day, switch over to hydrocortisone 20-25 mg every morning. The short half-life of hydrocortisone gives time for HPA system to recover. 8 am plasma cortisol should be measured monthly and if it less than 10 µg/dl, it indicates continued HPA suppression. If it is more than 10 µg/dl, hydrocortisone can be withdrawn.

Similarly, an ACTH test can be performed. Following ACTH if plasma cortisol increases > 20 µg/dl, it indicates a recovered HPA axis. If 8 am cortisol is greater than 10 µg/dl, but the response to ACTH is still blunted, steroid coverage for major illness will be necessary as long as the ACTH test yields a subnormal response.

Adrenal Crisis

It is a medical emergency and may be the first manifestation of hypoadrenalism.

It occurs in patients with chronic adrenal insufficiency often precipitated by infection, trauma, surgery or bilateral adrenal haemorrhage (Waterhouse-Friderichsen syndrome).

Clinical Features

Fever, dehydration, nausea, vomiting, hypotension with electrolyte imbalance (hyperkalaemia, hyponatraemia and hypercalcaemia occasionally).

Management

1. IV fluids (2-3 litres of 5% dextrose saline) as quickly as possible and monitor fluid balance with central venous pressure recording.
2. Hydrocortisone 100 mg IV is given initially and it should be repeated 100 mg 6th hourly till the patient stabilises.
3. Treatment of underlying precipitating cause.
4. Taper steroid to maintenance dose.
5. Mineralocorticoid replacement with fludrocortisone 0.1 mg orally daily after stopping saline infusion.

Pheochromocytoma

It is a relatively rare benign tumour arising from chromaffin cells of the sympathoadrenal system. It is a rare cause of hypertension accounting for < 0.1% of patients with sustained diastolic hypertension.

The majority of pheochromocytoma arise from adrenal medulla (90%). Other sites of origin are organ of Zuckerkandl, aortic bifurcation (8%), rarely from extra adrenal sites in the abdomen, chest (< 2%), neck (< 0.1%) and left atrial region.

It occurs at all ages with a peak incidence in the 3rd and 4th decade. There is equal frequency in both sexes (in adults). 90% of the tumours are benign and 90% are unilateral.

Multiple tumours (adrenal and extra adrenal) are common in children than adults.

It is called as 10% tumour because, 10% are bilateral, 10% malignant, 10% extra adrenal, 10% familial, 10% multiple and 10% occur in children.

Pathophysiology

They are encapsulated, vascular tumours of about 5 cm in diameter and weigh < 70 gm. There is no correlation between the size of the tumour and rise in plasma catecholamine levels or the clinical features. Most pheochromocytomas secrete both epinephrine and norepinephrine (predominant). Some tumours secrete dopamine.

Epinephrine is predominantly secreted in association with multiple endocrine neoplasia.

Clinical Features

Symptomatic episodes may occur as often as 25-30 times/day or as infrequently as once every few months. The duration of attack is usually less than one hour but may extend to as long as one week.

Common Symptoms

Headache	(90%)
Sweating	(60%)
Palpitations	(70%)
Nervousness	(40%)
Weight loss	(40%)
Nausea and vomiting	(30%)
Chest and abdominal pain	(30%)

Anxiety and fear of death (angor animi) occur in majority of the patients.

Signs

Patient may present with paroxysmal or persistent hypertension or postural hypotension. Hyperglycaemia or impaired glucose tolerance is common. Pallor, tremor, Raynaud's phenomenon and manifestations of coexisting diseases (GIT ganglioneuromatosis, neurofibromas, Cushing's syndrome) can also be present.

Attacks are precipitated by pressure in the vicinity of the tumour, anxiety, exercise, micturition, alcohol ingestion, general anaesthetics, beta blockers, nicotine, phenothiazines, morphine, metoclopramide, hydralazine, droperidol and atropine.

Syndromes Associated with Phaeochromocytoma

Multiple endocrine neoplasia (MEN)
MEN-I   Hyperparathyroidism
             Hyperpituitarism
             Zollinger-Ellison syndrome
             Hyperadrenalism (cortex)
             Hyperthyroidism
             Ectopic hyperinsulinism, hyperglucagonism and increased release of human pancreatic polypeptide
             Phaeochromocytoma (rarely)
MEN-II   Medullary carcinoma of thyroid
             Adenoma or hyperplasia of parathyroid
             Bilateral adrenal hyperplasia
             Pheochromocytoma

MEN-III or II B   Medullary carcinoma of thyroid
                    Mucosal neuromas
                    Thickened corneal nerves (slit lamp examination)
                    GIT ganglioneuromas
                    Marfanoid habitus
                    Pheochromocytoma.

Other Associated Syndromes

- Neurofibroma (NF) with cafe-au-lait spots (von Recklinghausen's disease NF, pheochromocytoma and somatostatin rich duodenal carcinoid tumour
- von Hippel-Lindau disease (cerebroretinal hemangioblastoma)
- Acromegaly

Investigations

1. *Single voided (spot) urinary metanephrine*: This correlates with 24 hours urine test and is particularly useful when urine is collected following an attack.
2. *24 hours urine test for total metanephrine*: This is the most reliable screening test. However, false positive tests are common in patients taking chlorpromazine, benzodiazepines or sympathomimetics.

   Normal metanephrine levels in urine
Total	< 1.3 mg/24 hours
Normetanephrine	< 0.9
Metanephrine	< 0.4

3. 24 hours urinary free catecholamines (epinephrine, norepinephrine or dopamine).

   Normal values
Total	< 100 μg/24 hours
Norepinephrine	< 75 μg/24 hours
Epinephrine	< 25 μg/24 hours

4. Plasma catecholamine levels before and after the attack.

Normal value (Plasma)		*Diagnostic value*
Norepinephrine	< 500 pg/ml	> 1500 pg/ml
Epinephrine	< 100 pg/ml	> 300 pg/ml

5. Vanillylmandelic acid levels in urine: Normally present upto 1.5-6.5 mg/day; > 8 mg/day is diagnostic. It is the least reliable of all tests.
6. Tumour localisation by CT scan, Meta-131-Iodo Benzyl Guanidine (MIBG) scintigraphy or MRI. Central venous blood sampling can assist in localization of tumour when all other measures fail (Figs 9.27 to 9.30).

Management

Acute medical therapy for severe hypertension.
a. Bedrest with head end of the bed elevated.

status of glycaemic control. Since the half-life of serum protein is short (20 to 25 days), this estimation gives an idea about the glycaemic status in the previous 2 to 3 weeks only.

Normal fructosamine level—0.9 to 1.5 ng/dl; > 1.5 ng/dl—abnormal.

Uncontrolled Diabetes Mellitus and Recurrent DKA

Noncompliance is a major cause of recurrent keto-acidosis in children.

Hypoglycaemia

Most episodes are predictable and preventable. But children are usually unaware of hypoglycaemic symptoms. The combination of alcoholic beverages with insulin produces very severe hypoglycaemia. Abnormal counter regulatory response in diabetic patients may account for prolonged hypoglycaemia.

Fasting Hyperglycaemia

Somogyi Phenomenon (Rebound effect): This is hypo-glycaemia induced hyperglycaemia due to increased secretion of counter regulatory hormones.

If the insulin dose is increased beyond the amount required for any given portion of the day, there is counter regulatory hormone response, resulting in hypergly-caemia. Reduction of insulin is advised in such situations.

Dawn Phenomenon: Many patients with IDDM demonstrate early morning (4–8 AM) hyperglycaemia that is aggravated again by intake of food during breakfast (but not due to it). It may either be due to increased hepatic glucose production or decreased peripheral utilization or both. In this condition, an excess of insulin is needed to control hyperglycaemia.

Early morning blood sampling at 3 am is necessary to differentiate both the conditions.

Type 2 Diabetes Mellitus

It is the most common type of diabetes accounting for 85–90% of the cases.

Risk Factors

1. Family history of DM
2. Obesity
3. Physical inactivity
4. Previously identified IGT
5. History of gestational DM
6. Delivery of large baby(> 4 kg)
7. Hypertension
8. HDL level < 35 mg/dl
9. TGL level > 250 mg/dl
10. Polycystic ovary syndrome
11. Acanthosis nigricans
12. History of vascular disease.

Pathophysiology

The characteristic pathophysiologic abnormalities of Type 2 DM are:
1. Impaired insulin secretion.
2. Peripheral insulin resistance.
3. Excessive hepatic glucose production.

There are 3 phases of development.

I phase (euglycaemia with increased insulin levels): Plasma glucose remains normal despite demonstrable insulin resistance because insulin levels are elevated.

II phase (post-prandial hyperglycaemia with increased insulin levels): Insulin resistance tends to worsen so that despite elevated insulin concentrations, glucose intolerance becomes mainfest by post-prandial hyperglycaemia.

III phase (overt diabetes with declining insulin levels): Insulin resistance does not change but insulin secretion declines resulting in fasting hyperglycaemia and overt diabetes.

Resistance to insulin in Type 2 diabetes is at post-receptor level. The substance responsible for this is termed amylin.

Clinical Features

Patients are usually obese; symptoms begin gradually (polyuria, polydipsia, polyphagia); patient may present with unhealed wounds, fungal infections, pruritus vulva or balanitis; patient can have frequent changes in refractory error and may have early development of cataract; patient may be asymptomatic also.

Rule out diabetes in tuberculous patients above 40 years and also in mothers who have babies born with a weight of more than 4 kg (macrosomia).

General Characteristics Type 1 and 2 DM

Features	Type 1 DM	Type 2 D
1. Genetic locus	Chromosome 6	Multifactorial
2. Age of onset	<30 yrs	>30 yrs
3. Body weight	Lean	80% obese, 20% lean
4. P. Insulin	Low or absent	Normal or high
5. P. Glucose	High, suppressible	High, resistant
6. Acute complications	DKA	NKHS
7. Insulin therapy	Essential	Early may not require Late may require
8. Sulphonylurea	Unresponsive	Responsive
9. Autoantibodies	Present	Absent
10. Early death without treatment	Yes	No
11. Associated disorder	Autoimmune diseases	Insulin resistance Hypertension Hyperlipidaemia Polycystic ovary

Diagnosis

A. According to National Diabetes Data Group (NDDG), Type 2 DM is Diagnosed when a Patient

(i) Is not ketosis prone under basal conditions does not require exogenous insulin for short-term survival

(ii) Random blood sugar > 200 mg/dl on two occasions

(iii) Has a fasting plasma glucose > 126 mg/dl or a sustained elevation of plasma glucose concentration ≥ 200 mg/dl after an oral glucose load of 75 gm at two hours.

B. Patients with Impaired GTT

10–50% of patients with impaired glucose tolerance develop Type 2 DM over a period of 10 years.

Diagnostic criteria for impaired GTT are:
Impaired glucose tolerance (IG) is defined by a 2-hour oral glucose tolerance test where the plasma glucose is > 140 mg/dl but < 200 mg/dl

Impaired fasting glucose is defined by a fasting plasma glucose of 110 mg/dl or greater but < 126 mg/dl/.

IFT and IGT are associated with insulin resistance and they are prone for micro/macrovascular complications and might end up with overt DM type 2.

Patients with impaired glucose tolerance are at an increased risk for atherosclerosis.

Patients with impaired glucose tolerance need further evaluation at a later date since they are potential diabetics.

It is treated with diet therapy, exercise, biguanides and sulphonylureas like glypizide and gliclazide. IGT is an important marker of skin disorders, neuropathy and hyperglycaemia in pregnancy.

C. Intravenous Glucose Tolerance Test

Preparation: Patient is given 3 days of unrestricted diet containing at least 150 gm of carbohydrate and has normal physical activity. Physical exertion should be avoided for 1 day prior to the test. Test should not be done in patients with intercurrent illness.

Fasting is advised for atleast 10 hours to a maximum period of 16 hours. Water alone is permitted. Smoking should be avoided.

Time of start of test (glucose infusion): 7.30–10 A.M.

Glucose dose: 0.5 g/kg upto 35 g 25% glucose diluted in normal saline and infused manually or by a pump in 3 minutes ± 15 seconds.

Two baseline samples and samples at 1, 3, 5, and 10 minutes after the test are taken. It is done for patients who cannot take oral glucose.

Glucose is present in urine and there is confusion with the diagnosis of diabetes in the following conditions.

Renal Glycosuria

The most common cause of glycosuria is a low renal threshold for glucose, which commonly occurs temporarily in pregnancy and is a much more frequent cause of glycosuria than diabetes in young people. Renal glycosuria is a benign condition and is not accompanied by the classical symptoms of diabetes.

Alimentary (Lag Storage) Glycosuria

In some individuals, an unusually rapid and transitory rise of blood glucose occurs following a meal. The concentration of glucose exceeds the normal renal threshold and it is present in the urine. This response following a meal or a dose of glucose is known as a 'lag storage' or alimentary glycosuria. It may occur in normal people or after gastric surgery (due to rapid gastric emptying leading to an increased rate of absorption into the blood stream), and also in patients with hyperthyroidism or hepatic disease. This type of blood glucose curve is usually benign and is unrelated to diabetes. The peak blood glucose concentration is abnormally high and the value two hours after oral glucose is normal.

Potential Diabetics

These are persons with a normal OGTT, who have an increased risk of developing diabetes for genetic reasons. E.g. individual who has a first degree relative with diabetes.

Latent Diabetics

These are persons who have a normal OGTT but who are known to have given an abnormal result under conditions imposing a burden on pancreatic β cells. E.g. Pregnancy, infection, myocardial infarction, steroid therapy.

Treatment

1. Diet Planning

Diet control is an endogenous insulin preserver.

a. Primary therapeutic goal is weight loss in obese individuals; Reduction in weight eliminates the need for oral hypoglycaemic drugs or insulin, especially if normal body weight is achieved. Consistency in composition and timing of meals is important particularly for patients using fixed insulin regimens or oral hypoglycaemic drugs.

b. Hypocaloric diets:
Caloric calculations is done for ideal body weight. Total calories should be kept ideally between 1000–1200 kcal/day;
For obese individuals, 20 kcal/kg ideal body weight
For normal adults (sedentary), 30 kcal/kg ideal body weight
For normal adults (manual worker) and growing children, 40 kcal/kg ideal body weight.

Carbohydrates: Carbohydrate should constitute 50–60% of total calories. Concentrated sugars are avoided except in the treatment of hypoglycaemia. Nibbling of foodstuff rather than gorging is recommended to slow the rate of carbohydrate absorption.

Fibers: About 25 gm of fibers per 1000 kcal is advised. Complex high-fiber carbohydrates (bran, whole grain cereals, breaks, legumes, vegetables and whole fruit) are recommended. Soluble fibres like guar 15 gm/day should be consumed.

Proteins: The total protein content of the diabetic meal plan should be 25–30%.

Fats: Total fat content should be between 25–30% of total calories. Skimmed or low fat milk is advised; only 2–3 eggs per week are allowed. Margarine should be taken instead of butter. Red and brown meat should be taken in reduced amounts. Fish and skimmed milk based cheeses can be taken.

Meal plan: Total calories have to be consumed as three major meals and three snacks in between major meals (breakfast 30%, midmorning snacks 10%, lunch 20%, evening snacks, 10% dinner 20% and bedtime snacks 10%).

General dietary considerations:
a. Hunger, fasting or over feeding should be avoided
b. Start with 1000 k cal/day for a 1 year old and increase by about 100 kcal/year thereafter upto adolescence. In adolescence, boys may need upto 3000 k cal/day for covering regular athletic activity when needed. Late adolescent males and young adult males require about 2200–2500 kcal/day.
c. Girls need calorie restriction at about 10–12 years because of early puberty, so that meal plans are increased to about 1800–2000 kcal/day until this stage and then decreased to 1100–1700 kcal/day according to metabolic needs.

d. Ice-cream can be liberalized because of its protein and fat content, especially when given in association with 30–90 minutes of continuous activity.
e. "Cheat" days are allowed 3 to 4 times during a year counter balancing with insulin and activity.
f. Avoid excessive sodium and alcohol. Alcohol inhibits hepatic gluconeogenesis, potentiates hypoglycaemic action of oral drugs. It may cause lactic acidosis. When used with sulfonylureas it causes disulfiram like reaction. The calorie content of alcohol is also high (empty calories)
g. Judicious use of artificial sweeteners are recommended.
   Artificial sweeteners like sorbitol and fructose are rich in energy and are not very useful. Their total intake should not exceed 50 g/day.
   Non-nutritive sweeteners like saccharin, aspartame, sucramate and acesulphane K are widely used; they provide less energy without loss of palatability.
h. In patients with hyperlipidaemia, lipid lowering agents can be given only on failure of diet therapy (step 1 and step 2). (refer chapter on hyperlipidemia).

Type of lipid	Minimal goal (mg/dl)	Ideal goal (mg/dl)
Total cholesterol	< 200	170
LDL	< 130	100
Non-HDL cholesterol	< 160	130

2. Exercise

Isotonic exercises like brisk walking, swimming or cycling are recommended.

a. Exercise potentiates beneficial effects of diet and other therapy. Aerobic exercises for 30–45 minutes/day, 5 times per week should be advocated. The rest period between exercise should not exceed 48 hours. Exercise is less effective in poorly controlled diabetics. In these individuals, exercise potentiates existing hyperglycaemia.
b. Vigorous exercise in those patients who have neither decreased their insulin nor increased their carbohydrate intake, might result in hypoglycemia. Hence, insulin should be reduced by 20–25% on the day of strenuous exercise. If he has already injected the usual dose, 20–30 gm of carbohydrate should be ingested prior to exercise, unless there is 2+ glycosuria or significant hyperglycaemia.
c. Feet and joints should be monitored after exercise especially if there is evidence of peripheral neuropathy.

d. If autonomic neuropathy is present, heart rate will not increase during exercise; there is also increased risk of cardiac arrhythmias and postexercise orthostatic hypotension.

e. Exercise regimen should start with warm up stretching, for 10 minutes, aerobic exercise for 30 to 45 minutes, and cool down stretching for 5 to 10 minutes.

f. When there is a persistent increase in blood sugar > 250 mg/dl, despite diet control and mild exercise regimens, vigorous exercise may be best avoided till blood sugar begins to fall.

g. Screen for CVS disease (ECG, stress test) before starting exercise regimen.

h. Avoid isometric exercises (bull worker, weight lifting).

Exercise and energy expenditure per hour:
a. Mild exercise
   One hour standing—120 kcal/hr
   Lying down—70 kcal/hr
   Sitting—80 kcal/hr
   Walking (2.5 mph)—180 kcal/hr.
b. Moderate exercise
   Swimming (0.25 mph)—250 kcal/hr
   Fast walk (3.75 mph)—250 kcal/hr.
c. Vigorous exercise
   Tennis—350 kcal/hr
   Cycling (10 mph)—600 kcal/hr
   Running (10 mph)—800 kcal/hr.

3. Drug Therapy

In obese individuals, drug therapy is advocated when intensive therapy with diet modification and exercise fails. Drugs are given when fasting plasma glucose is > 140 mg/dl and post prandial level is > 250 mg/dl inspite of regular exercise and diet control or when there are symptoms of hyperglycaemia, persistent ketosis, hyperosmolality or hyperlipidaemia.

A. Oral Antidiabetic Agents

I. Insulin secretagogues:

(i) *Sulfonylureas*
Sulfonylureas act by stimulating release of insulin from the pancreatic β cell. It upregulates the insulin receptors and magnifies the effect of available insulin. The hypoglycaemic effect is due to the reduction in hepatic release of glucose and diminished insulin resistance. Sulfonylureas reduce fasting blood glucose by approximately 70–80 mg/dl.

They are effective in lean diabetics and should not be prescribed in obese patients as first line of therapy; they are already hyperinsulinemic and treatment with suffonylureas aggravate this thereby increasing weight. In obese, sulfonylureas are tried only when vigorous diet, biguanides and exercise program have failed.

Extrapancreatic actions of sulfonylureas
I. *Liver*
   A. *Direct effects*
      1. Increases fructose-2, 6-biphosphate
      2. Increases glycolysis
      3. Decreases gluconeogenesis
      4. Decreases oxidation of long-chain fatty acids
   B. *Potentiate insulin action*
      1. Increases hepatic glycogen synthase and glycogen synthesis
      2. Increases hepatic lipogenesis
   C. *Decreases hepatic extraction of insulin*
II. *Skeletal muscles*
   A. *Direct effects*
      1. Increases glucose transport
      2. Increases fructose-2, 6-biphosphate
   B. *Potentiation of insulin stimulation of carbohydrate transport*
III. *Adipose tissue*
   A. *Direct effects*
      1. Increases adenosine-3' 5'-monophosphate diesterase and inhibition of lipolysis
      2. Increases glycogen synthase
   B. *Potentiation of insulin-mediated glucose transport and translocation of glucose transport molecules.*
      • Chlorpropamide has a central action also and it is equivalent to ultra lente insulin. Its hypothalamic action has made it useful in diabetes insipidus.
      • Gliclazide has a smooth action resembling physiological insulin secretion.

Treatment response
Primary failure: About 15% of patients show inadequate response to sulfonylureas during the first month of treatment with maximal dosage. This is primary sulfonylurea failure. If hyperglycaemia (fasting plasma glucose > 140 mg% and post-prandial glucose > 250 mg/dl) persists even after 1 month of drug therapy while the patient is on strict diet therapy and exercise, primary failure is diagnosed and insulin may have to be started.

Secondary failure: Some patients (5–10%) show initial satisfactory response followed by recurrence of hyperglycaemia. This is called secondary failure. The causes for secondary failure are:
1. Non-adherence to either diet or sulfonylurea therapy.
2. Disease progression.

3. Loss of efficiency of the drug.
4. Intercurrent illness
5. Physical or mental stress.

Side effects of sulfonylurea therapy

a. Hypoglycaemia: This is prolonged and recurrent. Treatment and intense monitoring should be continued for at least a week.
b. Several drugs may potentiate the action of sulfonylureas sulfonamides, coumarin, phenylbutazone, phenytoin etc.
c. Sulfonylureas should not be used in patients with liver disease, renal disease, allergic reactions to sulfonylureas or during pregnancy.
d. Chlopropramide induces fluid retention by exerting ADH effect on distal tubules.
e. Patients may experience flushing after alcohol intake.

Selection of sulfonylureas

1. Second generation drugs are advantageous.
2. For elderly, glipizide is preferred since there is less incidence of hypoglycaemia with this drug. Glyburide (Glibenclamide) is preferred when there is fasting hyperglycaemia.
3. In renal insufficiency, drugs having dual route of excretion (liver and biliary) like glyburide or drugs with inactive liver metabolites like glipizide should be used.
4. Drugs should be started in small dosage and should be increased gradually based on self-monitoring of blood glucose.

(ii) Meglitinide

These are a new class of insulin secretagogues which modulates β cell insulin release by regulating potassium channels. The first member of the group is Repaglanide – 0.25 to 4 mg before each meal. It has very fast onset of action with peak effect within 1hr of ingestion. Duration of action is 4-5 hrs. Because of the rapid onset and short duration it is indicated for post-parandial glucose control.

Contraindication includes hepatic impairment. Since there is no sulphur in the structure, it can be used in patients with sulfonylurea allergy.

(iii) Nateglinide

It is a D phenylalanine derivative which acts directly on β cells to stimulate early insulin secretion.
Dose: 120 mg orally taken 10 mts before each meal

Leads to insulin secretion within 15 mts and return to baseline in 3-4 hrs. It is effective in control of postprandial hyperglycaemia.

II. Insulin sensitisers:

(i) Biguanides

The drugs under this group are phenformin and metformin. These are drugs of choice for obese type II diabetes. They have no effect on insulin secretion. They improve peripheral tissue sensitivity to insulin thereby enhancing peripheral utilization of glucose. They suppress hepatic production of glucose by reducing gluconeogenesis. They do not cause weight gain and rather facilitate weight loss (due to anorexic effect). The drug also decreases triglycerides, especially when they are elevated. It also increases glucose transporters in insulin sensitive cells.

Biguanides can be given orally alone or with insulin. Primary failure is 5–20% and secondary failure is 5–10%, Starting dose of metformin is 500 mg/day with meals upto 3 gm/day in 2–3 doses.

They should be avoided in patients with renal or hepatic insufficiency, in alcoholics, in cardiopulmonary insufficiency and in other known risks for lactic acidosis. They should not be used in pregnancy. Absorption is decreased by guargum. Cimetidine delays its renal clearance. Biguanide can be used along with sulfonylureas and the combination has an additive glucose lowering effect.

Metformin should be withheld for one day prior to contrast studies with iodinated dyes and it can be restarted 48 hours after the contrast study (If renal function is normal).

(ii) Thiazolidinediones

They improve insulin sensitivity in muscle, liver and adipose tissue. There is reduced hepatic glucose production also. It seems to reduce plasma triglyceride levels and increases HDL cholesterol levels. There is no hypoglycemia, as they do not affect pancreatic insulin secretion. Patients with little pancreatic insulin reserve do not respond adequately. Hence it is used in type 2 DM it also prevents the progression from IGT to type 2 DM. They can be combined with other oral hypoglycemic agents or insulin.
Pioglitazone 15-45 mg OD
Rosiglitazone 2-8 mg OD

There should be frequent hepatic monitoring for idiosyncratic hepatic injury.

Contraindications
Liver disease
CCF—class III and IV

5. Bicarbonate may be needed when pH is < 7.2
6. *Insulin treatment:*
   Regular insulin 5–10 units IV, should be given when glucose is > 600 mg/dL and smaller doses are given later.
   Insulin can also be given as an infusion or intra-muscular injection. Insulin requirement is less when compared to DKA.

Lactic Acidosis

Patients with DM are vulnerable for disease like MI, sepsis, etc. Lactic acidosis is common in them and also during treatment with biguanides.

This is differentiated from DKA by plasma ketone levels and enzyme assays for lactate, acetoacetic acid, β hydroxy butyrate.
Lactic acidosis occurs in 2 general settings.
Type A—Vascular collapse + tissue hypoxia
Type B—No vascular collapse + No tissue hypoxia

Placenta is the only site where there can be lactic acidosis even in the presence of increased oxygen supply.

Lactic acidosis: Metabolic acidosis (pH < 7.2) with serum lactate > 5 mmol/L.

Causes

Group A (with Tissue Hypoxia)

Shock from any cause (septic shock, myocardial infarction, haemorrhage)
Respiratory failure
Cardiac failure
Poisoning with cyanide or carbon monoxide
Vigorous exercise (benign)
Convulsions.

Group B (without Tissue Hypoxia)

Diabetes mellitus
Hepatic failure
Severe infection
Pancreatitis.

Drugs
   Phenformin
   Sorbitol
   Metformin
   Fructose
   Salicylates
   Sodium nitroprusside
   INH
   Epinephrine and norepinephrine.

Toxins
   Ethanol
   Methanol.

Congenital enzyme defects
Glucose-6-phosphatase
Fructose 1, 6 biphosphatase
Pyruvate carboxylase
Pyruvate dehydrogenase
Leukaemia, lymphoma, solid tissue tumours (malignant).

Treatment

1. Treat the cause
2. Dichloroacetate has been tried
3. Bicarbonate is given for severe acidosis.

Long-term Complications of Diabetes

Diabetic Retinopathy

This is the most common cause for blindness in adults between 30 and 65 years.

The lesions can be broadly divided into
1. Simple/background retinopathy
2. Preproliferative retinopathy
3. Proliferative retinopathy.

Earliest change is increase in permeability of the capillaries which progresses to the formation of saccular and fusiform aneurysms.

Background Retinopathy Without Maculopathy

It constitutes
a. Venous dilatation
b. Peripheral microaneurysms, small blot haemo-rrhages, small hard exudates

Lesions in Background Retinopathy

1. Increased capillary permeability
2. Capillary closure and dilatation
3. Microaneurysm (outpouching of capillaries)
4. Arteriovenous shunts
5. Dilated veins
6. *Haemorrhages (dot and blot):* It occurs in deeper layers of the retina and hence are round and regular; flame shaped haemorrhage is common in patients with hypertension.
7. *Cotton wool spots:* These are microinfarcts, i.e. non-perfused areas surrounded by a ring of dilated

capillaries; a sudden increase in number is a bad prognostic sign.

8. Hard exudates: These are due to leakage of protein and lipids from damaged capillaries (Fig. 9.35).

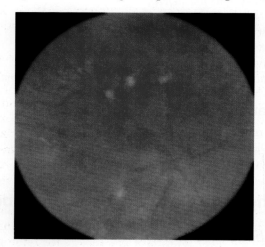

Fig. 9.35: Flame shaped haemorrhages and hard exudates— hypertension with diabetes

Macular oedema should be suspected when loss of visual acuity is not corrected by glasses.

There is no immediate threat to vision. Hypertension, DM, should be controlled. Smoking and alcohol should be avoided. Regular fundus examination every 6–12 months is recommended.

Preproliferative Retinopathy

It constitutes
a. Venous loops and beading
b. Clusters/sheets of microaneurysms
c. Small blot haemorrhages and/large retinal haemorrhages.
d. Intraretinal microvascular abnormalities
e. Multiple small exudates
f. Macular oedema and decreased visual acuity
g. Perimacular exudates ± retinal haemorrhages of any size.

This stage imposes mild threat to loss of vision. Rapid reduction of blood sugar results in development of soft exudates and haemorrhages and hence sugar has to be reduced gradually.

Proliferative Retinopathy

It constitutes
   Preretinal haemorrhage
   Neovascularization
   Fibrosis
   Exudative maculopathy.

This stage is an emergency and urgent ophthalmological review is mandatory.

Proliferative retinopathy is more common in insulin treated patients than in those not treated with insulin.

The lesions are (Figs 9.36 to 9.38):
1. New vessel formation (due to retinal hypoxia secondary to capillary or arteriolar occlusion; new vessels form from mature vessels on the optic disc or the retina in response to areas of ischaemic retina)
2. Formation of retinal scar (retinitis proliferans)
3. Vitreal haemorrhage
4. Retinal detachment.

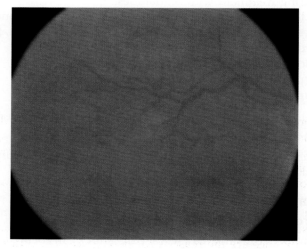

Fig. 9.36: Diabetic proliferative retinopathy— peripheral

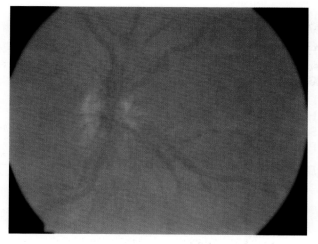

Fig. 9.37: Diabetic proliferative retinopathy well seen over the optic disc

The last two are serious complications of proliferative retinopathy causing sudden loss of vision in one eye.

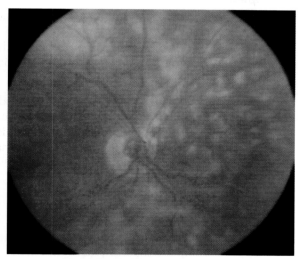

Fig. 9.38: Proliferative retinopathy—
Photocoagulation with laser

Risk Factors for Diabetic Retinopathy

Common in young males; uncommon < 10 years regardless of the duration of Type 1 DM; frequency of retinopathy increases after 13 years. Changes occurring in puberty (like increase in insulin like growth factor I, growth hormone and sex hormones) BP and poor glycaemic control are thought to be responsible for increase in incidence of retinopathy. Increased insulin resistance, inadequate insulin dosage, poor compliance are the reasons for poor glycaemic control in post-pubertal teenagers.

Patients develop cataract at an early age.

Rubeosis Iridis

There is development of new vessels on the anterior surface of iris and it may obstruct anterior angle of eye leading to glaucoma.

Treatment

1. Photocoagulation is the mainstay of treatment of diabetic retinopathy. It can be of two types namely xenon arc-white light, and laser beam (monochromatic blue or green light). It decreases the incidence of haemorrhage and scarring and is always indicated for neovascularisation.

   It is also used in the treatment of microaneurysms, haemorrhages and macular oedema even if the proliferative stage has not begun. Over a 2-week period, thousands of lesions (photocoagulation) are produced to diminish retinal demands for oxygen, thus decreasing the stimulus for neovascularization.

2. Pars plana vitrectomy is utilized for treatment of nonresolving vitreal haemorrhage and retinal detachment (retinal tears, detachment, cataract, recurrent vitreal hemorrhage, glaucoma, infection, loss of the eye are complications of the surgery).

3. Duration and degree of glycaemic control of diabetes are the most important risk factors for retinopathy. Patients usually have no visual symptoms until serious late complications develop, which have no effective treatment. Hence, regular screening for retinopathy is mandatory in all diabetics.

4. Extracapsular extraction of lens with intraocular lens implantation is done for cataract. This surgery is also indicated when adequate assessment of fundus is precluded or when laser therapy to retina is prevented by presence of the cataract.

Limited Joint Mobility (LJM, Diabetic Hand Syndrome)

This is common in 15–30% of adolescents with Type 1 DM; A subset of those are 400–600% at greater risk of developing complications associated with hyperglycaemia. Patient keeps the hands together in prayer

Anatomical Classification of Neuropathy

Structure	Disorder	Etiology	Signs and symptoms
A. Nerve root	Radiculopathy	Probably vascular	Pain and sensory loss along a dermatome
B. Mixed spinal or cranial nerve	Mononeuropathy	Probably vascular	Pain, weakness, loss of reflexes, sensory loss
C. Nerve terminals	Polyneuropathy	Metabolic	Glove and stocking sensory loss; minimal weakness, absent reflexes
D. Nerve terminal? Muscle?	Diabetic amyotrophy	Unknown	Anterior thigh pain; proximal muscle weakness
E. Sympathetic ganglion	Autonomic neuropathy	Unknown	Postural hypotension, anhidrosis, impotence gastropathy, bladder atony, nocturnal diarrhoea

position; there is sclerodermatous, tight, waxy skin; fifth finger is involved early (cannot extend fully).

Diabetic Neuropathy

This is the most frequently encountered chronic complication of diabetes. The neuropathic disorder includes manifestation of the somatic and/or autonomic parts of the nervous system.

Classification (Fig. 9.39)

1. Anatomical Classification
2. Clinical Classification
   a. Bilaterally symmetrical peripheral polyneuropathy
      (i) Sensory polyneuropathy
      (ii) Mixed sensory motor polyneuropathy
      (iii) Motor polyneuropathy.
   b. Symmetrical or asymmetrical proximal motor neuropathy
   c. Mononeuropathy (simplex or multiplex)
      (i) Cranial nerves
      (ii) Peripheral nerves.
   d. Abdominal polyradiculopathy
   e. Autonomic neuropathy.

Factors Involved in the Aetiology and Pathogenesis of Diabetic Neuropathy

A. *Metabolic*
   1. Hyperglycaemia
      a. Sorbitol accumulation
      b. Myo-inositol depletion
      c. Sodium-potassium ATPase deficiency
      d. Protein glycosylation
   2. Lipid disturbances
B. *Vascular*
C. *Others*
   1. Mechanical factors
   2. Stress
   3. Autoimmunity

4. Hereditary
5. Hypoglycaemia.

Small Fibre Neuropathy (C –fiber)
- Neuropathy of symptoms
- Pain and paresthesias – burning, lancinating, pins and needles, tingling, numbness, coldness
- Feet more affected than hands
- Acute < 6 months, Chronic > 6 months to years
- Decreased autonomic function – decreased sweating and dry skin
- Impaired blood flow – cold feet
- Motor power and deep reflexes are intact
- Risk of foot ulceration and gangrene
- Early detection of impairment of touch and pricking sensation by monofilament and Waardenberg wheel tests
- Topical application of capsaicin and clonidine are useful.

Large Fibre Neuropathy
- Neuropathy of signs
- Impairment of vibration and position sense
- Delta type deep seated gnawing pain similar to toothache
- Sensory ataxia – (Waddling like duck)
- Wasting of small muscles of hands and feet
- Shortening of Achilles tendon – pesequinus
- Increased blood flow – hot foot
- Charcot's neuro-arthropathy of different joints.

Classification of Autonomic Neuropathy in Diabetic Patients According to Systems Involved

1. Gastrointestinal disorders
   Esophageal dysfunction
   Stomach atony
   Gallbladder atony
   Small intestinal dysfunction
   Large intestinal atony
   Anorectal dysfunction

Different types of Diabetic Neuropathy

Features	Large fibre	Small fibre	Proximal motor	Acute mononeuropathy	Pressure palsies
Sensory loss	0 - +++	0 - ±	0 - ±	0 - ±	++
Pain	+ - ++	+ - +++	+ - +++	+ - +++	±
Tendon reflex	N - ↓↓↓	N - ↓	↓↓	Normal	Normal
Motor deficit	0 - +++	0	+++	++	++

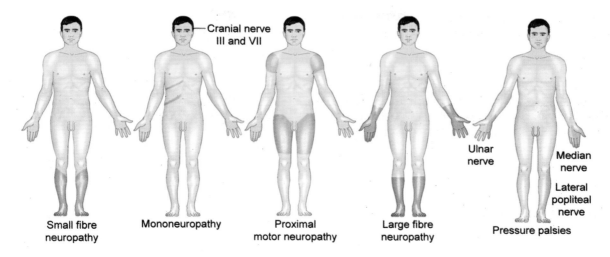

Fig. 9.39: Diabetic neuropathy

2. Genitourinary disorders
   Bladder atony
   Impotence
   Retrograde ejaculation of semen into the bladder
   Loss of testicular sensation
3. Cardiovascular disorders
   Orthostatic hypotension
   Heart rate abnormalities
   Painless myocardial infarction
4. Respiratory control and airway tone disturbances
5. Peripheral autonomic disorders
   Sudomotor and piloerector dysfunction
   Vasomotor disturbances
   Peripheral oedema
   Orthostatic hypotension
6. Endocrine disorders
   Hypoglycaemia
   Defective epinephrine and glucagon
      counterregulatory response
   Defective central perception
   Norepinephrine (vascular) deficiency
   Pancreatic polypeptide disturbances
   Renin disturbances
7. Lacrimal gland disorders
8. Pupillary disorders
9. Special complications related to neuropathy
   Diabetic foot disease
   Neuropathic arthropathy (Charcot's joint)
   Pseudotabes and pseudosyringomyelia
   Entrapment neuropathies
   Loss of visceral pain sense
   Increased mortality (associated with autonomic neuropathy).

Tip Therm Test

TIP THERM is an early diagnostic testing device for symmetrical polyneuropathy which measures temperature sensitivity of the skin. TIP THERM is made of special polymer and metal alloys. The polymer side feels warmer and the metal alloy side cooler due to the thermal conductivity property of the materials.

Diabetic neuropathy can lead to the diabetic foot syndrome, resulting in ulceration. This distal symmetrical polyneuropathy involves both large and small nerve fibres. The large myelinated (Aα, Aβ) fibres detect vibration and sensation. The small myelinated(Aδ) and unmyelinated C fibres can detect thermal sensation. Studies show abnormal small fibre function is usually affected before large fiber function

While temperature discrimination can be tested anywhere, it is best tested on the dorsal foot (Fig. 9.40). If sensation is not felt on the foot dorsum, try the test on

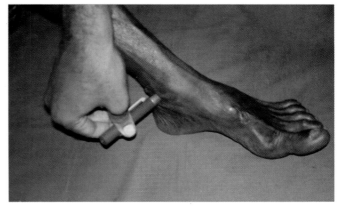

Fig. 9.40: Tip therm test

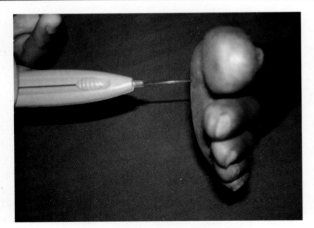

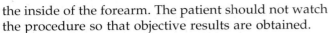

Fig. 9.41: Monofilament test

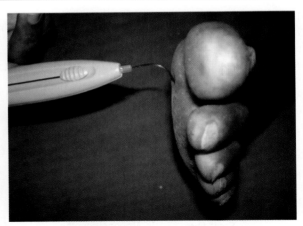

Fig. 9.42: Monofilament test

the inside of the forearm. The patient should not watch the procedure so that objective results are obtained.

It was shown to have 100% specificity and 97.3% sensitivity in diagnosing diabetic neuropathy compared to biothesiometer testing:

Note: Testing vibratory sensation using 128 MHZ tuning fork at the base of the great toe and also the ability to sense touch with a monofilament (size of the mono-filament- S 07/10g) are useful tests to detect moderately advanced diabetic neuropathy.

Monofilament Test

Early loss of protective sensation can be detected in the foot of the diabetic patients by using the 10 g mono-filament (Fig. 9.41).

Ten sites are chosen and the monofilament is applied with enough pressure to bend the filament for the duration of not less than 2 seconds (Fig. 9.42). It is tested for three times at each site and it is enough if he answers correctly in 2 out of 3 applications. Failure to feel the monofilament in more than 4 sites denotes loss of protective sensation. The risk of ulcer formation is greater. This test is 95% sensitive and 80% specific.

Management of the Diabetic Neuropathies
General Measures

a. Improvement in diabetic control
b. *Aldose reductase inhibitors:* Sorbitol accumulation has a role in the pathogenesis of diabetic neuropathy and cataract; this sorbitol pathway can be shutdown by aldose reductase inhibitors.
c. Relief of contributory factors like alcohol, ischaemia, hyperlipidemia, malnutrition, uraemia, neurotoxic drugs.

d. *Relief of nerve entrapment:* Constricting apparel, anti-inflammatory agents, surgical decompression, symptomatic drug treatment.
e. Treatment of painful neuropathy:
   (i) Ibuprofen, sulindac are used; narcotic analgesics are not useful.
   (ii) Tricyclic antidepressants, phenothiazines (imipramine or amitriptyline 50–150 mg/day + fluphenazine 1 mg every 8 hours is used in the treatment of various neuropathic cachexia.
   (iii) Carbamazepine—upto 200 mg every 8 hours (prevents generation of action potentials)
   (iv) Capsaicin—topical application works by depleting the nociceptive neurotransmitter substance 'P' in unmyelinated sensory nerve terminals.
f. Autonomic neuropathy
   (i) Gastroparesis—metoclopramide, cholinesterase inhibitors, domperidone, erythromycin
   (ii) Diabetic diarrhoea—clonidine, codeine, loperamide, diphenoxylate, kaopectate, cholestyramine, broad spectrum antibiotics, octreotide 50-75 µgm tid S/C
   (iii) Constipation—laxatives, metoclopramide
   (iv) Orthostatic hypotension—fludrocortisone, salt loading, sympathomimetics.
   (v) Diabetic cystopathy—cholinergics
   (vi) Retrograde ejaculation—brompheniramine maleate
   (vii) Gustatory sweating—anticholinergics, clonidine.

Supportive Measures, Prosthesis, Surgery

Foot care, foot wear
Foot and leg braces

Elastic stockings
Physical therapy
Small meals, gastroenterostomy
Bladder massage (crede), self-catheterisation, bladder neck resection
Orthopaedic surgical measures
Penile prosthesis
Anaesthetic precautions.

Treatment for Diabetic Erectile Dysfunction

Nonhormonal Therapy

Sildenafil citrate, a Phosphodiesterase 5 inhibitor is used at a dose of 50–100 mg (25 mg for men over 55 yrs) 1 hr before intercourse. It is contraindicated in patients with coronary artery disease and those taking nitrates.

α_2 blockers (yohimbine)

Tadalafil: It is very similar to sildenafil. It is a selective inhibitor of cyclic guanosine monophosphate (CGMP) and a specific phosphodiesterase 5 inhibitor (PDE 5). It is used in the dose of 10-20 mg one hour prior to sexual activity and the effect persists for 24 hours. Patients on nitrates or alpha blockers should avoid taking this drug.

Hormonal Therapy

Hypogonadotrophic hypogonadism—parenteral testosterone 200 mg IM.

Hyperprolactinaemia or pituitary tumour—cessation of causative medications, bromocriptine, extirpative surgery.

Noninvasive Therapy

Vacuum erection devices
Intracavernosal injection of vasoactive agents (papaverine, phentolamine, PG-E).

Invasive Therapy

Penile prosthesis
Microvascular arterial bypass surgery.

Diabetic Foot

It is a complication of diabetes due to an interplay of a number of disturbances like large vessel disease, neuropathy, infection, poor wound healing and possibly small vessel disease also (microangiopathy).

- Sensory loss results in unrecognized trauma from poorly fitting shoes, thermal or hot water burns, penetrating objects, toe nail cutting, etc.
- Motor defects causing foot deformities, produce abnormal pressure points on weight bearing areas.

Autonomic neuropathy results in poor arteriolar constriction and dilatation.

- Poor vasodilatation in response to heat or infection in combination with impaired sweating may compromise the local tissue microenvironment.
- Anhidrosis causes dry skin with fissures and cracks, predisposing to secondary infection.
- Denervation hypersensitivity (vasoconstriction in response to cold) may contribute to the development of diabetic foot ulcers.
- Hence, peripheral neuropathy is viewed as a primary underlying disturbance of diabetic foot lesions and vascular insufficiency is an important secondary factor.
- The ulcers are painless, with a punched out appearance. Foot is characteristically warm and pulses are easily felt. Secondary infection is common and may lead to wet gangrene. X-ray may show underlying osteomyelitis with sequestra and destruction of bone.
- Repetitive stress of walking results in interosseous atrophy causing cocked up toes and thinning of fat pad over metatarsal head.

Foot infections in diabetic patients are classified into two categories.

1. *Non-limb-threatening infections* (superficial, lack systemic toxicity, minimal cellulitis less than 2 cm, ulceration not extending fully through the skin, lack of significant ischemia) *S. aureus* is the major pathogen involved.
2. *Limb threatening infections* (extensive cellulitis, lymphangitis, ulcers penetrating through the skin into the subcutaneous tissues, prominent ischemia).

Polymicrobial infections are common. *Staphylococcus aureus*, group B streptococci, enterococcus, and facultative gram-negative bacilli along with anaerobes are commonly implicated.

Clinical Features of Diabetic Foot

Primarily neuropathic	Primarily ischaemic
Warm	Cold
Bounding pulses	Absent pulses
Diminished sensation	Sensation intact
Pink skin	Skin blanches on elevation
Anhidrosis	-
Callous formation	-
Cracks and fissures	-
Painless ulceration	Painful ulceration
Digital ulceration	Digital gangrene
Charcot's joints	-
Wasting of interosseous muscles	-
Clawed toes	-
Neuropathic oedema	Oedema associated with cardiac decompensation

Management

1. *General instructions:* Patients are advised not to smoke. They should not walk on hard surfaces or sandy beaches especially with barefeet. They should not use adhesive tapes or chemicals for removing corns/callosities. They should wear properly fitting stockings. Shoes should be comfortable at the time of purchase. Leather shoes are preferred and they are best tried in the afternoon when feet are largest. Shoes with pointed tips should be avoided. They should cut their nails straight across using a nail cutter. Regular chiropody should be done every week to debride the lesion.
2. Relieve high pressure area with bed rest and special footwear.
3. If there is cellulitis, admit the patient and start on IV antibiotics (benzylpenicillin 600 mg/6 h IV and flucloxacillin 500 mg/6 h IV ± metronidazole 500 mg/8 h IV or cefazolin IV).
   For mild infections, oral clindamycin or cephalexin or cloxacillin for 2 weeks can be given.
4. IV antimicrobial therapy is recommended for 10-12 weeks in the presence of osteomyelitis.

Absolute Indications for Surgery

a. Abscess or deep infection
b. Spreading anaerobic infection
c. Osteomyelitis
d. Severe ischaemia-gangrene/rest pain
e. Suppurative arthritis.

Newer Treatment

1. Platelet derived growth factor topical application for diabetic ulcer
2. Living human skin equivalents – by tissue engineering technique.

Diabetic Nephropathy (DN)

About 50% of end stage renal disease are due to diabetic nephropathy. About 35% of patients with IDDM develop this complication. In NIDDM, prevalence varies from 15–50%.

There are 2 distinct pathologic patterns.
1. *Diffuse glomerulosclerosis:* This consists of widening of glomerular basement membrane and mesangial thickening.
2. *Nodular glomerulosclerosis:* There is deposition of PAS positive material in the periphery of glomerular tufts, (the Kimmelstiel-Wilson lesion) In addition, there is hyalinization of afferent and efferent arterioles, 'capsular drops' in Bowman's capsule, fibrin caps and occlusion of glomeruli. Kimmelsteil-Wilson nodular glomerulosclerosis and capsular drops are pathognomonic of diabetic nephropathy.

Stages in Diabetic Nephropathy

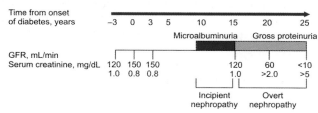

Time curve of diabetic nephropathy

Stage I   Glomerular hyperfiltration and renomegaly
Stage II   Early glomerular lesions (expansion of mesangial matrix and thickening of glomerular basement membrane). Occurs 18–36 months after onset of IDDM.
Stage III Microalbuminuria stage (incipient DN) with persistent hypertension of > 140–160/90 mm Hg.
           Albumin excretion is in the range of 30–300 mg/day.
           Albumin Excretion Rate (AER)—20–200 µg/min.

Microalbuminuria is due to ↓ concentration of anionic heparan sulfate-proteoglycan in the glomerular basement membrane. Diagnosis is by finding an AER > 15 µg/min (30 mg/d) in 2–3 samples collected in a 6 month period.

Persistent leakage of protein greater than 500 mg/day is predictive of subsequent macroproteinuria.

Stage IV   Clinical nephropathy (macroproteinuria)
           Once macroproteinuria begins, there is a steady decline in GFR of about 1 ml/min/month.
Stage V   End Stage Renal Disease
           Azotemia develops usually after 10 years progressing to nephrotic syndrome and ESRD later.

Treatment

1. Angiotensin—converting enzyme inhibitors are useful in slowing progression of diabetic nephropathy, especially in microalbuminuric stage. They are useful in hypertensive patients with be diabetes.

   If proteinuria persists after 3 months of therapy, the drug dose is increased until either the

at a lower level. After a feed there is an increase in blood glucose concentration closely followed by a rise in blood insulin concentration. This response is exaggerated in obese than in lean subjects. Fifty per cent of the insulin undergoes degradation in the liver and the rest, circulate and act on 3 specific receptors on liver, muscle and adipose tissue.

Hypoglycaemia is better tolerated by females. They do not develop symptoms till the blood glucose falls to 35–40 mg/dl.

Ten per cent of glucose is converted to glycogen and stored in the liver.

Hormonal Response to Hypoglycaemia

a. *In Normal Persons:* Levels of epinephrine, norepinephrine and glucagon increase quickly whereas levels of cortisol and growth hormone increase slowly during hypoglycaemia. This response is brought about by sensitising glucose receptors in hypothalamus and it continues for 8–10 hours.
b. *In Type I Diabetes:* First 5 years after the onset of Type 1 DM, glucagon response to hypoglycaemia is lost. After 10 years, the epinephrine response is also lost even in the absence of autonomic neuropathy. The other counter regulatory hormones continue to act. This results in absence of recognition of hypoglycemic symptoms produced by epinephrine and they become more prone for hypoglycaemia when on insulin therapy. Because of this, patients suffer from "hypoglycaemia unawareness" due to impaired, glucagon, epinephrine and autonomic nervous system response.
c. *In Type 2 Diabetes:* Levels of counter regulatory hormones remain normal.

Signs and Symptoms of Hypoglycaemia

1. *Adrenergic Symptoms* (Increased activity of the autonomic nervous system, triggered by a rapid fall in glucose level):
   Weakness, sweating, tachycardia, palpitations, tremor, nervousness, irritability, tingling of mouth and fingers, hunger, nausea, vomiting.
2. *Neuroglucopenic Symptoms* (due to decreased activity of CNS, requires an absolutely low level of glucose):
   Headache, hypothermia, visual disturbances, mental dullness, confusion, amnesia, seizures, coma.
3. Relationship between plasma glucose and signs of hypoglycaemia.
   90 – 75 mg%   Inhibition of insulin secretion
   75 – 60 mg%   Glucagon, epinephrine and GH secretion

60 – 45 mg%   Cortisol secretion, cognitive dysfunction
45 – 30 mg%   Lethargy
30 – 15 mg%   Coma, convulsions
<15 mg%   Permanent brain damage and death

Fasting Hypoglycaemia
Causes

Most common cause is treatment by insulin or sulfonylureas in a known diabetic.

The causes can be remembered by the pneumonic EXPLAIN.

Ex   Exogenous drugs—alcohol binge, insulin, sulfonylureas, quinine, salycylates, sulfonamide
P   Pituitary insufficiency
L   Liver failure and inherited enzyme defects (glucose-6-phosphatase, pyruvate carboxylase, fructose 1, 6-diphosphatase, glycogen synthetase, etc.)
A   Addison's disease
I   Increased insulin secretion
        Islet cell tumor
        Ectopic insulin secretion
N   Nonpancreatic neoplasm

Other causes are:
1. Renal failure
2. Insulin autoantibodies
3. Insulin receptor autoantibodies
4. Sepsis
5. Falciparum malaria
6. Congestive heart failure.

Fasting hypoglycaemia is gradual and prolonged. The adrenergic response is reverted by glucose or meal.

1. Drugs

Insulin is the most common drug causing hypoglycaemia. Sulfonylurea agents are the next common. Many other drugs potentiate the action of sulfonylureas. They are sulfonamides, chloramphenicol, clofibrate, dicuomarol, quinine, MAO inhibitors, phenylbutazone, and oxytetracycline.

Salicylates, pentamidine, propranolol may cause hypoglycaemia when taken alone.

Treatment

a. Blood should be taken for determination of glucose, insulin, C-peptide and sulfonylureas.
b. Treatment should be started before biochemical results arrive. The response is dramatic.

c. Initial treatment 50 ml of 50% glucose followed by constant IV glucose infusion until the patient is able to eat a meal. Hepatic glycogen repletion is not effective with small quantities of IV glucose and hence the importance of meal is stressed.
d. Hypoglycaemia from sulfonylureas may last for prolonged periods upto a few days and relapses are common. If glucose infusion is stopped early, patient may lapse back into coma. The prolonged effect of hypoglycemia may be due to drug interactions, hepatic or renal disease.
e. In hypoglycaemia due to insulin, glucagon (1 mg subcutaneously) can be given. In addition to stimulating hepatic glycogenolysis, it stimulates insulin secretion and hence it should not be given for sulfonylurea induced hypoglycaemia.
f. Patients who fail to regain consciousness may have cerebral oedema and they require treatment with mannitol or dexamethasone.

2. Factitious Hypoglycaemia

This is an unusual form of drug induced hypoglycemia. Patients surreptitiously take insulin or occasionally sulfonylureas.

Hypoglycaemia may be induced by exogenous/ endogenous insulin. It is differentiated by detecting high levels of C peptide in endogenously induced hypoglycaemia.

3. Ethanol

Ethanol produces hypoglycaemia by the following mechanism. It inhibits gluconeogenesis and occurs commonly in malnourished chronic alcoholic in whom glycogen stores in the liver are depleted.

4. Non β-Cell Tumour

Non β-cell tumors associated with hypoglycaemia are:
a. Large mesenchymal tumours (50%)
b. Hepatocellular carcinomas (25%)
c. Adrenal carcinomas (5–10%)
d. Gastrointestinal tumours (5–10%)
e. Lymphomas (5–10%)
f. Miscellaneous tumours (kidney, lung, anaplastic carcinomas, carcinoid).

The mechanism of hypoglycaemia is unclear. In rare instances, production of insulin or insulin like growth factor II (IGF-II) may be the cause.

Adrenal Carcinomas

Although rare, these are associated with hypoglycaemia commonly. Removal of the adrenal tumour is the treatment of choice.

Frequent feeding and glucocorticoids are also found to be helpful.

5. Hepatic Failure

In hepatic failure, hypoglycaemia occurs only when the liver is severely compromised (fulminant hepatic failure). Hourly blood glucose monitoring is mandatory and prompt correction should be done till the liver regenerates.

Hypoglycaemia occurring in this situation is a bad prognostic sign.

6. Adrenal Insufficiency

In this situation, decreased cortisol synthesis results in decreased gluconeogenesis and decreased hepatic glucose production.

Treatment

IV glucose as a bolus + 100 mg cortisol bolus followed by maintenance dose of steroids.

7. Beta Cell Tumour (Insulinomas)

These are rare tumours. Correct diagnosis is important as they are curable and if undetected for long periods of time, may develop neuropsychiatric sequelae. Glucose levels fall slowly and adrenergic response is often lacking (hypoglycaemia unawareness). They tend to present with confusion, transient neurologic syndromes, visual disturbances, personality changes, convulsions, coma and may lead to death. Weight gain is common in

Differential Diagnosis of Insulinoma and Factitious Hyperinsulinism

Test	Insulinoma	Exogenous insulin	Sulfonylurea
Plasma insulin	High (upto 200 mU/mL)	Very high (more than 100 mU/mL)	High
Insulin/glucose ratio	High	Very high	High
Proinsulin	Increased	Normal or low	Normal
C-peptide	Increased	Normal or low	Increased
Insulin antibodies	Absent	± Present	Absent
Plasma or urine sulfonylurea	Absent	Absent	Present

some of the patients. It is commonly associated with multiple endocrine neoplasia Type I.

This condition is diagnosed by the presence of Whipple's triad (fasting hypoglycaemia, symptoms of hypoglycemia, and immediate recovery after IV glucose) along with increased C-peptide and insulin levels and absent insulin antibodies or plasma/urine sulfonylureas.

Diagnostic Tests for Insulinomas

1. *Suppression of insulin secretion by fasting:* Fasting in normal subjects results in proportional fall of glucose and insulin (I/G ratio decreases).

In insulinoma, insulin is not suppressed and Insulin (microunit/mL)/Glucose (mg/mL) ratio increases. Ratios above 0.3 are diagnostic. Blood samples for glucose and insulin are drawn after the overnight fast and then every 2–4 hours after that. About two-thirds of patients will have hypoglycaemia symptoms within 24 hours of food deprivation. Another 25% will experience symptoms in the next 24 hours. The third day of fasting is required in 5% of patients who have insulinomas.

Protocol for 72 Hours Fast
a. Onset is time of last food.
b. Nothing by mouth except noncaloric beverages.
c. Patient should be active during waking hours.
d. Measure plasma glucose, insulin, C-peptide every 6 hours, every hourly when blood glucose is < 60 mg/dl.
e. End fast if plasma glucose is 45 mg/dl or less and when patient has symptoms.
f. At the end of fast, measure plasma glucose, insulin, C-peptide, sulfonylurea and ketone bodies.
g. Give glucagon 1 mg IV and measure plasma glucose every 10 minutes for 3 times.

2. *Measurement of proinsulin content along with insulin content* by radioimmunoassay of the fasting plasma is done. In insulinoma, proinsulin constitutes > 20% of insulin.

Ratio of insulin to proinsulin in normal individuals is 6 : 1. In insulinoma, the ratio is 1 : 1 whereas in sulfonylurea induced hypoglycaemia, the ratio is 10 : 1.

3. *C-Peptide Level:* It increases in equimolar concentration as that of insulin.

4. *Glucagon test:* After an overnight fast, give glucagon 1 mg IV and if the peak insulin response is more than 130 μu/ml, the test is positive.

5. *Localisation of tumour by CT, MRI, radionuclear scan* is done if the tumour is more than 2 cm in size. If the tumour is less than 2 cm in size, pancreatic arteriography and CT with contrast can be used.

Treatment

Medical: Acute treatment is by giving IV glucose infusion till plasma levels of glucose reach normal range. Drugs which act by increasing blood glucose level.
a. Oral diazoxide 300–1200 mg/day along with a diuretic (thiazide) to compensate for salt retaining property of diazoxide
b. Phenytoin
c. Chlorpromazine
d. Propranolol
e. Verapamil
f. Octreotide (100–600 mg/day subcutaneously).

Drug of choice for metastatic islet cell carcinoma is streptozotocin and doxorubicin or L-asparaginase or mithramycin.

Surgical: Surgery is the definitive treatment. Detectable tumours can be resected. If there is no detectable tumour, stepwise distal pancreatectomy is done until frozen section or blood glucose shows that all the tumour is removed.

8. Renal Failure

Poor dietary intake, decreased gluconeogenesis, and increased peripheral utilisation of glucose are the reasons for hypoglycaemia.

Treatment

Frequent feeding and glucocorticoids (15–20 mg predni-solone) sometimes. In patients with end stage renal disease, hypoglycaemia is a poor prognostic sign and the patients may die within 1 year.

9. Insulin Autoantibodies

Occasionally a patient may spontaneously develop antibodies to insulin even though he has never received insulin which leads to hypoglycaemia. This is due to binding of large amounts of endogenous insulin with subsequent release of free insulin at inappropriate time. Unusual cause for hypoglycaemia may be as a part of endocrine syndrome as occurs in rheumatoid arthritis, systemic lupus erythematosus, or Graves' disease.

10. Insulin Receptor Autoantibodies

This occurs usually in females. Patients have a syndrome of insulin resistance and acanthosis nigricans. Patients have raised ESR, anti-DNA antibodies, increased gamma globulin and decreased complement levels.

Male Osteoporosis

The incidence of osteoporosis in men is increasing due to the increased longevity of the population. The late onset of osteoporosis in men (10 years behind that of women) is due to higher initial bone mass in early life and absence of sudden loss of gonadal hormones as occurs in menopause in women.

Management

a. Good calcium and vitamin D intake
b. Regular physical exercise
c. Avoid smoking and excessive alcohol
d. Testosterone replacement for hypogonadism
e. Bisphosphonates like alendronate has been shown to increase bone mass and reduce incidence of fractures.
f. Management of concurrent medical disorders.

Paget's Disease

- Focal skeletal disorder – rapid disorganized bone remodeling affecting one or more bones – Characterized by increased bone turn over(osteoclastic activity) and increased but disorganized osteoid formation(osteoblastic activity)
- Incidence – 3% of population older than 50 years
- Family history – 15-30%
- Often affects pelvis, femur, spine and skull
- Bone pain, deformity and degenerative arthritis
- Sometimes extensive multi-focal involvement of many bones can occur
- Enormously elevated serum alkaline phosphatase value as a result of increased bone turn over.

Clinical Features

- Bone pain due to micro-fractures
- Muscular strain and accelerated osteoarthritis
- Joint deformity due to periarticular bone involvement
- Enlargement of head – due to involvement of skull
- Reduction in height
- Narrowing of cranial ostia and compression of cranial nerves
- Nerve root compression due to vertebral involvement
- Otosclerosis – hearing loss
- Hypercalcaemia and hypercalciuria with nephrolithiasis – due to prolonged immobilization
- High output cardiac failure – increased blood flow to the affected bones
- Osteogenic sarcoma – late complication and sudden accentuation of bone pain at a specific site denotes the possibility

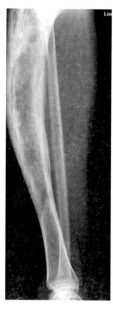

Fig. 9.46: Paget's disease—tibia

Investigations

- Elevated serum alkaline phosphatase
- Increased ^{99m}Tc bone scanning activity
- Characteristic X- ray finding – local radiolucency – more commonly affecting one region of skull 'Osteoporosis Circumscripta'
- X-ray tibia of lower limb (Fig. 9.46).

Management

1. Adequate hydration and mobilization to avoid hypercalcaemia
2. Pain relief – ibuprofen, COX-2 inhibitors
3. Mild disease (serum alkaline phosphatase < 3 times) Tiludronate 400 mg/day for 3 months or Etidronate 400 mg/day for 6 months
4. Moderate to severe disease Risedronate 30 mg/day for 2-3 months Alendronate 40 mg/day for 6 months

The effectiveness of therapy is monitored by measurement of serum alkaline phosphatase (SAP) and it must be monitored every 3 months. Therapy can be repeated when the SAP level increases above normal by 25%.

In very severe disease Pamidronate single dose 60 mg IV in 500 ml normal saline or dextrose over 4 hours for rapid response. Repeat the course weekly once for 1 month if the response is not adequate.

Calcitonin: Reserved for patients who cannot tolerate bisphosphonates.

Injection salmon calcitonin 100 U/day SC followed by 50 U SC three times/week for maintenance. It causes suppression of SAP. Use nasal form for milder disease.

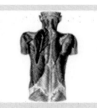

SYMPTOMS

JOINTS

PAIN

SWELLING
(acute/chronic
mono/polyarticular
symmetrical/asymmetrical)

MORNING STIFFNESS

LOSS OF FUNCTION

WEAKNESS

DEFORMITY

INSTABILITY

CHANGES IN SENSATION

SYSTEMIC SYMPTOMS

FEVER
RASH

FATIGUE
WEIGHT LOSS

HAIR LOSS

MUCOSAL ULCERS
(oral/genital)

DIARRHOEA

URETHRITIS

COLDNESS OF FINGER

DRY EYES/MOUTH
RED EYES

SIGNS

SYSTEMIC EXAMINATION

Inspect,

Rash
(malar area, over eyelids
generalised, over back
hair, scalp, axilla, gluteal
cleft, under the breast)

Photosensitivity
Microstomia
Ulcers
(mucosa-ocular/oral/genital
fingertips)
Iritis/Scleritis
Nodes/Nodules
Sclerodactyly
Raynaud's phenomenon
Pallor
Nail/hair changes

Hepatosplenomegaly
Prox. muscle weakness
Mononeuritis
Fundus changes

JOINT EXAMINATION
(including spine ex.)

Inflammatory signs in
joint

Pattern of joint
involvement

Muscle wasting
Attitude of limbs
deformity
Range of movements
Crepitus
Stress tests

Arthritis

Classification

A. Monoarthritis

Acute | Septic arthritis
| Gout
| Pseudogout
| Traumatic arthritis
Chronic | Psoriasis
| Ankylosing spondylitis
| Rheumatoid arthritis
| Tuberculosis
| Sarcoidosis
| Osteoarthritis

B. Polyarthritis

Asymmetric
Acute | Rheumatic fever
| Reactive arthritis
Chronic | Psoriatic arthritis
Symmetric
Acute | Hepatitis B, serum sickness
Chronic | Rheumatoid arthritis
| Systemic lupus erythematosis
| Osteoarthritis

C. Axial Arthritis

Ankylosing spondylitis
Reiter's syndrome
Tuberculosis
Brucellosis
Cervical or lumbar spondylosis.

Rheumatoid Arthritis

It is a chronic inflammatory, destructive and deforming symmetrical polyarthritis associated with systemic involvement. The individuals with HLA-D4 and HLA-DR4 are more prone to rheumatoid arthritis. The female: male ratio is 3 : 1.

Criteria for the Diagnosis

(i) Morning stiffness (more than one hour for more than six weeks)
(ii) Arthritis involving three or more joint areas (with or without soft tissue involvement lasting more than six weeks)
(iii) Arthritis of hand joints (wrist, MCP or PIP joints more than six weeks)

(iv) Symmetrical arthritis (at least one area lasting for six weeks)
(v) Rheumatoid nodules
(vi) Rheumatoid factor
(vii) Radiographic changes.

Diagnosis of rheumatoid arthritis is made when four or more criteria are present.

Pathogenesis

a. Synovitis (synovial cell hyperplasia, hypertrophy with CD4 lymphocytic infiltration and synovial effusion)
b. Pannus formation
c. Cartilage loss
d. Fibrosis
e. Bony erosion, deformity, fibrous and bony ankylosis
f. Muscle wasting
g. Periarticular osteoporosis.

Triggering Factors

1. Infection
2. Vaccinations
3. Physical trauma
4. Psychological stress.

Clinical Features

1. Fatigue
2. Weakness
3. Vague arthralgias
4. Myalgias
5. Joint stiffness.

The other joint manifestations are swelling, warmth, tenderness, and synovial thickening without erythema.

The joints most commonly involved are:
a. Finger joint (40%)
b. Shoulder joint (20%)
c. Foot joint (20%)
d. Wrist joint (15%).

Other joints involved in chronic rheumatoid arthritis are:
1. Temporomandibular joint (malalignment of teeth with mal occlusion)
2. Cervical joints C_1 C_2 (atlanto axial dislocation—quadriplegia)
3. Crico-arytenoid (sensation of foreign body, hoarseness, weak voice and stridor)
4. Sternoclavicular
5. Acromioclavicular

6. Glenohumeral
7. Elbow (extension defects, epicondylitis and olecranon bursitis-ulnar deviation), hand (swan neck deformity, button-hole deformity)
8. Hip and knee (Morant-Baker's cyst)
9. Talocalcaneal, midtarsal, metatarsophalangeal.

Course
It is variable.

It can be slowly progressive with oligoarthritis or rapidly progressive erosive arthritis with marked deformity with downhill course.

The following features, exclude rheumatoid arthritis
1. Butterfly rash—SLE
2. High concentration of LE cells
3. Polyarteritis nodosa
4. Dermatomyositis
5. Scleroderma
6. Chorea ⎱
   Erythema marginatum ⎰ Rheumatic fever
7. Tophi-Gout
8. Arthritis associated with bacterial or viral infections
9. Positive AFB
10. Reiter's syndrome
11. Shoulder hand syndrome
12. Hypertrophic pulmonary osteoarthropathy
13. Neuroarthropathy
14. Homogentisic acid in urine
15. Sarcoidosis
16. Multiple myeloma
17. Erythema nodosum
18. Leukaemia and lymphoma
19. Agammaglobulinaemia
20. Distal interphalangeal joint of hand and feet (Fig. 10.1).

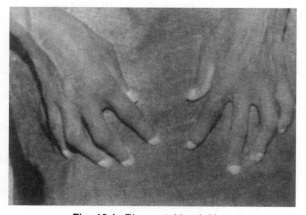

Fig. 10.1: Rheumatoid arthritis—sparing of distal IP joints

Nonarticular Manifestations of Rheumatoid Arthritis

Respiratory System

1. Pleurisy with or without effusion
2. Pneumothorax
3. Rheumatoid nodule (Caplan's)
4. Interstitial fibrosis
5. Pneumonia
6. Chronic bronchitis or bronchiectasis
7. Pulmonary hypertension.

Cardiovascular System

1. Pericarditis
2. Endocarditis
3. Cardiomyopathy
4. Conduction defects
5. Cardiac arrhythmias
6. Infiltration of valves (mitral incompetence and aortic incompetence)
7. Myocardial infarction (due to coronary vasculitis).

Gastrointestinal System

1. Xerostomia
2. Parotid enlargement
3. Dysphagia
4. Mesenteric artery occlusion.

Renal System

1. Pyelonephritis
2. Analgesic nephropathy
3. Amyloidosis.

Lymph Nodes

Local and generalised lymphadenopathy.

Ocular

1. Episcleritis, scleritis (Fig. 10.2)
2. Keratoconjunctivitis sicca
3. Scleromalacia perforans.

Ear

Defective hearing (involvement of ossicular chain).

Muscle

1. Weakness and atrophy
2. Myopathy (steroid, chloroquine)
3. Tenosynovitis.

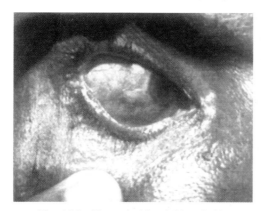

Fig. 10.2: Rheumatoid arthritis-scleritis

Skin

1. Dermal atrophy
2. Leg ulcers
3. Nail dystrophy
4. Nodules
5. Pyoderma gangrenosum.

Bones

1. Periarticular osteoporosis

Central Nervous System

1. Cervical dislocation (quadriplegia)
2. Peripheral neuropathy (sensory and motor)
3. Autonomic neuropathy (reduced sweating, cold hands, and palmar erythema)
4. Entrapment neuropathy.
   a. Elbow-ulnar
   b. Carpal tunnel—median
   c. Knee—lateral popliteal
   d. Tarsal tunnel—posterior tibial.

Haematological

1. Anaemia
   a. normocytic hypochromic
   b. megaloblastic ($\downarrow$ folic acid)
2. Haemolytic anaemia
3. Serum Fe—low
4. Iron binding capacity—normal
5. Raised ESR
6. Neutropenia ⎫
   Pancytopenia ⎬ Felty's syndrome
   Splenomegaly ⎭
7. Eosinophilia (vasculitis, nodules)
8. Hyperviscosity syndrome

It is due to increased rheumatoid factor. The manifestations are dizziness, diplopia, dyspnoea and bleeding tendency.
9. Vasculitis
   a. Dermal infarction
   b. Cranial-cerebrovascular accidents
   c. Coronary-myocardial infarction
   d. Mesenteric-gut gangrene
   e. Peripheral-digital gangrene
   f. Vasa nervosum-neuropathy.

Variants of Rheumatoid Arthritis

1. *Felty's syndrome:* It is characterised by splenomegaly, neutropenia, pancytopenia and lymphadenopathy
2. *Still's disease (rheumatoid arthritis occurring in children):* It is characterised by mono or polyarthritis, fever, maculopapular rash, hepatosplenomegaly, lymphadenopathy, and leucocytosis. The rheumatoid factor and antinuclear antibody are negative. It mostly occurs in juvenile age group. The joint deformity is rare but growth retardation is present.
3. *Sjögren's syndrome:* It is characterised by enlargement of lacrimal and salivary glands, xerostomia, kerato conjunctivitis sicca, leucopenia, lymphocytosis, and eosinophilia. The rheumatoid factor is positive and there is eosinophilia.

Comparison of Rheumatoid Arthritis and Osteoarthritis

Characteristics	Rheumatoid arthritis	Osteoarthritis
Age	Any age group	Middle/old age
Inflammation	Prominent	Mild
Disease cause	Autoimmunity	Trauma
Onset	Rapid with swelling	Gradual
Bone density	Decreased(osteoporosis)	Increased
Stiffness	Morning stiffness	Due to joint damage
Synovial space	Thickened and Increased	Decreased
DIP - Joint	Never involved	Involved

Investigations

1. Complete blood count (anaemia, thrombocytosis, $\uparrow$ ESR)
2. Increased acute phase proteins (C-reactive protein)
3. Increased plasma viscosity
4. Serum proteins
   a. Albumin $\downarrow$
   b. Gammaglobulins $\uparrow$

Synovial Fluid

	Colour	Viscosity	Clarity	Cell Count/mm³	Other Tests
Normal	Colourless	Very high	Clear	0–200	
Osteoarthritis	Colourless	High	Clear	400–4000	
* Rheumatoid arthritis	Yellow	Low	Cloudy	4000–40000	Low complement
Seronegative inflammatory arthritis	Yellow	Low	Cloudy	4000–40000	Normal complement
Gout/Pseudo-gout	Variable	Low	Variable	2000–40000	Crystals—monosodium urate, calcium pyrophosphate dihydrate under polarising microscope
Septic arthritis	Yellow	Low	Very turbid	> 50000	Gram stain, culture and GLC (gas liquid chromatography)

* Poor mucin precipitation

c. α_2 globulin $\uparrow$
d. IgG, IgM, IgA $\uparrow$

5. *Serological tests*
   Rheumatoid factor: Rheumatoid factors are immuno-globulins of the IgG or IgM class which react with the Fc portion of IgG. It is produced by plasma cells and lymphocytes in subsynovial tissue and draining lymph nodes. It is detected by
   a. *Rose Waaler test:* It is more specific and is said to be positive when more than 1 : 32
   b. *Latex test:* It is sensitive, but less specific and said to be positive when more than 1 : 20. The above two tests are used to detect IgM rheumatoid factor.
6. Radiological features of rheumatoid arthritis
   a. Early: soft tissue swelling
        periarticular osteoporosis
        periosteitis
        erosions—periarticular and subarticular cysts
   b. Late: narrowed joint spaces
        articular surface irregularity
        osteoporosis
        subluxation
        ankylosis
        secondary osteoarthritis
7. Antinuclear antibody is positive in 20 to 50%.
8. LE cell is positive in 10 to 20%.
9. Pleural fluid analysis
   a. Low glucose
   b. Increased LDH
   c. Low complement
10. Synovial fluid analysis.

Management

A. *Goals*
1. Education and motivation.
2. Disease modification through the suppression of inflammation and the immunologic process which is active systemically and in the joints and other tissues.
3. Maintenance of joint function and prevention of deformities.
4. Repair of joint damage if it will relieve pain or facilitate function.

B. *Systemic and Articular Rest*
1. Short bed-rest is recommended for about an hour in the midmorning and midafternoon.
2. Splints: The wrist splints are particularly useful during bouts of acute wrist synovitis and for management of carpal tunnel syndrome.

C. *Physiotherapy*
1. *Regular Exercise*
   a. Exercise is most successful after heat application.
   b. A fifteen minute early morning shower or a bath at 98–100 °F will help decrease morning stiffness.
   c. Static quadriceps exercises should be performed to strengthen the muscular, ligamentous, and tendinous support of the knees.
2. *Joint Protection*
   The principles of joint protection are maintenance of muscle strength and range of motion, avoidance of positions of deformity, the use of the strongest joints possible for a given task, and the utilization of joints in the most stable anatomic planes.

D. *Drug therapy*

Group I: Nonsteroidal Anti-inflammatory Drugs (NSAIDs)

a. Aspirin
b. Indomethacin
c. Fenamides
d. Propionic acid compounds

e. Sulindac (clinoryl)
f. Tolmetin
g. Piroxicam
h. Diclofenac
i. COX2 inhibitors

Choice of NSAIDs

The general approach is to choose an NSAID and treat for 2–4 weeks, the usual time period needed to define the drug's efficacy and side effect profile.

Salicylates

Aspirin (acetylsalicylic acid): Aspirin is the initial treatment of choice of rheumatoid arthritis.

Dose: 3–4 grams per day

Preparations

1. Plain tablets (inexpensive, cause gastritis, standard tablet dose 325 mg)
2. Buffered tablets (formulated with the insoluble calcium and magnesium antacids)
3. Enteric-coated tablets (the coating remains intact until tablet reaches small intestine)
4. Timed-release tablets (encapsulated aspirin particles, delayed absorption, more sustained plasma levels)
5. Sodium salicylate (enteric-coated) preparations preferred, less potent analgesic than aspirin)
6. Choline salicylate (very soluble, liquid form, negligible gastric bleeding)
7. Choline magnesium trisalicylate (trilisate).

Toxicities

1. *Common:* Dyspepsia, gastrointestinal bleeding, and peptic ulceration.
2. *Tinnitus or deafness:* It is the earliest indication of salicylate toxicity in adults and is reversible with a small (i.e. 1 or 2 tablets) decrease in daily dosage.
3. *Central nervous system symptoms:* Headache, vertigo, nausea, vomiting, irritability, and psychosis (elderly).
4. At high serum levels (25–35 mg/dl), especially in juvenile patients, salicylates may cause mild, acute, reversible hepatocellular injury, as demonstrated by a rise in serum enzymes.
5. Platelet adenosine diphosphate (ADP) release, adhesiveness, and aggregation are inhibited for as long as 72 hours after a single 300-mg dose of aspirin, probably as a result of irreversible acetylation of platelet membrane proteins.

Other Nonsteroidal Anti-inflammatory Drugs (NSAIDs)

These agents are equipotent to aspirin and exert anti-inflammatory action by modifying prostaglandin metabolism.

Indomethacin

Dose: 25–50 mg tid

Drug interactions
Probenecid prolongs action
Furosemide decreases action
Antacids delay absorption

Toxicity
Dyspepsia
GI bleeding
Gastric and ileal ulcer
Drowsiness
Depression
Seizures
Neuropathy
Interstitial nephritis
Hepatitis
Retinopathy
Blood dyscrasias.

Propionic Acid and Other Compounds

1. Ibuprofen (brufen)
2. Ketoprofen
3. Fenoprofen
4. Flurbiprofen
5. Naproxen.

Brufen

Dose: 200–400 mg tid.
• It is less toxic and less effective than aspirin and well tolerated.
• Piroxicam. 10–20 mg dose once daily.

Cyclo-oxygenase – 2 inhibitors
They have selectivity for COX 2 enzyme. GI symptoms and ulcerations are reduced. Platelet function is not impaired. The anti-inflammatory and analgesic efficacy is same as that of traditional NSAIDs.

Partially selective
Aceclofenac	100-200 mg /day
Meloxicam	7.5-15 mg/day
Nabumetone	500-1500 mg/day

Highly selective

Celecoxib	100-200 mg BD
Roficoxib	12.5-50 mg/day

Methotrexate

Methotrexate is the first choice in the management of moderate and severe rheumatoid arthritis. It is non-oncogenic and it acts rapidly in 4-6 weeks and is comparatively less toxic. It can be used along with NSAIDs. It is given in a dose of 7.5 mg PO weekly once along with breakfast. The dose can be increased upto 15 mg once a week.

Group II

Disease modifying agents (DMARDs): This group of drugs take a long time (6–12 weeks) for their actions to commence and so in the induction phase, NSAIDs must be given to reduce pain and their dose should be tapered subsequently.
1. Gold
2. Penicillamine
3. Chloroquine
4. Sulphasalazine

Indications

1. Failure of conservative management (even after 3 months with NSAIDs and general measures)
2. Rapidly progressive erosive arthritis.

Indications for 'gold' therapy: It is reserved for patients who continue to have active synovitis or who develop erosions on a conservative regimen of NSAIDs, rest, and physiotherapy.

Contraindications: It is contraindicated in patients with a history of previous severe skin, bone marrow, or renal reactions to gold.

Dose: Start with 10 mg per wk and then increase upto 50 mg per wk. Maintain with 50 mg once in 2 wks. It can be given orally or intramuscularly.

Toxicities
a. Bone marrow depression
b. Renal failure
c. Stomatitis and oral ulcer
d. Skin rash
e. Neuropathy
f. Hepatotoxicity
g. Ocular toxicity.

Chloroquine

Indications: Failure to respond to conservative regimen of rest, salicylates, other NSAIDs or gold.

Contraindications: Patients with significant visual, hepatic, or renal impairment or with porphyria, in pregnant women, and in children.

Dose: Chloroquine 250 mg OD;
          Hydroxy chloroquine 200 mg BD.

Toxicity
a. Keratopathy
b. Retinopathy
c. Neuropathy
d. Myopathy.

Penicillamine

It is particularly of value in the therapy of extra articular manifestations of rheumatoid arthritis (rheumatoid vasculitis, Felty's syndrome).

Dose: 600–1200 mg per day.

Toxicity
1. Taste impairment, anorexia, nausea and dyspepsia
2. Bone marrow aplasia
3. Polyarteritis
4. Nephrotic syndrome
5. Ocular and lingual ulceration
6. Skin rashes
7. Avoid in penicillin allergy.

Sulphasalazine

It is metabolized by the colonic bacteria into 5 amino salycilic acid and sulpha pyridine of which sulpha pyridine has more important anti-inflammatory role in rheumatoid arthritis.

Dose: Started at 500 mg/day and slowly increased to 1gm BD over a period of 4 weeks.

Toxicity
a. Rash
b. Depression
c. Megaloblastic anaemia
d. Leukopenia.

Group III (Highly Toxic)

1. Corticosteroids, * ACTH
2. Leflunomide
3. Azathioprine
4. Cyclophosphamide
5. Cyclosporine
6. Levamisole.

*Preferable in children since it does not interfere with growth. The drug of choice is prednisolone.

Corticosteroids

Indications

1. Along with DMARDs in the initial phase, if NSAIDs are not adequate to relieve the distressing symptoms, a short course of 7.5 mg of prednisolone can be added and tapered subsequently.
2. Failure to control the disabling symptoms.
3. Elderly patients in acute conditions.
4. Life-threatening conditions (severe pericarditis, poly-arteritis or scleritis).

Dose: Prednisolone 10–15 mg per day.

Toxicities

1. *Endocrine*
   a. Moon face
   b. Truncal obesity
   c. Hirsutism
   d. Impotence
   e. Menstrual irregularity
   f. Suppression of HPA axis
   g. Growth suppression.
2. *Metabolic*
   a. Negative Ca, K, N balance
   b. Sodium and fluid retention
   c. Hyperglycaemia
   d. Hyperlipoproteinaemia.
3. *Musculoskeletal*
   a. Myopathy
   b. Osteoporosis
   c. Avascular necrosis.
4. *Skin*
   a. Acne, striae
   b. Skin atrophy
   c. Bruising
   d. Impaired wound healing.
5. *Immunological*
   a. Suppression of delayed hypersensitivity
   b. Reactivation of TB
   c. Susceptibility to infection.
6. *Gastrointestinal*
   a. Peptic ulceration
   b. Pancreatitis.
7. *Cardiovascular*
   a. Hypertension
   b. Congestive cardiac failure.
8. *Ocular*
   a. Glaucoma
   b. Posterior subcapsular cataracts.
9. *CNS*
   a. Changes in mood and personality
   b. Psychosis
   c. Benign intracranial hypertension.

Leflunomide

It inhibits autoimmune T cell proliferation and production of antibodies by T cells. It also blocks TNF dependent nuclear factor kappa B activation.

Dose: 20 mg/day

Contraindications: Hypersensitivity, pregnancy, lactation, concurrent vaccination with live vaccines, uncontrolled infection, children < 18 years.

Toxicity: Elevation of liver enzymes, diarrhoea

Azathioprine

It is oncogenic.

Cyclophosphamide

It is effective for the treatment of rheumatoid vasculitis.
Cyclosporine (under trial)

Levamisole

It is an immunomodulator and can be given in a dose of 150 mg single weekly dose.

Toxicity

a. Skin rash
b. Dyspepsia
c. Leucopenia
d. Agranulocytosis (hence the drug is used with caution).

Group IV (Cytokine Antagonist)

TNF α Antagonist

Anti TNF α drugs produce a very good response when combined with methotrexate.

1. *Infliximab*
   It is a chimeric monoclonal antibody that binds with high affinity and specificity to human TNF α.
   Dose: 3 mg/kg at 0, 2 and 6 weeks and thereafter at intervals of 4 or 8 weeks intravenously.
   Toxicity: nausea, headache, rash, cough, upper respiratory infection, formation of human antichimeric antibodies, antinuclear antibodies and anti-dsDNA antibodies.

2. *Etanercept:*
   It is a recombinant fusion protein capable of binding to two TNF α molecules. It has an earlier onset of action than methotrexate.
   Dose: 25 mg subcutaneously twice weekly.
   Toxicity: Injection site reactions and development of anti-nuclear and anti-dsDNA antibody

3. *Adalimumab:*
   It is a fully human monoclonal antibody against TNF α.
   Dose: 20–80 mg S/C every 2 weeks

IL 1 Receptor Antagonist

1. *Anakinra*
   It is an interleukin 1 receptor antagonist. It can be combined with TNF α blockers.

Medical Synovectomy

Yttrium$_{90}$ silicate is used for larger joints (knee) and Erbium 159 acetate for smaller joints. Joints should be immobilized for 72 hours to prevent the spread to adjacent lymph nodes. It is contraindicated in patients below 45 years.

Surgical

a. Synovectomy
b. Arthroplasty
c. Osteotomy
d. Arthrodesis.

Rehabilitations

1. *Physical*
   a. Bath aid
   b. Toilet aid
   c. Dressing aid
   d. Walking aid
   e. Household aid
   f. Wheel chair
   g. Beds
   h. Reading, writing aids.
2. *Occupational.*

Causes of Death

1. Intercurrent infection
2. Cervical cord lesion
3. Arteritis
4. Cardiac failure
5. Renal failure
6. Amyloidosis
7. Iatrogenic
   a. Peptic ulcer
   b. Pyelonephritis
   c. Steroid toxicity.

Poor Prognostic Factors

1. Increased duration of morning stiffness
2. High titre of rheumatoid factor
3. ↑ ESR
4. Mode of onset (insidious onset of disease)
5. Weak hand grip
6. ↑ed feet-walking time
7. Systemic involvement—active more than one year without remission.

8. Associated vasculitis, Rheumatoid nodules
9. Involvement of cervical joints.
10. Protracted anaemia.

Seronegative Arthritis

These are a group of diseases in which an inflammatory arthritis, characterised by persistently negative tests for IgM rheumatoid factor is variably associated with a number of other common articular, extra-articular and genetic features.

Ankylosing Spondylitis

- Ankylosing spondylitis (AS) is an inflammatory disorder of unknown cause that primarily affects the axial skeleton.
- The disease usually begins in the second or third decade of life.
- Onset of the disease in adolescence correlates with a worse prognosis and more severe hip involvement.
- Men are affected approximately 3 times more than women. The disease in women tends to progress less frequently to total spinal ankylosis.
- Ankylosing spondylitis shows a striking correlation with the histocompatibility antigen HLA-B27.

Clinical Features

- Sacroilitis is usually one of the earliest manifestation of AS.
- The initial symptom is usually a dull pain, insidious in onset, felt deep in the lower lumbar or gluteal region, accompanied by low-back morning stiffness of up to a few hours' duration that improves with activity and returns following prolonged periods of inactivity.
- In some patients, bony tenderness over costosternal junctions, spinous processes, iliac crests, greater trochanters, ischial tuberosities, tibial tubercles, and heels may be present.
- Arthritis in the hips and shoulders may occur.
- Peripheral arthritis, if present, is usually asymmetric.
- Constitutional symptoms such as fatigue, anorexia, fever, weight loss, or night sweats may occur.
- Acute anterior uveitis, can antedate the spondylitis (Fig. 10.4).
- Attacks are typically unilateral and tend to recur.
- Loss of spinal mobility, with limitation of anterior flexion, lateral flexion, and extension of the lumbar spine, is seen (Fig. 10.3).

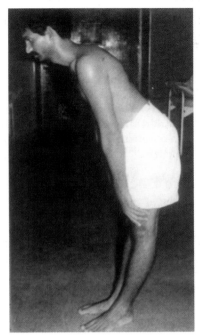

Fig. 10.3: Ankylosing spondylitis-limitation of spinal forward flexion

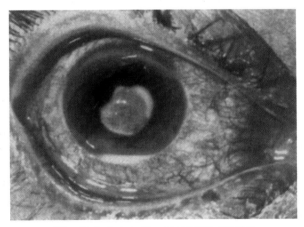

Fig. 10.4: Ankylosing spondylitis-anterior uveitis with hypopyon

The Schober Test

It is a useful measure of forward flexion of the lumbar spine. The patient stands erect, with heels together, and marks are made directly over the spine 5 cm below and 10 cm above the lumbosacral junction. The patient then bends forward maximally, and the distance between the two marks is measured. The distance between the two marks increases 5 cm or more in the case of normal lumbar mobility and less than 4 cm in the case of decreased lumbar mobility.

There is limitation of chest expansion (Normal chest expansion is 5 cm or greater).

As the disease progresses, the lumbar lordosis is obliterated with accompanying atrophy of the buttocks. The thoracic kyphosis is accentuated. If the cervical spine is involved, there may be a forward stoop of the neck. Hip involvement with ankylosis may lead to flexion contractures.

The progression of the disease may be followed by
• Measuring the patient's height (the patient's height decreases with progression of the disease due to exaggerated thoracic kyphosis and forward stooping of the neck).
• Chest expansion (chest expansion decreases with disease progression, and produces a restrictive lung disease, culminating in type 1 respiratory failure).
• Schober test.
• Occiput-to-wall distance when the patient stands erect with the heels and back flat against the wall (this distance increases with increasing involvement of the cervical spine by the disease due to increasing forward stoop of the neck).

Complications that can arise are spinal fracture, which can occur with even minor trauma to the rigid, osteoporotic spine. Involvement of the cervical spine can lead to quadriplegia. Cauda equina syndrome is another complication of long-standing spinal disease.

Pulmonary involvement, is characterized by slowly progressive upper lobe fibrosis.

Cardiovascular involvement may manifest as aortic insufficiency or cardiac conduction disturbances (including third degree heart block).

Prostatitis occurs with increased frequency in men.

Investigations

• Elevated ESR and C-reactive protein.
• Mild normochromic, normocytic anaemia.
• Elevated serum alkaline phosphatase.
• Elevated IgA levels.

Radiographic Findings

The earliest changes in the sacroiliac joints demonstrable by plain X-ray show blurring of the cortical margins of the subchondral bone, followed by erosions and sclerosis. Progression of the erosions leads to 'pseudo-widening' of the joint space and later the joints may become obliterated with onset of bony ankylosis.

X-ray of the spine shows a characteristic appearance of a 'bamboo spine' (ossification of interspinous ligaments). There is diffuse osteoporosis of the vertebral column. Erosion of vertebral bodies at the disc margin leads to 'squaring' of the vertebra.

Modified New York criteria for diagnosis of ankylosing spondylitis:
1. A history of back pain.
2. Limitation of motion of the lumbar spine.
3. Limited chest expansion.
4. Definite radiographic sacroiliitis.

Under these criteria, the presence of radiographic sacroiliitis plus any one of the other three criteria is sufficient for a diagnosis of definite ankylosing spondylitis.

The detection of HLA B27 is useful only as a diagnostic adjunct, since the presence of B27 is neither necessary nor sufficient for the diagnosis, but it can be helpful in patients who have not yet developed radiographic sacroiliitis.

Treatment

*   There is no definite treatment for ankylosing spondylitis. An exercise programme may be designed in order to maintain functional mobility. Anti-inflammatory agents may be given to achieve sufficient relief of symptoms
*   Indication for surgery in patients with ankylosing spondylitis is severe hip joint arthritis, when total hip arthroplasty may be done
*   Attacks of acute anterior uveitis are usually effectively managed with local glucocorticoid administration in conjunction with mydriatic agents
*   Methotrexate and sulphasalazine may be beneficial in some cases
*   *Infliximab* (Chimeric Human/Mouse Anti-TNF-2 monoclonal antibody)
    It is given in a dose of 5 mg/kg IV infusion, repeated at 2 weeks, 6 weeks and then at 8 weeks interval.
*   *Etanercept* (Soluble P75 TNF-α receptor-IgG fusion protein)
    It is given in a dose of 25 mg SC bid.
    Both the above drugs have shown rapid, profound and sustained reductions in all clinical and lab measures of disease activity.

Diffuse Idiopathic Skeletal Hyperostosis (DISH)

*   DISH occurs in the middle age and elderly
*   Usually asymptomatic and may have stiffness
*   Ligamentous calcification and ossification
*   'Flowing Wax'-appearance on the anterior bodies of the vertebra as a result of anterior spinal ligament calcification

*   Intervertebral disc spaces are preserved
*   Sacroiliac and apophyseal joints appear normal.

Reiter's Disease

It is characterised by a triad of seronegative oligoarthritis, conjunctivitis and nonspecific urethritis, 1–3 weeks following bacterial dysentery or exposure to sexually transmitted disease. Arthritis occurring alone following sexual exposure or enteric infection is known as reactive arthritis.

Arthritogenic Bacteria in Reactive Arthritis

1. Salmonella
2. Shigella
3. Campylobacter
4. Yersinia
5. Chlamydia.

Clinical Features

1. It presents with monoarthritis of a knee or an asymmetrical inflammatory arthritis of interphalangeal joints.
2. Patients can have heel pain, Achilles tendinitis or plantar fasciitis with presence of circinate balanitis. The presence of rash of keratoderma blennorrhagica is diagnostic of Reiter's disease in the absence of classical triad.
3. Skin lesions are faint macules, vesicles and pustules on the hands and feet to marked hyperkeratosis with plaque like lesions spreading to scalp and trunk.
4. Dystrophy of nail and massive subungual hyper keratosis may be seen.
5. Ocular involvement (mild bilateral conjunctivitis) subsides spontaneously within a month. Iritis can occur in 10% of cases.
6. Symptomatic urethritis (mild dysuria and clear sterile discharge) is seen in most cases.
7. Self-limiting arthritis is seen in all cases
8. The extra-articular features are:
    a. Conjunctivitis
    b. Iritis
    c. Aortic regurgitation
    d. Cardiac conduction defects
    e. Peripheral neuropathy.

Investigations

1. Raised ESR
2. Normocytic, normochromic anaemia and polymorphonuclear leukocytosis are present in peripheral smear
3. Rheumatoid factor and ANA are negative

4. HLA-B27 is seen in more than 70% of cases
5. Periarticular osteoporosis, reduction of joint space and erosive changes are the radiological features
6. Low viscosity inflammatory effusion with leucocyte count of 50,000/cumm and sterile on culture are seen in synovial fluid analysis.

Treatment

1. Rest
2. Analgesics
3. Local corticosteroids are useful in the case of iritis
4. The nonspecific urethritis is treated with a short course of tetracycline.

Psoriatic Arthritis

It is a seronegative inflammatory arthritis and associated with characteristic changes in the nails (pitting and transverse ridges). It occurs in about 1/1000 of the general population and in 7% of patients with psoriasis.

Clinical Features

- Asymmetrical oligoarthritis (70%)
- Sacroiliitis/spondylitis (40%)
- Symmetrical seronegative arthritis (15%)
- Distal interphalangeal joint arthritis (15%)
- Arthritis mutilans.

Extra-articular Features

1. Scaly skin lesions are seen over extensor surfaces (scalp, natal cleft and umbilicus)
2. The nail changes are pitting, onycholysis, sub-ungual hyperkeratosis and horizontal ridging.

Investigations

1. Normochromic normocytic anaemia
2. Raised ESR
3. Test for RF and ANA are negative
4. The terminal IP joint involvement and relative periarticular osteoporosis are seen.

Treatment

1. Analgesics (NSAIDs)
2. Sulphasalazine and gold are used in persistent symptomatic cases without exacerbation
3. Chloroquine and hydroxychloroquine are used
4. Retinoid etretinate 30 mg/day is effective for both arthritis and skin lesions

5. Photochemotherapy with methoxy psoralen and long wave ultraviolet light (PUVA) are used for severe skin lesions
6. Methotrexate can also be given.

Prognosis

It has better prognosis than rheumatoid arthritis.

Systemic Lupus Erythematosus (SLE)

It is a multisystem connective tissue disease of unknown cause in which tissues and cells are damaged by pathogenic autoantibodies and immune complexes.

It is more common in women of child bearing age (male: female is 1 : 9).

Aetiology and Pathogenesis

1. There is disturbance of immune regulation.
2. Genetic factors are involved (HLA-B8 and DR3)
3. Involvement of environmental factors (sunlight).
4. *Drugs:* oestrogens, oral contraceptives, quinidine, INH, hydralazine, chlorpromazine, practolol, methyldopa, phenytoin, a interferon and procainamide (most frequent).
5. Infection is thought to be one of the aetiological factors.
6. Immunologically-mediated tissue damage, also results.
7. Miscellaneous: Ingested alfalfa sprout and chemicals like hydrazines, hairdyes are also implicated.

Autoantibodies in SLE

Antinuclear antibodies	(95%)
Anti-DNA-histone (and LE cells)	(70%)
Anti-DNA-(single strand)	(70%)
Anti-DNA-(double strand)	(70%)
Anti-RNA	
Anti-Sm	(30%)
Anti-UI-RNP	(40%)
Anti-Ro/SS-A	(30%)
Anti-La/SS-B	(10%)
Anti-cardiolipin	(50%)
Anti-erythrocyte	(60%)
Anti-lymphocyte	(70%)
Anti-platelet	(50%)
Anti-neuronal	(60%)
Anti-MA	
Anti-PCNA	

Criteria for the Diagnosis of SLE

1. Malar rash

2. Photosensitivity
3. Oral/nasopharyngeal ulcers
4. Arthritis involving >2 peripheral joints
5. Serositis – pleura/pericardium
6. Renal involvement
7. Neurological manifestations – seizure/psychosis
8. Haematological disorders
   Leucopenia - < 4000/μL
   Lymphopenia - < 1500/μL
   Thrombocytopenia - < 1,00,000/μL
9. Immunological markers
   Antinuclear/antiphospholipid/Anti ds DNA/
   Anti Sm

For diagnosis 4 or more criteria should be present either serially or simultaneously.

WHO - Classification of Lupus Nephritis

Grade	Histological changes
I	No histological changes
II	Proliferative changes confined to the mesangium
III	Proliferative changes 10-50% of glomeruli
IV	Proliferative glomerulonephritis >50% of glomeruli
V	Membranous changes with various degree of proliferation
VI	End stage scarred glomeruli

Investigations

1. Elevated ESR
2. *Peripheral smear:* normocytic, normochromic anaemia of chronic disease, leucopenia and thrombocytopenia.

3. Coombs' test may be positive (hemolytic anaemia)
4. *Anti-nuclear antibodies (ANA):* Detection of ANA is more sensitive for diagnosing SLE. They can be detected by indirect immunofluorescence in the serum of more than 90% of patients.
   Conditions with positive ANA
   a. SLE
   b. Polymyositis
   c. Rheumatoid arthritis
   d. Scleroderma
   e. Sjögren's syndrome
   f. Myasthenia gravis
   g. Fibrosing alveolitis
   h. Chronic liver disease
   i. Polyarteritis
   j. Leukemia.
5. *Antibodies to double stranded DNA (anti-dsDNA):* These are more specific for the diagnosis of SLE and can be detected by radio-immunoassay.
   A recent increase in anti-DNA double strand (ds DNA) antibodies indicates a flare. Antibodies to Sm are also specific for SLE and assist in diagnosis and Sm antibodies do not usually correlate with disease activity.
6. *Evidence of activation of classical complement pathway* (High levels of anti-DNA antibodies, low C_3 and C_4) are seen.
7. *Organ biopsies and lupus band test* (immunofluorescence at the dermoepidermal junction of normal skin due to the presence of immune complexes,

Clinical Features

System Involved	Manifestations
1. Skin	Fixed, erythematous rash over malar regions (Butterfly rash) (Fig. 10.5), discoid rash, alopecia, diffuse maculopapular rash, urticaria, erythema multiforme, lichen planus like lesions, photosensitivity, psori form lesions (subacute cutaneous lupus), oral ulcers, vasculitis
2. Renal	Proteinuria, nephrotic syndrome, focal, proliferative glomerulonephritis, hypocomplementemia and renal failure.
3. Nervous system	Meninges, spinal cord, cranial and peripheral nerves are involved. Patients can have cognitive dysfunction, organic brain syndromes (psychosis, neurosis), pseudotumour cerebri, extrapyramidal and cerebellar involvement. Hypothalamic dysfunction causes inappropriate ADH secretion.
4. Vascular	Thrombosis can occur due to vasculitis, antibodies against phospholipids (lupus anticoagulant, anti cardiolipin antibodies), and immune complex mediated destruction.
5. Hematological	Anaemia of chronic disease, leucopenia, mild thrombocytopenia.
6. Cardiopulmonary	Pericarditis, pericardial effusion, constrictive pericarditis, myocarditis (arrhythmias, CCF) sudden death due to MI, and Libman-Sachs' endocarditis causing MR or AR. Pleurisy and pleural effusion are common. Lupus pneumonia, interstitial fibrosis, pulmonary hypertension and ARDS can occur.
7. Gastrointestinal	Nausea, diarrhoea, vague discomfort, lupus peritonitis, vasculitis of intestine, intestinal perforation, GI motility disorders and intestinal pseudo obstruction.
8. Ocular	Retinal vasculitis, conjunctivitis, episcleritis and blindness can occur (fundus shows sheathed, narrow retinal arterioles and cystoid bodies) (Figs 10.6 and 10.7).
9. Musculoskeletal system	Myopathy, myositis and ischaemic bone necrosis are common; Arthritis, arthralgia which can be transient or persistent leading to chronic inflammatory arthritis and tenosynovitis causing deformities and contractures.
10. Systemic	Fatigue, malaise, fever, anorexia, and weight loss can occur.

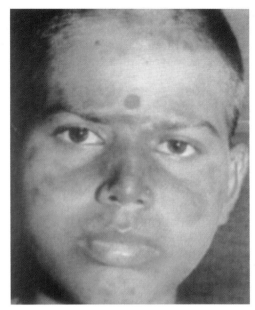

Fig. 10.5: Butterfly rash in SLE

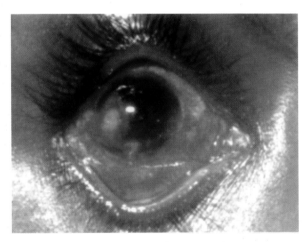

Fig. 10.6: SLE—Sclerokeratitis

complement components and immunoglobulins) are also diagnostic.

8. *Lupus anticoagulants:* This is an anticardiolipin antibody detected either by a prolongation of the partial thromboplastin time which is not correctable by the addition of normal plasma, or by a prolongation of dilute prothrombin time. These are detected by ELISA also and are responsible for thrombocytopenia and recurrent abortions especially in the first trimester.

Lupus anticoagulants also occur in other immunological disorders, HIV infection, or in association with drugs like chlorpromazine, procainamide, and hydralazine.

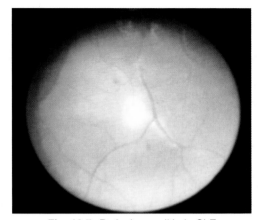

Fig. 10.7: Retinal vasculitis in SLE

Pregnancy and SLE

The disease flares up during pregnancy, more so, around 6 weeks postpartum.

Pregnant women are prone for preeclampsia due to multiple placental infarctions. They are also prone for recurrent abortions. Child may be born with transient rashes, congenital complete heart block due to transmission of maternal anti-Ro antibodies across the placenta (*neonatal lupus*).

Treatment

a. No intervention of pregnancy is needed.
b. Low dose aspirin should be given daily along with high dose steroids and subcutaneous heparin twice daily in full anticoagulating doses.

Dexamethasone and betamethasone are inactivated by placental enzymes and hence preferred.

Tests that can Confirm Clinical Diagnosis and Predict Severity

Specific for SLE

Anti-dsDNA
Anti-sm.

Nonspecific

ANA (most sensitive)
Anti-Ro
Direct Coombs' test
VDRL (due to anti-cardiolipin antibodies)
PTT
Anticardiolipin
Hematocrit
WBC count
Platelet count

- Skin involvement is in the form of folliculitis, erythema nodosum, acne like exanthem, and vasculitis.
- Involvement of eyes may be in the form of posterior uveitis, iritis, retinal vessel occlusion and optic neuritis.
- Patients can have superficial and deep vein thrombosis, and SVC obstruction.
- CNS involvement causes benign ICT, multiple sclerosis like picture, pyramidal signs and psychiatric disturbances.
- Pulmonary artery vasculitis presents with dysponea, cough, chest pain, haemoptysis and infiltrates on chest X-rays
- The arthritis is not deforming and affects the knees and ankles.

Investigations

1. Elevated ESR
2. Elevated C reactive protein
3. Antibodies to oral mucosa.

4. *Pathergy test:* This is an abnormal inflammatory response to scratch or intradermal saline administration, which is not seen in normal individuals.

Diagnostic Criteria

In addition to recurrent oral ulcers if the patient has any two of the following criteria, the diagnosis is confirmed.
1. Genital ulcers
2. Skin lesions
3. Eye lesions
4. Pathergy test.

Treatment

- For mouth ulcers, topical steroids as paste or mouth wash.
- Analgesics for arthritis
- Aspirin 150 mg/day for thrombophlebitis
- Prednisone 1 mg/kg/day for uveitis
- In refractory cases, azathioprine in a dose of 2–3 mg/kg/day or cyclosporine A in a dose of 5–10 mg/kg/day can be tried.

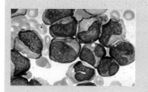

SYMPTOMS

LOCAL
SYSTEMIC
    NONMETASTATIC
    METASTATIC

COMMON PRESENTATIONS
CHILDREN
Anaemia/fever/purpura
   - Leukaemias
Mass in abdomen
   - Nephroblastoma/
     Leukaemia
Childhood cataract
   - Retinoblastoma
ADULT MALE
Dry and persistent cough
with/without hemoptysis
   - Ca. lung
New and persistent mass
   - Lymphomas/sarcomas
Painless testicular swelling
   - Testicular malig.
Painless jaundice
   - Malignant obstruction
Worsening of jaundice in
a cirrhotic
   - Hepatocellular car.
ELDERLY MALE
Painless hematuria
   - Urogenital tumours
Bladder symptoms
   - Prostatic ca.
Altered bowel habits/abd. pain
unexplained iron def. anaemia
   - GI malignancy
Chronic backache
   - Secondries/myeloma
Nonhealing ulcer anywhere
   - Basal/squamous cell ca.
Hyperpigmented itchy lesion
   - Melanoma
ADULT FEMALE
Breast mass/nipple discharge
   -Carcinoma breast
Post menopausal bleeding PV
post coital bleeding
   -Carcinoma cervix
Abdominal mass
   -Ovarian tumours

THE PHYSICAL EXAMINATION

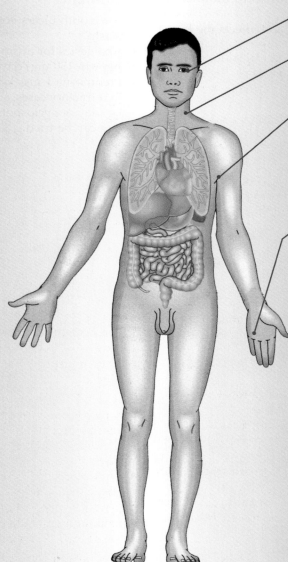

GENERAL EXAMINATION
Cachexia
Mental status
Pallor
Icterus
Clubbing
Pedal oedema
Lymph node enlargement
External markers of
malignancy
   Acanthosis nigricans
   Erythema gyratum repens
   Dermatomyositis
   Cushingoid features
   Circinate erythema
   Acquired icthyosis
   Pachydermoperiostitis
   Sweet's syndrome
   Vitiligo
   Hyperkeratosis
   Migratory thrombophlebitis
   Glucaganoma syndrome, etc.

VITAL SIGNS

LOCAL EXAMINATION

SYSTEM EXAMINATION
Cardiovascular system
Respiratory system
Gastrointestinal system
Nervous system

WORKING DIAGNOSIS

PERFORMANCE STATUS

INVESTIGATIONS
   Diagnosis
   Staging
   Assessing prognosis

EXPLANATION TO
THE PATIENT/RELATIVES
(about therapeutic options
and complications)

TREATMENT/FUTURE PLAN

Basic Concepts

Oncology is the study of tumours. Neoplasia means abnormal new growth, which may be benign or malignant.

Cancer is the term used to describe a wide variety of malignant diseases. Cancer is second only to coronary artery disease as the most common cause of death. Nearly all cancers originate from a single cell.

Genes and Cancer

Cancer is a genetic disease. Cancer arises because of alterations in the DNA , which can be as a result of either random replication errors due to exposure to carcinogens or faulty DNA repair process.

Proto-oncogenes promote normal cell growth. Over activation of proto-oncogenes by point mutation, amplification or dysregulation results in the formation of *oncogenes.*

Genes that normally restrains cell growth are called tumour suppressors and unregulated cell growth occurs if their function is lost. Cancer can arise as a result of either over activation of oncogenes or loss of function of tumour suppressor genes. DNA repair genes can contribute to the development of malignancy through mutations involving oncogenes and tumour suppressor genes.

Tumour Suppressor Genes and Familial Cancers

Most of the genes responsible for the dominantly inherited cancer syndromes are tumour suppressor genes.

Mutations of Genes can Cause Cancer

Evidences that mutations can cause cancer include:
- Malignant tumours are clonal nature
- Some cancers show Mendelian inheritance.
- DNA from malignant cell can some time transform normal cell to malignant phenotype.
- Most tumours contain somatic mutations in oncogenes/tumour suppressor genes.
- Recurring sites of chromosome change are observed in cancers at the site of genes involved in cellular growth control.
- Most carcinogens are mutagens.
- Defects in DNA repair increase the probability of cancer.

Selected Tumour Suppressor Genes Responsible for Familial Cancer Syndromes

Gene	Chromosome	Syndrome
PTC	9	Basal cell nevus
BRCA 1	17	Familial breast/ovarian cancer
BRCA 2	13	Familial breast cancer
p16	9	Familial melanoma
APC	5	Familial polyposis coli
RB	13	Familial retinoblastoma
WT1	11	Familial Wilms tumour
EXT1	11	Hereditary multiple exostosis
p53	17	Li-Fraumeni (Sarcoma, breast cancer)
NF1	17	Neurofibromatosis type 1
NF2	22	Neurofibromatosis type 2
TSC2	16	Tuberous sclerosis
VHL	3	Von Hippel Lindau

Chromosomal Translocations can Cause Cancer

Translocation	Genes	Malignancy
(9:22)	ABL-BCR	CML
(3:21)	AML 1 EAP	AML
(11:14)	BCL 1 IgH	Mantle cell lymphoma
(14:18)	BCL2 IgH	Follicular lymphoma
(1:7)	LCK TCRB	T cell ALL
(4:11)	MLL ALL 1 HRX	ALL
(8:14)	myc	Burkitt's lymphoma, T cell ALL
(7:9)	TAN 1	T cell ALL
(14:19)	BCL 3 IgH	B cell CLL

Cell Biology of Cancer

Cancer is most common in tissues with rapid turnover especially those exposed to environmental carcinogens and whose proliferation is regulated by hormones.

Tissues with rapid turnover:
- Skin
- Bone marrow
- Gut.

Tissues with no turn over: They persist throughout life without dividing or being replaced. Neoplasia in such tissues is rare.
- Cardiac myocytes
- Lens fibres
- Sensory receptors for light and sound.

In cancer, cell growth is not regulated by external signals. (i.e. autonomous) and this leads to uncontrolled growth of abnormal cell.

A neoplasm can be benign or malignant.

Benign neoplasm: In benign lesions the uncontrolled growth of abnormal cells remain within the tissue of origin.

Oncogenes and Associated Human Tumours

Category	Proto-oncogene	Associated human tumours
Growth factors		
PDGF β chain	*sis*	Astrocytoma Osteosarcoma
Fibroblast growth factors	*hst-1*	Stomach cancer
	Int-2	Bladder cancer Breast cancer Melanoma
Growth factor receptors		
EGF- receptor family	*erb*-B1	Squamous cell ca lung
	erb-B2	Breast, ovary, lung and stomach cancer
	erb-B3	Breast cancer
CSF-1 receptor	*fms*	Leukaemia
	ret	MEN 2A, 2B, Familial medullary thyroid cancer
Proteins involved in signal transduction		
GTP- binding	*ras*	Number of cancers including lung, colon, pancreas and leukaemias
Nonreceptor tyrosine kinase	*abl*	CML, ALL
Nuclear regulatory proteins		
Transcriptional activators	*myc*	Burkitt's lymphoma
	N-*myc*	Neuroblastoma, small cell lung cancer
	L-*myc*	Small cell lung cancer
Cell cycle regulators		
Cyclins	*cyclin D*	Mantle cell lymphoma Breast, liver and esophageal Cancer
Cyclin dependent kinase	*CDK-4*	Glioblastoma, melanoma, sarcoma

Malignant neoplasm: The cardinal feature of malignant neoplasm is its capacity to invade tissues and leave the tissue of origin to disseminate and form metastases.

Histological distinction between benign and malignant diseases:
1. Pleomorphic cells.
2. Presence of aberrations in the nucleus.
3. Increased number of mitosis.
4. Evidence of invasion.

Classification of Cancers

Type	Tissue or cell of origin	Example
Carcinoma	Endoderm or ectoderm	Adeno ca colon, small cell ca bronchus
Sarcoma	Mesoderm	Osteosarcoma, fibrosarcoma
Leukemia	WBC	ALL
Lymphoma	Monocyte/macrophage	Hodgkin's disease

Carcinogens

Carcinogens are agents that are thought to act as cancer initiators and/or promoters.

Carcinogens and Associated Cancers

Carcinogen	Associated cancer
Alkylating agents	AML, bladder cancer
Androgens	Prostate cancer
Aromatic amines	Bladder cancer
Arsenic	Lung and skin cancer
Asbestos	Lung, pleura and peritoneal cancer
Benzene	AML
Chromium	Lung cancer
Diethyl stilbesterol prenatally	Vaginal cancer
EBV	Burkitt's lymphoma
Estrogens	Endometrial and liver cancer
Ethanol	Liver, esophageal and head and neck cancers
H. pylori	Gastric cancer
HBV/HCV	Liver cancer
HIV	NHL, Kaposi sarcoma, Squamous cell carcinoma
HTLV 1	Adult T cell leukaemia, lymphoma
Immunosuppressive agents (Azathioprine, Cyclosporine and glucocorticoids)	NHL
Nitrogen mustard gas	Lung, head and neck and paranasal sinus carcinoma
Nickel dust	Lung, nasal sinus cancer
Phenacetin	Renal pelvic and bladder cancer
Polycyclic hydrocarbon	Lung and skin cancer
Schistosomiasis	Bladder cancer
Ultraviolet radiations	Skin cancer
Tobacco	Cancer of upper aerodigestive tract and bladder
Vinyl chloride	Angiosarcoma liver

Aetiology of Cancers

Cancer is a genetic disease. There are several other environmental factors that exert potent effects on gene. Certain viruses can cause human malignancies.

Viruses Causing Malignancy

Human Papilloma virus type 16 and 18	Cervical cancer
Hepatitis B and C viruses	Hepatoma
Epstein Barr virus	Nasopharyngeal carcinoma Lymphoma Burkitt's lymphoma,
Human T cell lymphotropic virus	T cell Lymphoma Leukaemia

Tumour Markers

Tumour marker	Cancer	Non-neoplastic conditions
Oncofetal antigens		
AFP	Hepatoma, Gonadal germ cell tumour	Cirrhosis, hepatitis
CEA	Adenocarcinoma of colon, pancreas, lung, breast, ovary	Pancreatitis, hepatitis, inflammatory bowel disease, smoking
Tumour associated protein		
Prostate specific Ag	Prostate cancer	Prostatitis, prostatic Hypertrophy
Monoclonal Ig	Myeloma	Infection, monoclonal gammopathy of uncertain significance
CA 125	Ovarian cancer, some lymphomas	Menstruation, peritonitis, Pregnancy.
CA 19-9	Colon, pancreas and breast ca	Pancreatitis, ulcerative colitis
CD 30	Hodgkin's disease, Anaplastic large cell lymphoma	
CD 25	Hairy cell leukaemia, Adult T cell leukaemia/ lymphoma	
Enzymes		
Prostatic acid phosphatase	Prostate cancer	Prostatitis, prostatic hypertrophy
Neuron specific enolase	Small cell carcinoma	
LDH	Lymphoma, Ewing's sarcoma	Hepatitis, haemolytic anaemia, etc.
Hormones		
HCG	Gestational trophoblastic disease, Gonadal germ cell tumour	Pregnancy
Calcitonin	Medullary carcinoma thyroid	
Catecholamines	Pheochromocytoma	

Esophageal Cancer

- Excessive alcohol consumption
- Cigarette smoking
- Ingested carcinogens like nitrates, smoked opiates, fungal toxins in pickled vegetables.
- Mucosal damage from physical agents like hot tea, chronic achalasia, radiation induced strictures
- Host susceptibility
  - Plummer-Vinson syndrome
  - Tylosis palmaris et plantaris
- Barrett's esophagus
- Dietary deficiency of Molybdenum, zinc and vitamin A
- Coeliac sprue

Gastric Carcinoma

Dietary nitrates are converted into carcinogenic nitrites by bacteria.

Exogenous sources of nitrate converting bacteria
- Bacterially contaminated food
- *H. pylori* infection

Endogenous factors favouring growth of nitrate converting bacteria
- Decreased gastric acidity
- Prior gastric surgery
- Atrophic gastritis/pernicious anaemia

Higher incidence of gastric cancer is reported in individuals with blood group A.

Neurologic Paraneoplastic Syndromes

Syndrome	Features	Antibody Target	Neoplasm/Percentage
Brain			
Limbic encephalitis	Onset: subacute Confusion Memory loss Temporal lobe seizures	Hu	SCLC, testicular cancer, breast, colon, bladder, lymphoma
Brainstem encephalitis	Vertigo Cerebellar: ataxia, nystagmus Ocular: diplopia, gaze palsies	Hu	SCLC
Cerebellar degeneration	Cerebellar: ataxia, dysarthria	Yo Tr Glutamate receptors	Ovary, uterus, SCLC, Hodgkin's lymphoma
Opsoclonus/myoclonus	Involuntary eye movements: rapid, random directions Ataxia Encephalopathy	Ri (NOVA) Hu Neurofilament	Neuroblastoma, lung, breast
Spinal cord			
Necrotizing myelopathy	Weakness: paraplegia or quadriplegia Sensory loss: spinal level Urinary incontinence	Not known	SCLC, lymphoma
Peripheral nerve			
Neuronopathies			
Sensory neuronopathy	Onset: subacute Sensory loss; diffuse, asymmetric, numbness/paresthesias, dysesthesia/pain Sensory ataxia: pseudoathetosis ± encephalomyelitis	Hu	SCLC (90% of cases), breast, ovary, prostate
Motor neuronopathy	Onset: subacute Weakness: arms > legs Usually asymmetric	Not known	Lymphoma
Axonal neuropathies			
Sensorimotor neuropathy	Distal motor and sensory loss Most common paraneoplastic neuropathy, especially with >15% weight loss Axonal neuropathy	None	Many neoplasms
Mononeuritis multiplex	Weakness and/or sensory loss in the distribution of multiple nerves Onset: acute to subacute	Not known	Cryoglobulinaemia, leukaemia, lymphoma
Neuromyotonia (Isaacs)	Weakness: distal and proximal Stiffness Fasciculations	Voltage-gated potassium channels	Thymoma
Amyloid neuropathy	Distal symmetric axonal loss: small > large Autonomic symptoms prominent	Not known	Multiple myeloma
Autonomic neuropathies			
Enteric neuropathy	Gastroparesis Intestinal pseudo-obstruction Esophageal achalasia Dysphagia	Hu	Thymoma, SCLC
Demyelinating neuropathies			
Anti-MAG	Sensory > motor Distal, symmetric Gait disorder Tremor	Myelin-associated glycoprotein (MAG)	MGUS, IgM M-protein in 85%

Contd...

Contd...

Syndrome	Features	Antibody Target	Neoplasm/Percentage
	Slowly progressive NCV: Long distal latencies, Conduction block uncommon		
Multifocal motor neuropathy	Slowly progressive Motor Distal > proximal Asymmetric NCV: Motor conduction block Motor axon loss (late)	G_{M1} ganglioside	MGUS, IgM M-protein in 20%
Anti-sulfatide	Slowly progressive Sensory > motor Distal, symmetric Demyelinating or axonal	Sulfatide	MGUS, IgM M-protein in 90% with demyelinating neuropathy
POEMS	Sensorimotor neuropathy Symmetric Mixed demyelinating and axonal	Not known	Multiple myeloma, IgG or IgA M-protein in 90%
CIDP	Chronic or relapsing Motor > sensory Distal and proximal weakness Usually symmetric NCV: Conduction block, slow sensory and motor conduction velocities	β-Tubulin in 20%	MGUS, IgM or IgG M-protein in 15%, lymphoma
Neuromuscular junction			
LEMS	Weakness: proximal and distal Ocular: ptosis May improve with exercise Dry mouth Rapid repetitive stimulation: increment	Voltage-gated P/Q calcium channels	SCLC in 60% of cases, especially older and smoking history
Myasthenia gravis	Weakness Cranial: ocular, face, bulbar Respiratory, limbs, trunk Fatigue Slow repetitive stimulation: decrement	Nicotinic acetylcholine receptor	Thymoma in 10%, especially >30 years
Muscle			
Necrotizing myopathy	Males > 40 Rapid-onset weakness Necrosis on muscle biopsy May improve with treatment of cancer	Not known	Lung, breast, alimentary tract
Dermatomyositis	Females > 40 Proximal muscle weakness Skin rash	Not known	Ovarian, nasopharyngeal
Type II atrophy	Especially with weight loss > 15% Wasting > weakness	Not known	Many neoplasms
Myopathy with anti-decorin antibodies	> 50 years of age Proximal symmetric weakness Mildly elevated creatine kinase	Decorin	Waldenström's macroglobulinaemia, IgM M-protein
Rippling muscle disease	Cramps induced by touching muscle Muscle waves induced by percussion Electrically silent	Not known	Thymoma
Scleromyxedema	Skin papules Raynaud's phenomenon Proximal muscle weakness High creatine kinase Myopathic electromyography	Not known	MGUS, IgG or IgA M-protein

Management

Dexamethasone 4-8 mg IV or orally 6th hourly
Whole brain irradiation
For solitary lesions—surgery followed by radiotherapy
Intubation- hyperventilation-mannitol infusion (maintain PCO2 at 25-30 mmHg)
Stereotactic radiosurgery for inaccessible lesions.

Meningeal Carcinomatosis

Involvement of leptomeninges either by primary or metastatic tumour.

Causes

Lung cancer
Breast cancer
Melanoma
Acute leukaemia
Lymphoma.

Clinical Features

Headache, vomiting, gait abnormalities
Cranial nerve palsies, mental changes
Seizures, limb weakness, decreased deep tendon reflexes.

Investigations

CT/MRI before LP to rule out parenchymal metastasis
LP—CSF cytology, elevated protein level
MRI—Hydrocephalus/smooth or nodular enhancement of meninges.

Treatment

Intrathecal chemotherapy (methotrexate, cytarabine, thiotepa)
Local radiation therapy
IV arabinoside for meningeal lymphoma.

Intracerebral Leucocytostasis (Ball's Disease)

Potential fatal complication of acute leukaemia
More common with myelogenous leukaemia
It occurs when the peripheral blast cell count is more than 1 lakh/µL
Brain invasion with blast cell through endothelial damage results in haemorrhage.

Clinical Features

- Visual disturbance
- Ataxia, stupor
- Dizziness
- Coma, death.

Management

Whole brain irradiation
Aggressive antileukaemic therapy.

Seizures

Causes

Primary/metastatic tumour
Metabolic disturbance
Radiation injury
Chemotherapy related encephalopathy
CNS infections / cerebral infarction
Drugs—etoposide, busulphan, chlorambucil.

Management

Anticonvulsant therapy with phenytoin.

Spinal Cord Compression

Hematogenous spread of cancer to vertebral bodies.

Causes

- Lung cancer
- Breast cancer
- Prostate cancers
- Multiple myeloma.

Site of Lesion

Vertebral column more involved than other bones
- Thoracic spine—70%
- Lumbosacral spine—20%
- Cervical spine—10%

Clinical Features

- Localized back pain and tenderness
- Pain precedes neurological deficits
- Pain aggravated by coughing and sneezing
- Radicular pain—unilateral or bilateral
- Loss of bowel and bladder control
- Pain worsens when the patient is supine (in disc lesions pain is relieved in supine positions)
- Signs of cord compression.

Investigations

X-ray of spine
    Erosion of pedicles (winking owl sign)
    Increased interpedicular distance
    Vertebral destruction and collapse.
MRI spine
    Gadolinium enhanced MRI for intramedullary lesions
    In case of poor MR images, myelography or CT with myelography.

Management

High dose dexamethasone- 8 mg 6th hourly
Radiation therapy
Surgery and chemotherapy.

Malignant Effusions

Malignant Pericardial Effusion

Causes

Lung cancer
Breast cancer
Leukaemias and lymphoma
Radiation
Drug induced.

Radiation

1. Acute inflammatory effusive pericarditis (within months)
2. Chronic effusive pericarditis with thickened pericardium (upto 20 years after irradiation).

Clinical Features

Dyspnoea, cough , chest pain
Distended jugular veins
Hepatomegaly
Peripheral oedema
Paradoxical pulse and pulsus alternans
Friction rub and cardiac tamponade.

Management

Cardiac tamponade warrants immediate pericardiocentesis
Uncontrolled disease—pericardiocentesis with sclerosis
Sclerosis—30-60 mg Bleomycin instillation and withdrawal after 10 mts
Recurrent accumulation—subxyphoid pericardiotomy

Malignant Pleural Effusion

Caused by invasion by tumour or obstruction to lymphatic drainage.

Management

Drainage of pleural fluid followed by instillation of sclerosing agents
    Resistant effusion- pleurectomy.

Malignant Ascites

Cause

Peritoneal carcinomatosis
    Controlled by systemic chemotherapy and rarely intraperitoneal instillation of chemotherapeutic agent.

Airway Obstruction

Causes

Intraluminal tumour growth
Extrinsic compression.

Management

Obstruction proximal to larynx—tracheostomy is life saving
Distal obstructions—Laser treatment, photodynamic therapy and stenting
Emergency radiotherapy and glucocorticoids may open the airway.

Haemoptysis

Causes

Twenty per cent of patients with lung cancer
Metastasis from breast, colon, kidney, melanoma and carcinoid tumours.

Management

Blood transfusion,
Oxygen
Emergency bronchoscopy
Surgery/Nd: YAG laser therapy
Bronchial artery embolisation.

Intestinal Obstruction

Causes

Colorectal and ovarian cancers
Metastatic lesions of lung and breast cancers and melanoma.

Clinical Features

- Colicky pain
- Vomiting
- Constipation
- Abdominal pain
- Visible peristalsis
- High pitched bowel sounds
- Palpable tumour masses.

Investigations

- Plain X-ray abdomen erect:
  - Multiple air fluid level
  - Dilation of small or large bowel
- USG abdomen.

Prognosis

- Overall prognosis is poor
- Acute caecal dilation is a surgical emergency
- Median survival 3-4 months.

Management

- Nasogastric decompression
- Antispasmodics
- Surgery
- Self-expanding metal stents.

Urinary Obstruction

Causes

- Prostate/cervix cancer
- Radiation therapy for pelvic tumours.

Clinical Features

- Outlet obstruction results in bilateral hydronephrosis and renal failure
- Flank pain dysuria
- Proteinuria, haematuria
- Polyuria, anuria
- Rising urea and creatinine value.

Investigations

- Renal USG
- CT abdomen to identify retroperitoneal mass/lymphadenopathy.

Management

- Stents for ureteral obstructions

- Percutaneous nephrostomy for hydronephrosis
- Suprapubic cystostomy for bladder outlet obstruction.

Biliary Obstruction

Causes

- Pancreatic cancer
- Bile duct carcinoma
- Hepatoma
- Metastasis from gastric, colonic, breast and lung cancers.

Clinical Features

- High coloured/ light coloured stools
- Jaundice, pruritus
- Malabsorption leading to weight loss.

Investigations

- USG/CT abdomen
- Percutaneous transhepatic/Endoscopic retrograde cholangiopancreatography.

Management

- Stenting/surgical bypass
- Radiotherapy/chemotherapy.

Other Emergencies

- Lactic acidosis
- Hypoglycaemia
- Adrenal insufficiency
- Bone metastasis and spontaneous fractures
- Minimal change/membranous glomerulonephritis.

Metastatic Cancer of Unknown Primary Site

Biologic Behaviour

- Primary becomes apparent during the course of illness in 20%
- Primary diagnosed at autopsy in 60%
- Primary not traced even at autopsy in 20%
- Median survival 6-12 months.

Clinical Evaluation

Suggested clinical evaluation of patients with metastatic cancer of unknown primary site

- History: smoking history, asbestos exposure, abdominal pain

- Physical examination: lymph nodes, thyroid, skin;
- Men: prostate
- Women: breasts, pelvic examination
- Laboratory evaluation: stool evaluation for occult blood; urinalysis; complete blood count; liver function tests; calcium, electrolytes, creatinine; measurement of serum levels of hCG, AFP, CEA, and CA-125 (women); chest X-ray; abdominal and pelvic CT; mammography.

Pathological Evaluation or Biopsy

Possible pathologic evaluation of biopsy specimens from patients with metastatic cancer of unknown primary site:

Evaluation/findings	Suggested primary site or neoplasm
HISTOLOGY (HEMATOXYLIN AND EOSIN STAINING)	
Psammoma bodies, papillary configuration	Ovary, thyroid
Signet ring cells	Stomach
IMMUNOHISTOLOGY	
Leukocyte common antigen (LCA, CD45)	Lymphoid neoplasm
Leu-M1	Hodgkin's disease
Epithelial membrane antigen	Carcinoma
Cytokeratin	Carcinoma[a]
CEA	Carcinoma
HMB45	Melanoma
Desmin	Sarcoma
Thyroglobulin	Thyroid carcinoma
Calcitonin	Medullary carcinoma of the thyroid
Myoglobin	Rhabdomyosarcoma
PSA/prostatic acid phosphatase	Prostate
AFP	Liver, stomach, germ cell
Placental alkaline phosphatase	Germ cell
B, T cell markers	Lymphoid neoplasm
S-100 protein	Neuroendocrine tumour, melanoma
Gross cystic fluid protein	Breast, sweat gland
Factor VIII	Kaposi's sarcoma, angiosarcoma
FLOW CYTOMETRY	
B, T cell markers	Lymphoid neoplasm
ULTRASTRUCTURE	
Actin-myosin filaments	Rhabdomyosarcoma
Secretory granules	Neuroendocrine tumours
Desmosomes	Carcinoma
Premelanosomes	Melanoma
CYTOGENETICS	
Isochromosome 12p; 12q(-)	Germ cell
t(11;22)	Ewing's sarcoma, primitive neuroectodermal tumour
t(8;14)	Lymphoid neoplasm
3p(-)	Small cell lung carcinoma; renal cell carcinoma, mesothelioma
t(X;18)	Synovial sarcoma
t(12;16)	Myxoid liposarcoma
t(12;22)	Clear cell sarcoma (melanoma of soft parts)
t(2;13)	Alveolar rhabdomyosarcoma
1p(-)	Neuroblastoma

RECEPTOR ANALYSIS
Oestrogen/progesterone receptor Breast

MOLECULAR BIOLOGIC STUDIES
Immunoglobulin, bcl-2, T-cell   Lymphoid neoplasm
receptor gene rearrangement

Management Protocol

Presentations that dictate specific therapies in patients with CUPS. See Table on next page.

Principles of Cancer Therapy

The ultimate aim of cancer therapy is to totally eradicate the cancer. When eradication is not possible the next goal of cancer therapy is palliation . The palliative therapy aims to achieve amelioration of symptoms, preserve the quality of life and to prolong longevity.

There are 4 modalities of cancer therapy:
1. Surgery
2. Radiation including photodynamic therapy
3. Chemotherapy including hormonal treatment
4. Biologic therapy including immunotherapy.

Surgery

Surgical modality is useful in prevention, diagnosis, staging, and eradication of cancer. It is also useful in palliation and rehabilitation.

Prevention

- Resection of premalignant lesions- skin, colon, cervix, oral cavity
- Colectomy for ulcerative colitis and familial polyposis
- Thyroidectomy for MEN 2
- Orchiectomy for undescended testis
- Mastectomy and oophorectomy for familial breast and ovarian cancer.

Diagnosis

- Various types of biopsy procedures

Staging

- Laparotomy and lymph node sampling for lymphoma and intra-abdominal cancers
- Axillary lymph node for breast cancers

Clinicopathologic features	Suspected primary site	Suggested therapy
Squamous cell carcinoma, cervical node Carcinoma, axillary nodes (female)	Head and neck cancer	Radical neck dissection; radiotherapy ± chemotherapy
	Breast cancer	Breast radiotherapy or mastectomy, systemic adjuvant therapy
Peritoneal carcinomatosis (female)	Ovarian cancer	Debulking surgery, cisplatin-based chemotherapy
Pleural effusion, adenocarcinoma cells oestrogen and/or progesterone receptor positive	Breast cancer	Systemic therapy for metastatic breast cancer
Poorly differentiated cancer, age <50, lung or retroperitoneal or mediastinal mass or lymph nodes, elevated serum β hCG or AFP levels	Germ cell tumour (extragonadal)	Cisplatin/VP-16-based chemotherapy (controversial)
Bony metastases (male)	Prostate cancer	Androgen blockade (leuprolide plus flutamide)
Adenocarcinoma, liver metastases, elevated CEA level	Gastrointestinal malignancy	Surgical resection of liver lesion feasible; colonoscopy with resection (if appropriate) of tumours; 5-fluoro-uracil/leucovorin

Treatment

- Surgery is the best and most effective modality of cancer therapy
- Surgery cures 40% of cancer patients
- Surgical removal of tumor helps in preserving the organ function, e.g. Ca bladder and Ca larynx
- Debulking is helpful for subsequent effective therapy
- For hormonally responsive tumours—oophorectomy, adrenalectomy, orchiectomy.

Palliation

- Surgical procedures for malignant effusions
- Insertion of central venous catheters
- Surgical bypass for intestinal, urinary and biliary obstruction
- Caval interruption for recurrent pulmonary emboli.

Rehabilitation

- Orthopaedic procedures for early ambulation
- Reconstructive plastic surgery.

Radiation Therapy

- Tumour tissue is more sensitive to radiation than normal tissue.
- There are three ways of delivering radiation
  1. Teletherapy—radiation beams generated at a distance
  2. Brachytherapy—encapsulated sources of radiation directly implanted into tumor tissue
  3. Radionuclide therapy

- Hypoxic cells are relatively resistant to radiotherapy
- Non-dividing cells are more resistant than dividing cells
- A Rad (radiation absorbed dose) is 100 ergs of energy per gm of tissue
- Gy(Gray)- A Gy is 100 rads.

Teletherapy

Teletherapy is most commonly used
All radiation therapy is given for 5 days a week.

Curative Radiation Therapy

- Breast cancer
- Hodgkin's disease
- Head and neck cancer
- Gynaecological cancers
- Prostate cancers.

Palliative Radiation Therapy

- Control of brain metastasis
- Relief of bone pain from metastasis
- Relief of SVC obstruction
- Relief of spinal cord compression
- Prevention of meningeal involvement and brain metastasis.

Brachytherapy

- Brain tumour
- Cervical cancer

Radionuclide Therapy

- Iodine 131 for thyroid cancer
- Strontium 89 and Samarium 153 for bone lesions.

Radioimmunotherapy

- Delivering monoclonal antibodies attached to radio-isotopes
  E.g. iodine 131 labelled anti CD 20
  Yttrium 90 labelled anti CD20
  Both are active in B cell lymphoma.

Photodynamic Therapy

Cancer cells selectively absorb certain chemicals like porphyrins and Phthalocyanines. When laser light is delivered these cells generate free radicals and the cells die. This modality is used in skin, lung, ovarian, esophageal and colorectal cancers.

Toxicity of Radiation Therapy

This depends on the field of radiation.

General
  Fatigue, anorexia, nausea, vomiting

Local
  Mucositis
  Skin erythema
  Bone marrow toxicity
  Thyroid failure
  Cataracts
  Retinal damage
  Cessation of salivary secretion
  Taste and smell affection
  Testicular and ovarian affection
  Development of second solid tumours in the second decade.

Chemotherapy

It has several phases.

Induction
It is the chemotherapy used to achieve a complete remission.

Consolidation
Here chemotherapy is administered to patients who initially responded to treatment.

Maintenance
This refers to low dose outpatient treatment to prolong remission.

Adjuvant chemotherapy
This is given after surgical or radiological management of primary malignancy.

Classification of Anticancer Drugs

There are six main groups of drugs.
1. Antimetabolites: By inhibiting the folate metabolism, they interfere with synthesis of purines and pyramidines.
2. Alkylating agents: Addition of alkyl group to constituents of DNA interferes with replication and transcription of mRNA, leading to cell death.
3. Plant alkaloids: They inhibit cell division by binding to tubulin and disrupting the mitotic spindle.
4. Antibiotics: They act by intercalating between base pairs and DNA.
5. Taxanes: They act by stabilizing the mitotic spindle
6. Miscellaneous synthetic compounds
   Dacarbazine
   Cisplatin
   Procarbazine
   Hexamethylmelamine
   Hydroxyurea
   Mitozantrone.

Response to Treatment

Complete response/remission
  Malignancy with all its evidence is eradicated

Partial response
  Decreases in tumour mass by more than 50%.

Curability of Cancers with Chemotherapy

A. Advanced Cancers with Possible Cure

- Acute lymphoid and acute myeloid leukaemia (paediatric/adult)
- Hodgkin's disease (paediatric/adult)
- Lymphomas-certain types (paediatric/adult)
- Small cell lung carcinoma
- *Germ cell neoplasms*
  - Embryonal carcinoma
  - Teratocarcinoma
  - Choriocarcinoma
  - Seminoma or dysgerminoma
- Gestational trophoblastic neoplasia
- Ovarian carcinoma
- *Paediatric neoplasms*
  - Ewing's sarcoma
  - Peripheral neuroepithelioma

- Neuroblastoma
- Wilms' tumour
- Embryonal rhabdomyocarcinoma.

B. Advanced cancers possibly cured by chemotherapy and radiation

- Squamous carcinoma (head and neck)
- Squamous carcinoma (anus)
- Breast carcinoma
- Carcinoma of the uterine cervix
- Non-small cell lung carcinoma (stage III)
- Small cell lung carcinoma.

C. Cancers possibly cured with chemotherapy as adjuvant to surgery

- Breast carcinoma
- Colorectal carcinoma
- Osteogenic sarcoma
- Soft tissue sarcoma.

D. Cancers possibly cured with "high-dose" chemotherapy with stem cell support

- Relapsed leukaemias, lymphoid and myeloid
- Relapsed lymphomas, Hodgkin's and non-Hodgkin's
- Chronic myeloid leukaemia
- Multiple myeloma.

E. Cancers responsive with useful palliation, but not cure, by chemotherapy

- Bladder carcinoma
- Chronic myeloid leukaemia
- Hairy cell leukaemia
- Chronic lymphocytic leukaemia
- Lymphoma-certain types
- Multiple myeloma
- Gastric carcinoma
- Cervix carcinoma
- Endometrial carcinoma
- Soft tissue sarcoma
- Head and neck cancer
- Adrenocortical carcinoma
- Islet-cell neoplasms
- Breast carcinoma.

F. Tumor poorly responsive in advanced stages to chemotherapy

- Pancreatic carcinoma
- Biliary-tract neoplasms
- Renal carcinoma
- Thyroid carcinoma
- Carcinoma of the vulva

- Colorectal carcinoma
- Non-small cell lung carcinoma
- Prostate carcinoma
- Melanoma
- Hepatocellular carcinoma.

Therapy of Selected Cancers
Gastric Cancers

- Adenocarcinoma—localized lesions—early surgery
- Advanced unresectable—may benefit by chemotherapy and radiation
- Metastatic disease- palliation by chemotherapy.

Esophageal Cancer

- Squamous cell/adenocarcinoma
- Surgical resection of esophagus or chemo-radiation followed by resection
- Unresectable growth- chemotherapy and radiation.
- Metastatic disease- palliation by chemotherapy
- Obstructive complication- stenting.

Colon Cancer

- Adenocarcinoma—surgical resection
- Regional lymph node involvement- 5FU and Levamisole for 12 months
- Or 5 FU and Leucovorin for 6 months.

Rectal Cancer

- Recurs locally after surgery
- Postoperative radiation and 5FU are recommended.

Anal Cancer

- Chemotherapy and radiation offer high cure rates than surgical resection
- This modality preserves anal sphincter and fecal continence.

Breast Cancer

- Tylectomy—Lumpectomy and axillary lymph node dissection
- As effective as modified radical mastectomy
- Adjuvant chemotherapy- for patients with tumour size more than 1 cm or axillary node involvement or estrogen receptor (ER) negative cancer or has over expression of her-2 especially in premenopausal women.
- ER positive breast cancers- Tamoxifen 20 mg /day for 5 years.

Commonly Used Cancer Chemotherapy Agents

Drug	Examples of Usual Doses	Toxicity	Interactions, Issues
Direct DNA-Interacting Agents			
Alkylators			
Cyclophosphamide	400-2000 mg/m^{2}IV 100 mg/m^2 PO qd	Marrow (relative platelet sparing) Cystitis Common alkylator Cardiac (high dose)	Liver metabolism required to activate to phosphoramide mustard + acrolein MESNA protects against "high-dose" bladder damage
Mechlorethamine	6 mg/m^2 IV day 1 and day 8	Marrow Vesicant Nausea	Topical use in cutaneous lymphoma
Chlorambucil	1-3 mg/m^2 qd PO	Marrow Common alkylator	
Melphalan	8 mg/m^2 qd × 5, PO	Marrow (delayed nadir) GI (high dose)	Decreased renal function delays clearance
BCNU	200 mg/m^2 IV 150 mg/m^2 PO	Marrow (delayed nadir) GI, liver (high dose) Renal	
CCNU	100-300 mg/m^2 PO	Marrow (delayed nadir)	
Ifosfamide	1.2 g/m^2 per day qd × 5 + MESNA	Myelosuppressive Bladder Neurologic Metabolic acidosis Neuropathy	Isomeric analogue of cyclophosphamide More lipid soluble Greater activity vs testicular neoplasms and sarcomas Must use MESNA
Procarbazine	100 mg/m^2 per day qd ×14	Marrow Nausea Neurologic Common alkylator	Liver and tissue metabolism required Disulfiran-like effect with ethanol Acts as MAOI HBP after tyrosinase-rich foods
DTIC	375 mg/m^2 IV day 1 and day 15	Marrow Nausea Flulike	Metabolic activation
Hexamethylmelamine	260 mg/m^2 per day qd ×14-21 as 4 divided oral doses	Nausea Neurologic (mood swing) Neuropathy Marrow (less)	Liver activation Barbiturates enhance/cimetidine diminishes
Cisplatin	20 mg/m^2 qd ×5 IV 1 q3-4 weeks or 100-200 mg/m^2/ dose IV q3-4 weeks	Nausea Neuropathy Auditory Marrow platelets > WBCs Renal Mg^{2+}, Ca^{2+}	Maintain high urine flow; osmotic diuresis, monitor intake/output K$^+$, Mg^{2+} Emetogenic-prophylaxis needed Full dose if CrCl > 60 mL/min and tolerate fluid push
Carboplatin	365 mg/m^2 IV q3-4 weeks as adjusted for CrCl	Marrow platelets > WBCs Nausea Renal (high dose)	Reduce dose according to CrCl: AUC = dose/(CrCl + 25) to AUC of 5-7 mg/mL per min
Antitumour antibiotics			
Bleomycin	15-25 mg/d qd ×5 IV bolus or continuous IV	Pulmonary Skin effects Raynaud's Hypersensitivity	Inactivate by bleomycin hydrolase (decreased in lung/skin) O$_2$ enhances pulmonary toxicity Cisplatin-induced decrease in CrCl may increase skin/lung toxicity Reduce dose if CrCl < 60 mL/min
Actinomycin D	10-15 µg/kg per day qd ×5 IV bolus	Marrow Nausea Mucositis Vesicant Alopecia	Radiation recall
Mithramycin	15-20 µg/kg qd ×4-7 (hypercalcemia) or 50 µg/kg qod ×3-8 (antineoplastic)	Marrow Liver Renal Mucositis Hypocalcemia Nausea Vesicant	Acute hemorrhagic syndrome

Contd...

Contd...

Drug	Examples of Usual Doses	Toxicity	Interactions, Issues
Mitomycin C	6-10 mg/m² q6 weeks	Marrow Vesicant Hemolytic-uremic syndrome Lung CV-heart failure	Treat superficial bladder cancers by intravesical infusion Delayed marrow toxicity Cumulative marrow toxicity
Etoposide (VP16-213)	100-150 mg/m² IV qd ×3-5d or 50 mg/m² PO qd ×21d or up to 1500 mg/m²/of dose (high dose with stem cell support)	Marrow (WBCs > platelet) Alopecia Hypotension Hypersensitivity (rapid IV) Nausea Mucositis (high dose)	Hepatic metabolism-renal 30% Reduce doses with renal failure Schedule-dependant (5 day better than 1 day) Late leukemogenic Accentuate antimetabolite action
Teniposide (VM-26)	150-200 mg/m² twice per week for 4 weeks	Marrow Alopecia	
Amsacrine	100-150 mg/m² IV qd ×5	Marrow Mucositis Nausea CV-arrhythmia (avoid hypokalemia)	Decrease dose by 30% if liver or renal failure
Topotecan	20 mg/m² IV q3-4 weeks over 30 min or 1.5-3 mg/m² q3-4 weeks over 24 h or 0.5 mg/m² per day over 21 days	Marrow Mucositis Nausea Mild alopecia	Reduce dose with renal failure No liver toxicity
Irinotecan (CPT II)	100-150 mg/m² IV over 90 min q3-4 weeks or 30 mg/m² per day over 120 h	Diarrhoea: "early onset" with cramping, flushing, vomiting; "late onset" after several doses Marrow Alopecia Nausea Vomiting Pulmonary	Prodrug requires enzymatic clearance to active drug "SN 38" "Early diarrhoea" likely due to biliary excretion Late diarrhoea, use "high-dose" loperamide (2 mg q2-4 h)
Doxorubicin and daunorubicin	45-60 mg/m² dose q3-4 weeks or 10-30 mg/m² dose q week or continuous-infusion regimen	Marrow Mucositis Alopecia Cardiovascular acute/chronic Vesicant	Heparin aggregate; coadministration increases clearance Tylenol, BCNU increase liver toxicity Radiation recall
Idarubicin	10-15 mg/m² IV q 3 weeks or 10 mg/m² IV qd ×3	Marrow Cardiac (less than doxorubicin)	None established
Epirubicin	150 mg/m² IV q3 weeks	Marrow Cardiac	None established
Mitoxantrone	12 mg/m² qd ×3 or 12-14 mg/m² q3 weeks	Marrow Cardiac (less than doxorubicin) Vesicant (mild) Blue urine, sclerae, nails	Interacts with heparin Less alopecia, nausea than doxorubicin Radiation recall

Indirect DNA-Interacting Agents

Antimetabolites

| Deoxycoformycin | 4 mg/m² IV every other week | Nausea
Immunosuppression
Neurologic
Renal | Excretes in urine
Reduce dose for renal failure
Inhibits adenosine deaminase |

Contd...

Contd...

Drug	Examples of Usual Doses	Toxicity	Interactions, Issues
6-Mercaptopurine	75 mg/m^2 PO or up 500 mg/m^2 PO (high dose)	Marrow Liver Nausea	Variable bioavailability Metabolize by xanthine oxidase Decrease dose with allopurinol Increased toxicity with thiopurine methyltransferase deficiency
6-Thioguanine	2-3 mg/kg per day for up to 3-4 weeks	Marrow Liver Nausea	Variable bioavailability Increased toxicity with thiopurine methyltransferase deficiency
Azathioprine	1-5 mg/kg per day	Marrow Nausea Liver	Metabolizes to 6-MP, therefore reduce dose with allopurinol Increased toxicity with thiopurine methyltransferase deficiency
2-Chlorodeoxy-adenosine	0.09 mg/kg per day qd ×7 as continuous infusion	Marrow Renal Fever	Notable use in hairy cell leukaemia
Hydroxyurea	20-50 mg/kg (lean body weight) PO qd or 1-3 g/d	Marrow Nausea Mucositis Skin changes Rare renal, liver, lung, CNS	Decrease dose with renal failure Augments antimetabolite effect
Methotrexate	15-30 mg PO or IM qd ×3-5 or 30 mg IV days 1 and 8 or 1.5-12 g/m^2 per day (with leucovorin)	Marrow Liver/lung Renal tubular Mucositis	Rescue with leucovorin Excreted in urine Decrease dose in renal failure NSAIDs increase renal toxicity
5-Fluorouracil	375 mg/m^2 IV qd ×5 or 600 mg/m^2 IV days 1 and 8	Marrow Mucositis Neurologic Skin changes	Toxicity enhanced by leucovorin Dihydropyrimidine dehydrogenase deficiency increases toxicity Metabolizes in tissues
Cytosine arabinoside	100 mg/m^2 per day qd ×7 by continuous infusion or 1-3 g/m^2 dose IV bolus	Marrow Mucositis Neurologic (high dose) Conjunctivitis (high dose) Noncardiogenic pulmonary oedema	Enhances activity of alkylating agents Metabolizes in tissues by deamination
Azacytidine	750 mg/m^2 per week or 150-200 mg/m^2 per day ×5-10 (bolus) or (continuous IV)	Marrow Nausea Liver Neurologic Myalgia	Use limited to leukaemia Altered methylation of DNA alters gene expression
Gemcitabine	1000 mg/m^2 IV weekly ×7	Marrow Nausea Hepatic Fever/"flu syndrome"	
Fludarabine phosphate	25 mg/m^2 IV qd ×5	Marrow Neurologic Lung	Dose reduction with renal failure Metabolized to F-ara converted to F-ara ATP in cells by deoxycytidine kinase
Asparaginase	25,000 IU/m^2 q3-4 weeks or 6000 IU/m^2 per day qod for 3-4 weeks or 1000-2000 IU/m^2 for 10-20 days	Protein synthesis Clotting factors Glucose Albumin Hypersensitivity CNS Pancreatitis Hepatic	Blocks methotrexate action

Contd...

Contd...

Drug	Examples of Usual Doses	Toxicity	Interactions, Issues
Antimitotic agents			
Vincristine	1-1.4 mg/m² per week	Vesicant Marrow Neurologic GI: ileus/constipation; bladder hypotoxicity; SIADH Cardiovascular	Hepatic clearance Dose reduction for bilirubin >1.5 mg/dL Prophylactic bowel regimen
Vinblastine	6-8 mg/m² per week	Vesicant Marrow Neurologic (less common but similar spectrum to other vincas) Hypertension Raynaud's	Hepatic clearance Dose reduction as with vincristine
Vinorelbine	15-30 mg/m² per week	Vesicant Marrow Allergic/bronchospasm (immediate) Dyspnoea/cough (subacute) Neurologic (less prominent but similar spectrum to other vincas)	Hepatic clearance
Paclitaxel	135-175 mg/m² per 24-h infusion or 175 mg/m² per 3-h infusion or 140 mg/m² per 96-h infusion or 250 mg/m² per 24-h infusion plus G-CSF	Hypersensitivity Marrow Mucositis Alopecia Sensory neuropathy CV conduction disturbance Nausea-infrequent	Premedicate with steroids, H_1 and H_2 blockers Hepatic clearance Dose reduction as with vincas
Docetaxel	100 mg/m² per 1-h infusion q3 weeks	Hypersensitivity Fluid retention syndrome Marrow Dermatologic Sensory neuropathy Nausea infrequent Some stomatitis	Premedicate with steroids, H_1 and H_2 blockers
Estramustine phosphate	14 mg/kg per day in 3-4 divided doses with water >2 h after meals Avoid Ca^{2+}-rich foods	Nausea Vomiting Diarrhoea CHF Thrombosis Gynaecomastia	
Hormonal agents			
Tamoxifen	10 mg orally BD	hormone flare after 7-14 days of treatment (bone pain, erythema, hypercalcaemia) Endometrial cancer, DVT	Hormone flare does not require stopping therapy. Long-term administration is not associated with systemic antiestrogen effect
Gonadotropin agonists Leuprolide acetate and Goserelin acetate	given as monthly subcutaneous depot injection	flare up of symptoms	Signs of Neurologic dysfunction or urinary obstruction should be monitored
Progestational agents Megestrol acetate and Medroxyprogesterone	40 mg QID PO 10 mg OD PO	weight gain, fluid retention, hot flashe.	Also used in cancer cachexia

Contd...

Introduction

One of the most striking changes in the demography of the world has been the increased proportion of elderly individuals in the population.

The relevance of this to health and social services is that there is an exponential increase in disability, and mental and physical morbidity, in individuals over the age of 75 years.

Ageing

Ageing can be described, from a physiologic standpoint, as a progressive constriction of the homeostatic reserve of every organ system. This decline, referred to as homeostasis is evident by the third decade and is then gradually progressive. The rate and extent of this decline of each organ system of the body is influenced by genetic factors, environment, diet and personal habits (the rate of deterioration in organ function often can be reduced by factors such as regular exercise, or accelerated by bad habits such as cigarette smoking or heavy alcohol consumption).

Therefore, with advancing age, there may be a moderate decline in organ function. This remains unchanged in some elderly individuals, whereas in others it is so severe that it leaves them seriously incapacitated.

It should also be borne in mind that the effects of ageing are usually insufficient to interfere with the function of an organ under baseline conditions, but the changes may be sufficient enough to reduce the reserve capacity of the organ in presence of stress of a mild illness or unaccustomed exercise and precipitate a crisis.

The practical value in defining the characteristics of normal ageing is that this provides a baseline against which the signs and symptoms of disease in elderly patients can be assessed.

Multiple pathology is so common in old age that elderly individuals free from disease form a biological elite.

Postulated Mechanisms for Ageing

1. Ageing may be due to cumulative spontaneous somatic mutations.
2. Ageing may result from errors in protein synthesis.
3. Ageing may be a result of ongoing DNA rearrangements.
4. Ageing may be a result of damage by free radicals.

An abrupt decline in any system or function is always due to disease and not due to "Normal Ageing".

Some Physiological Effects of Ageing

1. Skin and Integuments

Changes within the connective tissue result in the skin losing its elasticity and becoming wrinkled. The appearance is similar to that associated with dehydration, so that the dehydration is easily missed in elderly patients.

A decline in the number of sweat glands in the elderly results in difficulty in regulation of body temperature especially in warm weather and they are susceptible to heat stroke.

There is diffuse loss of hair, and the hair also becomes finer. In some individuals there is depigmentation of hair (grey hair).

2. Musculoskeletal System

There is a decline in the number of anterior horn cells with ageing which results in muscle weakness and wasting. The process often is accentuated by the physical inactivity and may be minimised by taking regular physical exercise.

3. Smell and Taste Sensation

There is a decline in taste sensation and the sense of smell with ageing, resulting in decreased appreciation of flavour of food.

4. Joints

There is development of degenerative changes in the joints, especially the weight bearing joints like the knee joint, with ageing, resulting in osteoarthritis.

Degeneration of the cervical and lumbar vertebrae and their intervertebral discs may lead to the development of cervical spondylosis and lumbar spondylosis.

5. Immune Function

Ageing, poor nutrition and chronic ill health in many old people interact with each other to interfere with immune function. Results of this include an attenuated inflammatory response so that the local and systemic effects of infection are masked, leading to atypical presentation of infectious diseases. A reduced immune surveillance in the elderly predisposes them to the development of malignancy.

Characteristics of Disease in Old Age

There are differences of emphasis in the approach to old people compared with young people, due to

Signs and Symptoms of Age Related Physiological Changes and their Consequences and Disease States in the Elderly

Organ/system	Age-related physiological change	Symptoms/signs caused by age-related physiological change	Symptoms/signs caused by disease
1. General	a. Increased body fat	Increased volume of distribution of fat soluble drugs	Obesity
	b. Decreased total body water.	Decreased volume of distribution of water soluble drugs.	Anorexia
2. Eyes	a. Presbyopia	Decreased accommodation	
	b. Lens opacification	Increased susceptibility to glare	Decreased acuity of vision (cataract formation)
3. Ears	Decreased high frequency acuity	Difficulty in discriminating words if background noise is present	Deafness (sensorineural)
4. Endocrine	a. Impaired glucose tolerance	Stress hyperglycaemia	Diabetes mellitus
	b. Decreased thyroxine clearance and/or production	Decreased T_4 requirement in hypothyroidism	Thyroid dysfunction (hypothyroidism or hyperthyroidism)
	c. Decreased testosterone		
	d. Decreased vitamin D absorption and activation	Osteopenia	Osteoporosis; osteomalacia
5. Respiratory system	Decreased lung elasticity and increased chest wall stiffness	Ventilation-perfusion mismatch and decreased PO_2	Dyspnoea
6. Cardiovascular system	a Decreased arterial compliance and increased systolic blood pressure	Hypotensive response to volume depletion or loss of atrial contraction	Syncope
	b. Decreased β adrenergic responsiveness	Decreased cardiac output	Heart failure
	c. Decreased baroreceptor sensitivity and decreased SA node automaticity	Impaired blood pressure response to standing (postural hypotension)	Heart block
7. GIT	a. Decreased hepatic function	Delayed metabolism of drugs	Cirrhosis
	b. Decreased gastric acidity	Decreased calcium absorption on empty stomach	Osteoporosis; vitamin B_{12} deficiency
	c. Decreased colonic motility	Constipation	Fecal impaction (leading to urinary incontinence or spurious diarrhoea)
8. Renal	Decreased GFR	Impaired excretion of some drugs	Increased serum creatinine
9. Genitourinary system	a. Vaginal/urethral mucosal atrophy	Dyspareunia; asymptomatic bacteriuria	Symptomatic urinary tract infection
	b. Prostate enlargement	Increased residual urine volume	Urinary incontinence; urinary retention
10. Nervous system	a. Decreased brain catecholamine synthesis	-	Depression
	b. Decreased brain dopaminergic synthesis	Stiff gait	Parkinson's disease
	c. Decreased righting reflexes	Increased body swaying	Recurrent falls
	d. Decreased stage 4 sleep	Early morning awakening	Sleep apnoea
	e. Brain atrophy	Forgetfulness	Dementia; delirium

presence of certain characteristic features of disease in the elderly.

1. *Multiple aetiology and pathology:* Several disease processes may combine to produce a symptom in an elderly individual (e.g. recurrent falls may be due to the presence of a combination of postural hypotension, decreased righting reflexes, decreased visual acuity due to cataract and muscle weakness). This is in contrast to disease presentation in the young, whereby the same symptom may be due to any one of the above mentioned abnormalities.

In the elderly, therefore, treating each aetiology of the problem alone may do little good to the patient and treating all may be of great benefit.

2. *Non-specific presentation of disease:* Some presentations of disease are common in old age, in particular the 'geriatric giants' namely urinary incontinence, acute confusion, immobility and falls. Diseases may also present atypically in the elderly.
3. Many findings that are abnormal in young age may be relatively common in old people (bacteriuria, premature ventricular ectopics, isolated systolic hypertension, low bone mineral density, impaired glucose tolerance and uninhibited bladder contractions).
4. Rapid deterioration can occur if disease is untreated.
5. Complications are common.
6. More time is required for recovery.
7. There is impaired metabolism and excretion of drugs. Doses of drugs may need lowering.

Atypical Presentation of Disease in Elderly

The effect of age changes, impaired immunological function, poor nutrition, multiple pathology, sensory deficits, psychiatric disorders and intercurrent drug treatment interact to both modify and mask the typical symptoms and signs of disease in many elderly patients.

Giants of Geriatric Medicine

These refer to four of the most common causes of incapacity in elderly patients referred to a geriatric unit, namely acute confusion, urinary incontinence, immobility and falls.

1. Acute Confusion

Acute confusional state in an elderly patient usually is the result of organic disease, or a manifestation of drug toxicity (esp. sedatives, hypnotics, antiemetics, or anticholinergics).

2. Urinary Incontinence

Confusion and immobility associated with acute illness often result in urinary incontinence. This usually settles with resolution of the illness, but in a proportion of cases the incontinence persists.

A common neurological cause of chronic urinary incontinence is damage to the cerebral cortex with damage to normal bladder inhibition, so that the bladder has a small volume and increased tone, and empties frequently (uninhibited bladder). Disorders that are responsible for this are cerebrovascular disease, Alzheimer's disease or Parkinson's disease.

Spinal cord damage due to multiple sclerosis, trauma or a tumour, though less common in the elderly, can cause bladder dysfunction.

Damage to afferent parasympathetic fibres in disorders such as diabetic autonomic neuropathy gives rise to a large volume atonic bladder in which there is a continuous dribbling overflow incontinence.

Local causes of urinary incontinence may be due to pressure on the bladder due to faecal impaction, or prostatic enlargement.

Stress incontinence is often due to weakness of the pelvic floor muscles, especially in multiparous and postmenopausal women.

In postmenopausal women, atrophic changes in the vagina may be accompanied by similar abnormalities in the mucosa of the urethra and trigone due to lack of oestrogen resulting in urinary frequency and urge incontinence.

Drugs such as diuretics may cause incontinence.

Poor mobility and thereby a delay in reaching the lavatory may be the cause for incontinence.

Drugs that may Affect Continence

Medications	Examples	Effects on continence
NSAIDs	COX 2 inhibitors	Nocturnal diuresis due to fluid retention
Alcohol		Frequency, urgency, polyuria, sedation, delirium
Sedatives / Hypnotics	Benzodiazepines	Excess sedation, delirium
Narcotic analgesics	Morphine derivatives	Retention, fecal impaction, delirium, excess sedation
Anticholinergics	Dicyclomine, antihistamine	Retention -overflow
Antipsychotics	Haloperidol, thioridazine	Retention, rigidity, sedation
Antidepressants	Amitriptyline	Retention –overflow
Antiparkinsonians	Trihexyphenidyl	Retention-overflow
Calcium channel blockers	All dihydropyridines	Nocturnal diuresis due to fluid retention
Loop-diuretics	Furosemide, bumetanide	Polyuria, urgency, frequency
ACE inhibitors	Enalapril, lisinopril	Drug induced cough causing stress incontinence
Vincristine		Urinary retention

Disorders Presenting with Atypical Features in Elderly Patients

Disorder	Atypical presentation
Myocardial infarction	Confusion, weakness, fatigue, breathlessness and palpitations without chest pain. May also present with unexplained sweating, vomiting, postural hypotension or bowel urgency.
Bronchopneumonia	Confusion and rapid respiration, no pyrexia and minimal chest signs.
Appendicitis	Confusion, constipation or diarrhoea, no pyrexia and few localising signs.
Peptic ulcer	Anaemia, haematemesis or melaena without previous symptoms of dyspepsia.
Urinary tract infection	Confusion and urinary incontinence, no pyrexia or increased frequency or dysuria.
Dehydration	No thirst, and skin changes indistinguishable from those of ageing.
Hypothyroidism	Lethargy and general deterioration with no other characteristic symptoms and signs.
Thyrotoxicosis	Apathy, weight loss and cardiac signs (atrial arrhythmias) without anxiety, excess sweating or heat intolerance.
Diabetes mellitus	Asymptomatic until onset of complications, e.g. nephropathy, neuropathy or retinopathy.
Brain tumour	Confusion, drowsiness and focal neurological signs without headache or papilloedema.

In some patients urinary incontinence is a manifestation of anxiety, or an attention-seeking device.

Management

The mainstay of management of urinary incontinence is proper and adequate toilet training in which the patient is encouraged to develop the habit of regular emptying of the bladder.

Faecal impaction if present should be treated.

An oestrogen cream should be used where there is atrophic vaginitis.

If there is stress incontinence, exercises for the pelvic floor should be taught to the patient.

In men, prostatectomy may relieve overflow incontinence.

As a last resort, intractable urinary incontinence should be managed by devices such as catheters, urinals, incontinence pads or marsupial pants.

3. Immobility

Age related changes in the neurological and musculoskeletal system and a high prevalence of disorders such as stroke, Parkinson's disease, osteoarthritis and osteoporosis, interact to make poor mobility one of the most common problems to afflict elderly patients.

Since there often is little reserve capacity in skeletal muscles, even a short duration of bed-rest may render the patient immobile. It is therefore essential that an active rehabilitation programme be instituted as soon as possible after an episode of acute illness in order to prevent development of prolonged incapacitation.

4. Falls

There is an increased incidence of falls with advancing age.

Falls in the elderly usually have a plethora of causes. 50% are due to tripping or an accident.

About 10% are related to loss of consciousness or dizziness (due to vertebro-basilar insufficiency).

For the rest there is no clear cause.

Drug intake may be an important cause of falls (drugs causing postural hypotension, sedation or cardiac dysrhythmias).

Alcohol consumption may also cause falls in the elderly.

The consequences of falls in the elderly may be detrimental to the patient especially with development of fracture neck of femur or head injury resulting in subdural haematoma.

Prevention of falls in the elderly is very important as even a single fall can shatter the patient's confidence, even if no serious injury has been sustained.

Physiotherapy, which includes learning techniques to get up from the bed or floor and moving about carefully in the house may be of great benefit to the patient.

Postural Hypotension

Detection of presence of postural hypotension in the elderly is important as it is common in them and is also a common cause of falls and poor mobility.

Typical times of occurrence of postural hypotension are after meals, on exertion, and on getting up suddenly from the lying posture, especially at night. This may also manifest transiently with intercurrent illnesses (e.g. viral fever).

Postural hypotension may be due to venous insufficiency in the legs, autonomic neuropathy, drugs (diuretics, nitrates, antihypertensives, antidepressants, sedatives), or decreased baroreceptor response to pressure changes.

Risk factors for Fall and Possible Rehabilitation Measures

Risk factors	Medical intervention	Rehabilitation
Reduced visual acuity	Refraction, cataract surgery	Safety measures at home
Reduced hearing	Removal of wax , evaluation for hearing	Hearing aid if needed
Vestibular dysfunction	ENT / Neurological evaluation	Avoidance of drugs that affect the vestibular system
Dementia	Correct the treatable causes	Avoid sedation, home safety measures
Proprioceptive dysfunction	Correct vitamin B_{12} level, treat C. spondylosis	Correct size footwear, Walking aid
Postural hypotension	Screen the drugs consumed	Elevation of head end-bed
Sedatives	Use lowest effective dose	Slow and steady walk
Antihypertensives	Avoid postural hypotension	Check BP lying and standing
Musculoskeletal disorders	Neurological evaluation	Exercise and gait training

Some Adverse Reactions of Drugs Noticed in Geriatric Patients

	Drug	Side effects
1.	Sedatives and hypnotics	Confusional states, falls, incontinence
2.	Antiemetics and neuroleptics	Parkinsonian syndrome, confusional state, postural hypotension, tardive dyskinesia, drowsiness, susceptibility to hypothermia
3.	Diuretics	Dehydration, electrolyte imbalance, postural hypotension.
4.	NSAIDs	Dyspepsia, upper GI bleed, oedema, cardiac failure.
5.	Anticholinergics and antidepressants	Confusional states, urinary retention, constipation, dry mouth.

Some Drugs to be Avoided/Used with Caution in Disorders in the Elderly

	Disorder	Drugs to be avoided/used with caution
1.	Hypertension	Use vasodilators with caution as it can precipitate postural hypotension and stroke. β blockers and calcium channel blockers to be used with caution in presence of conduction defects and incipient cardiac failure. β blocker aggravates existing peripheral vascular insufficiency.
2.	CCF	Use diuretics with caution as it can cause dehydration and electrolyte imbalance.
3.	IHD	Use digoxin with care as digoxin toxicity may be precipitated especially when there is impaired renal excretion. Sublingual nitroglycerin to be administered in the lying posture as it may precipitate postural hypotension and falls if administered in the sitting or standing posture.
4.	Mural thrombus	Oral anticoagulants (warfarin) to be used with caution as there may be increased activity due to reduced plasma binding of the drug. Prolonged use of heparin may exacerbate pre-existing osteoporosis and produce pathological fractures.
5.	Bronchial asthma/COPD	Adrenaline must not be used as it can precipitate coronary vasospasm. Theophylline to be used with caution as impaired hepatic oxidation/ hydroxylation can increase plasma level of the drug to toxic levels. β agonists (salbutamol) to be given in minimal optimal dose as it may precipitate tachycardia and IHD. Prolonged administration of steroids to be avoided as it may result in exacerbation of pre-existing osteoporosis and electrolyte imbalance (hypokalaemia).
6.	Parkinson's disease	Avoid anticholinergics as it can precipitate glaucoma, urinary retention and confusional states.
7.	Cerebrovascular accidents	Antioedema measures to be used with caution as it may precipitate dehydration and electrolyte imbalance. Mannitol may precipitate renal failure and LVF when used in patients with impaired renal function.
8.	Diarrhoea	Fluid and electrolyte loss should be carefully monitored and their replacement must be meticulous. Hypovolemia and haemoconcentration can result in stroke, peripheral vascular occlusion and gangrene. Avoid use of antispasmodics or antimotility agents as they may produce paralytic ileus
9.	Constipation	Avoid prolonged use of laxatives as they may produce hypokalaemia
10.	Hypothyroidism	Replacement therapy with L-thyroxine should be initiated with minimal optimal dose and then gradually increased over 2–3 weeks. Initial high dose replacement may precipitate IHD.
11.	Hyperthyroidism/senile tremors	Initiate propranolol therapy with caution as its serum level may be increased due to decreased first pass metabolism through the liver.
12.	Psychiatric disorders	Antipsychotic drugs must be used with caution as they may cause falls and confusional states.

intake of vasodilator antihypertensive agents, leading to risk of postural hypotension.

3. *Aspirin and other NSAIDs:* Incidence of gastric irritation and upper GI bleed is increased with concurrent intake of alcohol and NSAIDs.
4. *Insulin:* There is an increased risk of developing severe hypoglycaemia in diabetic patient on insulin when there is an excessive intake of alcohol.
5. *Monoamine oxidase inhibitors:* Some alcoholic drinks contain tyramine and so there may be a risk of developing severe hypertension in patients taking MAO inhibitors and consuming alcohol.
6. *Oral contraceptives:* Women taking oral contraceptives eliminate alcohol slowly and so the effect of alcohol is prolonged.
7. *Metronidazole, chloral hydrate and disulfiram:* These drugs inhibit aldehyde dehydrogenase activity and lead to accumulation of acetaldehyde. When alcohol is also consumed along with any one of these drugs, the level of acetaldehyde rises markedly leading to facial flushing, tachycardia, hypotension, dyspnoea, nausea and vomiting.
8. *Warfarin:* Acute alcohol intoxication potentiates the hypoprothrombinaemic effect of warfarin leading to bleeding tendencies.

Psychological

1. Anxiety
2. Depression
3. Personality change
4. Misuse of other drugs
5. Cognitive impairment.

Social

1. Family problems, marital discord
2. Financial problems
3. Repeated road traffic accidents, driving offences
4. Employment (e.g. absenteeism, especially on monday, poor performance)
5. Sexual abuse.

Smoking

Cigarette smoke is a heterogenous aerosol produced by incomplete combustion of tobacco leaf. On an average, smokers lose more than one day of life every week.

Main stream smoke: Smoke emerging from mouthpiece during puffing

Side stream smoke: Smoke emitted between puffs at the burning cone and from the mouthpiece

Side stream smoke contains more of particulate matter especially carcinogens.

Contents of Cigarette Smoke

Carcinogens	Tar
	Polynuclear aromatic hydro-carbons
	β-napthylamine
	N-nitrosonornicotine
	Benzopyrene
	Trace metals—nickel, arsenic. polonium 210
	Nitrosamines, hydrazine, vinyl-chloride
Co-carcinogens	Phenol, cresol, catechol
Tumour accelerator	Indole, carbazole

Pharmacology of Cigarette Smoke

There are more than 4000 substances identified in cigarette smoke. They have antigenic, cytotoxic, mutagenic and carcinogenic properties.

Nicotine is a toxic alkaloid present in cigarette smoke which is both a ganglionic stimulant and a depressant.

Acute cardiovascular effects of nicotine are increase in
a. both systolic and diastolic BP
b. heart rate
c. force of myocardial contraction and excitability
d. myocardial oxygen consumption
e. coronary artery blood flow
f. peripheral vasoconstriction.

Major carcinogens found in cigarette smoke are polynuclear aromatic hydrocarbons, aromatic amines and nitrosamines. Co-carcinogens like catechol enhance the carcinogenecity.

Carbon monoxide is a toxic gas found in smoke (2-6%) and causes polycythaemia and CNS impairment. This is the major cause for COPD.

Smoking also causes chronic cough, sputum, dyspnoea, change in lung function tests, increase in incidence of pneumonia and inflammatory lung disease.

Characteristics of Smokers

Smokers drink more alcohol, coffee and tea than nonsmokers. Menopause comes earlier in smoking women. Smokers have impaired exercise performance, impaired immune system compared to nonsmokers. They show increase in hematocrit, WBC count and platelet count, there is decrease in leucocyte vitamin C levels, serum uric acid and albumin in smokers.

The ratio of HDL to LDL cholesterol is also reduced.

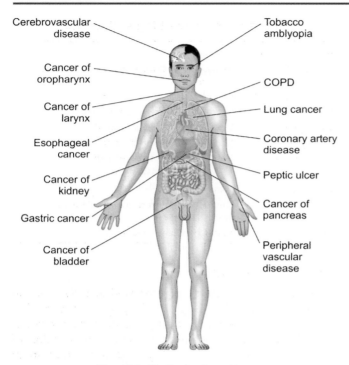

Fig. 13.2: Ill-effects of smoking

Labels on figure: Cerebrovascular disease, Cancer of oropharynx, Cancer of larynx, Esophageal cancer, Cancer of kidney, Gastric cancer, Cancer of bladder, Tobacco amblyopia, COPD, Lung cancer, Coronary artery disease, Peptic ulcer, Cancer of pancreas, Peripheral vascular disease

Clinical Correlations

Common disorders associated with smoking include atherosclerotic cardiovascular disease, cancer and COPD. The risk is dependent on duration, intensity and type of smoke exposure (Fig. 13.2).

Smoking and Cardiovascular Disease

- Smoking, hypertension, and hypercholesterolemia are three major risk factors for coronary heart disease (CHD). Presence of two out of the three risk factors may produce a 4-fold increase in CHD risk and 3 risk factors produces a 8-fold increase in CHD risk.
- CHD death rates are 60–70% greater in male smokers than in nonsmokers.
- Sudden death is 2–4 times more common in young male smokers.
- Women smokers also develop CHD especially when they take oral contraceptive pill also.
- Those who continue to smoke after acute MI are most likely to die from CHD than those who quit smoking. Smokers have an increased perioperative mortality than nonsmokers.
- Similarly, cerebrovascular disease and stroke is also common in smokers. In women smokers, subarachnoid haemorrhage is more common; oral contraceptives increase the risk in them.

- Peripheral vascular diseases like thromboangiitis obliterans (TAO) and arteriosclerosis obliterans are common in smokers.
- Hypertensives who smoke are at a greater risk of developing malignant hypertension and they die from complications of hypertension.

Smoking and Cancer

Smoking causes cancer of	
Oral cavity	Pancreas
Larynx	Kidney
Lung	Urinary bladder
Esophagus	Uterine cervix
Stomach	Myelocytic leukaemia

Smoking Index (SI)

SI = number of cigarette/day × total duration in years
SI < 100   Mild smoker
SI 101–300   Moderate smoker
SI > 300   Heavy smoker

Lung cancer is common if smoking index is more than 300.

Pack Year

No. of pack years = 1 packet of cigarette/day × number of years (one pack = 20 cigarettes).

The risk of developing lung cancer is 40 times more in patients who smoke 2 packs per day for 20 years.

Smoking and Respiratory Disease

Male smokers have 4-25 times higher mortality secondary to COPD than nonsmokers.

Prolonged cigarette smoking impairs ciliary movement, inhibits function of alveolar macrophages and leads to hypertrophy and hyperplasia of mucus secreting glands. It also inhibits antiproteases and causes polymorphs to release proteolytic enzymes acutely. The inhaled cigarette smoke increases airway resistance due to vagally mediated smooth muscle constriction by way of stimulating submucosal irritant receptors.

Abnormalities in pulmonary function tests, (measurements of elastic recoil, airflow in large and small airways and diffusing capacity) is common in smokers. There is increase in incidence of respiratory infections and deaths due to pneumonia and influenza. Postoperative respiratory complications, spontaneous pneumothorax are also common. Chronic pharyngitis, chronic laryngitis and chronic bronchitis occur more frequently in smokers.

Smoking and Gastrointestinal Disorders

In smokers, there are changes in hard and soft tissues of the mouth, discolouration of the teeth and there is decreased sensation of taste and smell.

Gastric, and duodenal ulcer disease is more prevalent in smokers both in males and females. Smoking impairs ulcer healing, favours recurrence of ulcers, inhibits pancreatic HCO^-_3 secretion and decreases the pressure of esophageal and pyloric sphincters. Inhibition of nocturnal acid secretion by H_2 blockers is also prevented by smoking.

Smoking and Depression

Prevalence of smoking is increased in those who have a major depressive disorder.

Smoking and Body Weight

There is an inverse association between smoking and body weight. Weight gain occurs after cessation of smoking.

Smoking and Pregnancy

Smoking delays conception and smoking during pregnancy affects the foetus. Babies born to mothers who smoke have a weight of about 170 gm less than the babies born to non-smokers. This is due to impaired uteroplacental circulation.

Spontaneous abortion, foetal death, neonatal death and sudden infant death syndromes are also common. The long-term physical growth and intellectual development of the child is also affected.

Passive Smoking

Since side stream smoke is diluted in a large volume of air, smoke exposure from involuntary inhalation is less than that associated with smoking.

Passive smoking is one of the causes for lung cancer in nonsmokers. Parental smoking is a cause for middle ear effusions, acute or chronic respiratory illness and asthma in children. Passive smoking may also cause coronary heart disease.

Smoking and Drugs

Tobacco smoke constituents induce hepatic microsomal enzyme systems which are important in the metabolism of drugs like propranolol, theophylline and propoxyphene and hence increase in dose in smokers is recommended.

Interaction of Smoking and Drugs

Benzodiazepines	Less sedation
Beta blockers	Reduced effect due to increased 1st pass clearance
Imipramine	Decreased serum concentration
Chlorpromazine	Decreased serum concentration
Clomipramine	Decreased serum concentration
Clozapine	Decreased serum concentration
Haloperidol	Decreased serum concentration
Oral oestrogens	Increased hepatic clearance
Heparin	Faster clearance
Insulin	Delayed absorption due to cutaneous vasoconstriction
Theophylline	Faster metabolic clearance

Type of Smoking

- Using low tar-nicotine cigarettes shows decrease in risk of developing lung and laryngeal cancers. The risk is the same for both high tar-nicotine cigarettes and low tar-nicotine cigarettes when the number of cigarettes smoked per day and the duration of smoking are more in the latter group.
- Using pipe, or cigar reduces the overall risk (the patients do not inhale more smoke since the alkaline pH of tobacco used in them is a potent irritant of respiratory tract).
- Death rates of cigar, pipe and cigarette smokers are more or less the same as far as carcinoma of oral cavity, larynx and esophagus are concerned. Otherwise there are more adverse health regarding cancer at other sites, CHD or COPD.
- Chewing tobacco or using snuff produces increased risk for oral cancers.
- Cessation of smoking produces immediate and long-term physical, psychological and economic benefits. The sense of smell and taste may improve within a few days of quitting the cigarette.
- One year after stopping, there is a decrease in risk for CHD; cessation also decrease risk for tobacco related cancers, cerebrovascular disease, MI, and COPD.

Cessation Process

Smokers should stop smoking in a stepwise process. First they think about quitting, then they decide to quit and later they should maintain an ex-smoker status.

Most successful quitters relapse and recycle through these stages 3–4 times before abstinence. Factors encouraging long-term cessation include decreased social acceptability, increased concern about health consequences and increased cost of tobacco.

Cessation Methods

Counselling, group therapy, behavioural training, hypnosis, and acupuncture are the methods tried.

Quitting 'cold turkey' is the method used by 80% of smokers.

Pharmacotherapy

1. Nicotine containing chewing gum 2 or 4 mg chewed over 20-30 minutes, repeated upto 60 mg/day.
2. Transdermal nicotine patch; started as high dose patch, 21 mg/day for 6 weeks followed by intermediate dose patch, 14 mg/day for 2-4 weeks followed by low dose patch, 7mg/day for 2-4 weeks.
3. Nicotine nasal spray; 2 sprays (equivalent to 1 mg) as needed not to exceed 5 doses/hr or 40 doses/day.
4. Nicotine inhalor. 6-16 cartridges/day for 12 weeks followed by tapering over 6-12 weeks.
5. Bupropion hydrochloride.

It acts by inhibiting neuronal reuptake of Dopamine and nor-adrenaline. The drug is started 1 week before quiting smoking at a dose of 150 mg orally OD for 3 days followed by 150 mg orally BD for 7-12 weeks, increases smoking cessation rate when used with behaviour modification programme and can be combined with nicotine replacement.

Contraindication:
  Seizure disorder
  Eating disorder like bulimia or anorexia nervosa.
  Administration of MAO inhibitors
  Head trauma
  CNS tumour
  Concomitant antidepressants or antipsychotics
  Hypersensitivity
  Concomitant alcohol or benzodiazepines should be avoided.
6. Second line therapies:
   i. Clonidine – initial dose 0.1 mg bid PO and increased to 0.15-0.75 mg/day PO or transdermal patch 0.1 to 0.2 mg for 3 to 10 weeks.
   ii. Nortriptyline 25 mg/day and increased upto 100 mg/day PO for 12 weeks.

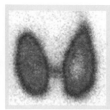
RESPIRATORY SYSTEM

CXR
Initial choice
picks up early lesions

CT
Imaging the hila/
mediastinum/pleura
HRCT-Bronchiectasis/ILD
Biopsies

PULMONARY ANGIOGRAPHY
Pulmonary vascular
disease
PHT/embolism

VP SCAN
PE

CARDIOVASCULAR SYSTEM

CXR
Initial choice
Cardiac enlargement
Valve calcifications

ECHO
Valvular/congenital
heart diseases
Quantification of LV function
clots/vegetations/effusions

ANGIOGRAM
CAD-diagnostic/therapeutic
Assessing the severity of
valvular/cong. heart disease

MR ANGIOGRAPHY
Angiography
Aortic diseases

NUCLEAR IMAGING
Assessing regional
myocardial blood flow
and cellular integrity of myocytes

NEUROLOGY

CT
CVA -initial choice
Tumours/abscesses
Traumatic conditions

MRI
Posterior fossa lesions
Spinal cord lesions
White matter lesions

X-RAY
Calcifications
Bony abnormalities

ABDOMEN

X-RAY
Acute abdomen
free intraperitoneal gas
dilated bowel/fluid levels

ULTRASOUND
Studying liver/spleen/
kidneys/ovaries/prostate
obstetric study

CT
Detailed study of masses
retroperitoneal structure

CONTRAST STUDIES (oral/IV)
To study intraluminal
pathology-stone/neoplasms
strictures/ulcers/hernia, etc.

MRCP
Noninvasive way to
investigate hepatobiliary and
pancreatic disorders

The Chest Film

The chest film is the mirror for many systemic disorders in addition to the information it reveals for respiratory and cardiovascular disorders. It normally shows anterior portion of 6±1 ribs and posterior portion of 9±1 ribs. More ribs/ intercostals spaces can be seen in COPD, bronchial asthma and emphysema.

The right hemi-diaphragm is higher than the left diaphragm by 3 cm in 95% of cases. This apparent elevation of the right diaphragm (not due to liver) is due to the downward displacement of the left side of diaphragm by the heart. The lateral costo-phrenic angles should be sharp and acute.

This angle is blunted or ill-defined in pleural effusion or hyperinflation. The cardio-thoracic ratio is the ratio of heart width to the chest width. It should be less than 50% in PA view since the heart is magnified in AP view.

The left hilum is higher than the right by 1 cm. The density is equal. Change in density denotes rotated film or tumour or lymph nodes.

Lateral views are useful to study the segment of the lung fields affected and also to note the cardiac chamber hypertrophy. The right hemi-diaphragm crosses through the heart shadow to the anterior chest wall and the left hemi-diaphragm ends at the posterior cardiac border in lateral views of the chest X-ray (Figs 14.1 to 14.3).

In left lateral view left ventricular hypertrophy is best visualized as it encroaches the spine and the right ventricular hypertrophy is well visualized as it encroaches the retro-sternal space. Barium swallow RAO view demonstrates the sickling effect of compression on oesophagus by the left atrium.

Comma shaped calcification of the aortic knuckle indicates atherosclerosis. Calcification of the ascending aorta is diagnostic of syphilis.

Increased translucency of lung fields:
1. Pneumothorax -Absent vascular marking with visible collapsed lung
2. Bullous change – emphysema
3. Pulmonary embolus – Westermark's sign
4. Hyperinflation in COPD
5. Pulmonary hypertension.

Abnormal opacities:
1. Consolidation: Opacity + Air bronchogram within it (Silhouette sign)
2. Collapse: Loss of volume causes shift of the normal landmarks (Mediastinum, Hila, Fissures, etc.)
3. Linear opacities: atelectasis, septal lines (Kerley B lines–interlobular lymphatics), tumour, lymphangitis carcinomatosis

4. Ring shadows: bronchiectasis, cavitating lesions, tumour, abscess, hydatid cyst, Pulmonary infarct (Triangular with a pleural base – Hampton's hump)
5. 'Coin' lesions: enormous conditions (always rule out tumour)

Rest of the details is dealt in depth in the chapter on respiratory system.

Plain Abdominal Film

In an emergency, plain X-ray of the abdomen is taken without prior preparation. Demonstration of gas underneath the diaphragm in the erect film denotes bowel perforation. Small bowel is recognized by its central position and valvulae conniventes which reach from one wall to other. Large bowel is peripheral in position with its haustration. Displacement of bowel denotes space occupying lesion (Tumour) or massive organomegaly (Figs 14.4 and 14.5).

Extra Luminal Gas

- In the liver or biliary system – gas forming infection, after ERCP, after passing stone
- In the genitourinary system – entero-vesical fistula, emphysematous pyelonephritis (Diagnostic of DM with *E. coli* infection)
- In the colonic wall—Pneumatosis coli/infective colitis
- In the sub-phrenic abscess.

Calcification in the Abdomen

- Egg-shell calcification in an aneurysm
- Calcified lymph nodes (TB – abdomen)
- Calculi gallbladder,
- Intra-renal or ureteric calculi,
- Pancreatic calculi (chronic pancreatitis)
- Uterus – myoma calcified, very rarely foetus
- Dermoid cyst which may contain teeth.

Soft Tissues

Note the kidney size (10-12 cm) and shape-parallel to the psoas line – length equal to 2-3.5 vertebral bodies (T12 to L2). The psoas lines are obliterated in retroperitoneal inflammation, haemorrhage or peritonitis.

Meteorism

Localised peritoneal inflammation can cause a localised ileus. It can be seen as a 'sentinel loop' of intra-luminal gas and can provide a clue to the site of pathology – such as cholecystitis, pancreatitis, appendicitis and diverticulitis. However, at times even localised infection can produce generalised ileus.

BRONCHOPULMONARY SEGMENTS

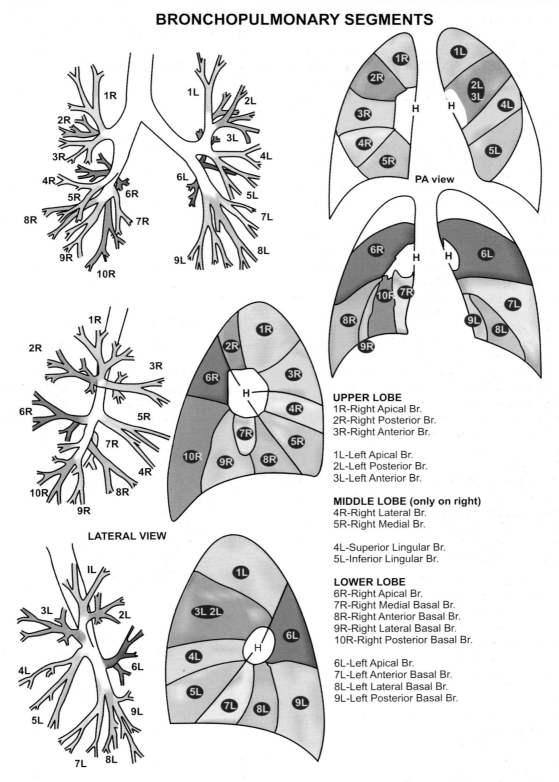

PA view

LATERAL VIEW

UPPER LOBE
1R-Right Apical Br.
2R-Right Posterior Br.
3R-Right Anterior Br.

1L-Left Apical Br.
2L-Left Posterior Br.
3L-Left Anterior Br.

MIDDLE LOBE (only on right)
4R-Right Lateral Br.
5R-Right Medial Br.

4L-Superior Lingular Br.
5L-Inferior Lingular Br.

LOWER LOBE
6R-Right Apical Br.
7R-Right Medial Basal Br.
8R-Right Anterior Basal Br.
9R-Right Lateral Basal Br.
10R-Right Posterior Basal Br.

6L-Left Apical Br.
7L-Left Anterior Basal Br.
8L-Left Lateral Basal Br.
9L-Left Posterior Basal Br.

Note: Take PA and respective lateral view to localise the exact segment since segments overlap

Fig. 14.1: Diagram of positions of segments seen in chest X-rays

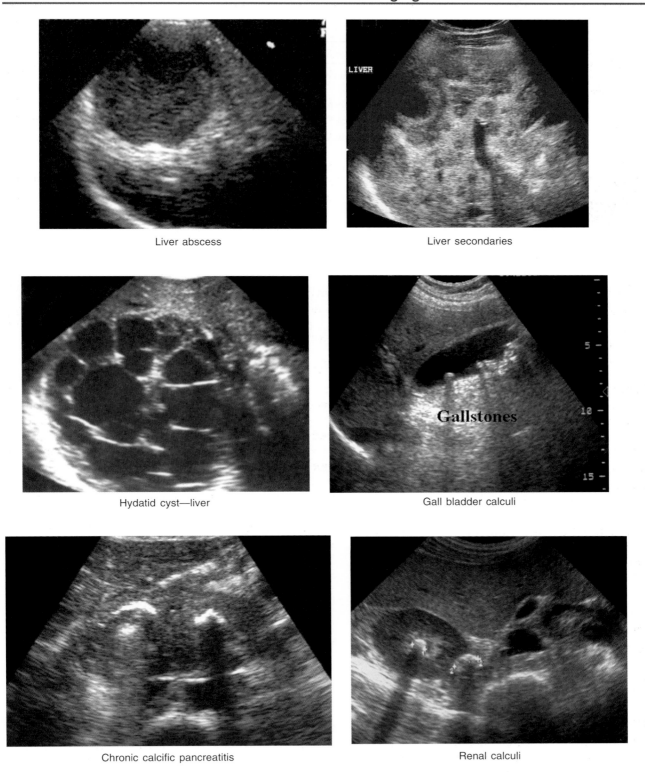

Liver abscess

Liver secondaries

Hydatid cyst—liver

Gall bladder calculi

Chronic calcific pancreatitis

Renal calculi

Fig. 14.18: Ultrasound: abdomen

Imaging Intensity—Ultrasound Abdomen

Organ	Hyperechoic	Hypoechoic	Anechoic
Liver	Stones, metastases, granulomas, cirrhosis, hemangiomas	Metastases, abscesses	Cysts, abscesses
Spleen	Hemangiomas, granulomas	Haematoma, Lymphoma, metastases	Cysts, abscesses
Gallbladder	Calculi, polyps	Carcinoma, empyema	Cholecystitis, abscesses
Kidneys	Calculi, lipoma, angioma	Abscesses, metastases, CA	Cysts, Dilated pelvi-calyceal system
Pancreas	Chronic pancreatitis, calculi	Acute pancreatitis, carcinoma	Abscesses, cysts, pseudocysts

4. Gallbladder – thickening of wall, polyp, gallstones
5. Pancreas –Pseudocysts, abscesses, tumour, calculi
6. Kidneys – enlarged or contracted, calculi, hydronephrosis, polycystic disease, mass lesions, adrenal mass lesions
7. Aneurysms of aorta and major vessels
8. Doppler studies of portal and splanchnic veins – to assess direction of flow and to rule out thrombosis
9. To monitor normal and abnormal pregnancy
10. To monitor fetal growth and development
11. Localization of placenta
12. To identify ectopic pregnancy
13. Ovarian mass lesions including PCOD
14. Uterine mass lesions
15. Testicular size, mass lesions, hydrocele.

Echocardiography

This non-invasive technique offers a wealth of anatomic and physiologic information of the heart. It is safe, painless, repeatable, inexpensive and it does not utilize ionizing radiation. All the modern equipments provide the following facilities:

1. M-mode
2. B-mode or two dimensional echocardiography
3. Pulsed Doppler
4. Continuous wave Doppler
5. Colour-flow imaging.

M-mode echocardiography: It gives an ice-pick view of the heart and it has many limitations. It allows measurements of chamber size, assessment of valve and wall motion. Cardiac structures closer to the transducer are displayed at the top of the record and the distant structures are displayed below (on trans-thoracic M mode echocardiogram –the anteriorly placed right sided structures are displayed on the top and the posteriorly placed left sided structures displayed on the bottom and the order is reversed in the trans-esophageal echocardiogram).

B-mode or two dimensional echocardiography:
• Useful in the diagnosis of congenital heart disease such as
  a. Septal defect
  b. Congenital valvular disease
  c. Relationship of great vessels to the cardiac chambers
  d. Foetal imaging for the antenatal diagnosis of congenital heart disease
  e. Mal-position of the heart
• To assess the cardiac chamber hypertrophy, dilatation, systolic and diastolic dysfunction, type of cardiomyopathy
• To assess the type of valvular lesion – congenital, rheumatic, degenerative
• To diagnose infective endocarditis – vegetation > 2 mm size
• To diagnose pericardial thickening, effusion and impending cardiac tamponade
• Useful for the evaluation and diagnosis of coronary artery disease (including stress echo and pharmacological stress test)
• Doppler echocardiography is used to assess the direction and velocity of blood flow in the heart and great vessels (to detect shunts, regurgitant lesions and quantify valvular stenosis)
• Colour flow data when superimposed on B-mode echocardiography provides more useful qualitative data. The colour coded mapping reveals red colour indicating flow towards and the blue away from, the transducer.

Thyroid Scan

• Useful to measure the size of thyroid enlargement and also to differentiate cyst, nodule/tumour.
• Not useful to differentiate benign and malignant nodule.

Orbit and Eye

• Aids in the localization of foreign bodies

- Assessment of retinal and choroidal detachment
- Assessment of retro-orbital mass lesions.

Large Veins and Arteries

- Assessment of blood flow in the limbs
- To assess the extent of thrombosis.

Special Techniques

- Trans-esophageal echocardiogram to assess mitral valve lesions and vegetations in infective endo-carditis
- Trans-vaginal to study uterine and ovarian lesion
- Trans-rectal to assess the lesions of prosate and rectum
- Intravascular ultrasound – to study the extent of plaque, and it has a clinical role in coronary angioplasty and stenting
- Endoscopic ultrasound – Assessment of depth of mucosal penetration in cancer and thus helpful in staging (Ca esophagus, stomach, colon and rectum).

Computerized Tomography (CT-Scan)

The X-ray beam moves around the patient in a circular path and the slices can be cut at various levels. The detailed images are constructed from X-ray absorption data with the help of the computer. CT scan is very useful in stroke patients to differentiate infarction from haemorrhage since the treatment modality is different. In major trauma with head injury CT scan is the most important investigation of choice.

CT scan is performed with or without contrast. Contrast CT is useful in abdomen, pelvis and brain. It helps in GI tract to delineate the bowel and in brain to assess the vascularity of mass lesions and in performing carotid or 4 vessel angiogram.

Density measurements are essential to differentiate cyst, tumour, and haematomas. It is expressed in "Hounsfield Units". (Water is 0, bone is +1000, air is -1000 Units, fat – 50 to –150 and it varies for other tissues depending on the density)

Skeletal system disorders are better imaged by CT-scan.

CT- Brain

CT scan is useful for the diagnosis and assessment of various lesions:
- Fracture involving skull vault or base
- Hydrocephalus – dilated ventricles with effaced sulci and thinned out cortex
- Infarction (area of low attenuation with or without mass effect) and haemorrhage (high density lesion)

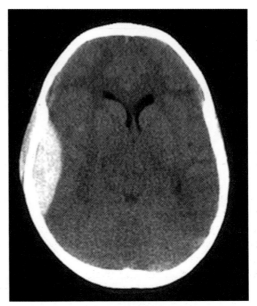

Fig. 14.19: Extradural hematoma

- Cerebral oedema due to stroke or different types of metabolic coma
- Mass lesions with or without midline shift
- High density extra-dural or sub-dural haematoma in acute phase (Fig. 14.19)
- Low density chronic sub-dural haematoma
- Various types of cerebellar lesions
- Multiple sclerosis and metastatic lesions
- Cerebral atrophy – Prominence of the sulci and atrophy of the gyri.

CT –Chest (Fig. 14.20)

- High resolution CT is investigation of choice to diagnose bronchiectasis
- Detecting and staging primary cancer of the lungs, pleura, and mediastinum
- To diagnose metastases of the lungs/pleura
- To detect infiltrative lung disease
- For the diagnosis of pulmonary emboli
- Evaluation of interstitial lung disease.

CT Coronary Angiography (Fig. 14.21)

- Multi-slice computed tomography scanners are used
- Coronary angiography is performed with 64 – slice technology
- 80 ml iodixanol is injected into an ante-cubital vein at a flow rate of 5 ml/s followed by a 50 ml saline chasing bolus
- The overall scan time is shorter than 15 seconds and the total period of study is less than 15 minutes

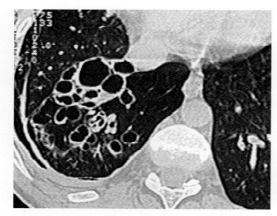

Bronchiectasis

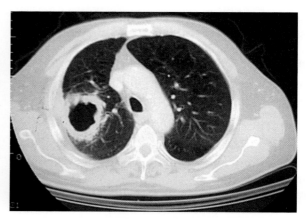

Cavitating bronchogenic carcinoma

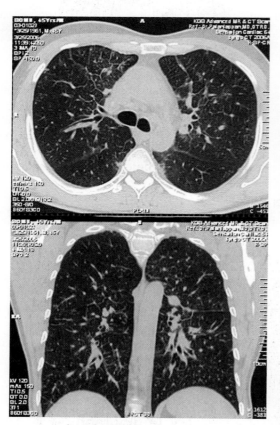

Lymphangitis carcinamatosa

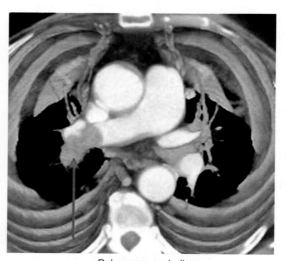

Pulmonary embolism

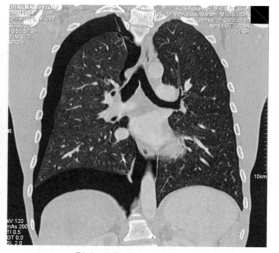

Right sided pneumothorax
Note: The ruptured BLEB in apex of lung
is indicated by arrows

Fig. 14.20: CT Chest (contd...)

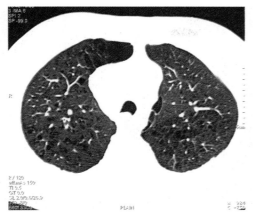

Centriacinar emphysema

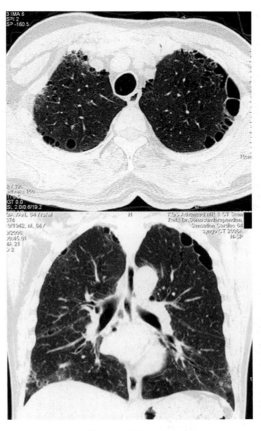

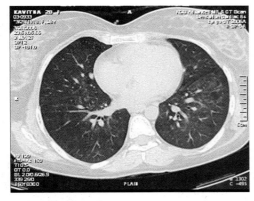

Pneumocystis pneumonia

Paraseptal emphysema

Fig. 14.20: CT Chest

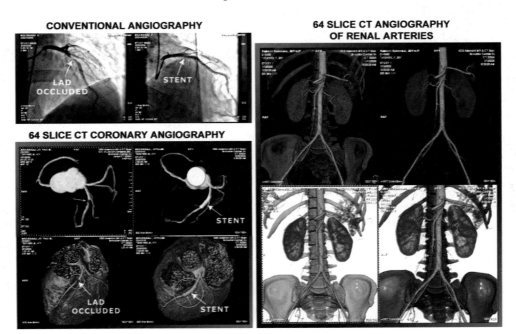

Fig. 14.21: 64 slice CT angiography

- A minimum of 10 slides should be made and stained immediately.

Dry Tap

1. Faulty technique
2. Hypoplasia/aplasia of bone marrow
3. Tightly packed marrow
4. Myelofibrosis.

Complications of Sternal Puncture

1. Injury to the underlying large vessel or heart in the sternal approach leading to fatal hemorrhage.
2. Pericardial tamponade
3. Mediastinitis
4. Pneumomediastinum.

Trephine Biopsy

The posterior iliac crest is the preferred site for performing trephine biopsy. The patient is placed in the right or left lateral position with the back comfortably flexed, and the medial expansion of the uppermost crest is chosen.

The skin overlying the crest is incised with a scalpel. The needle is then introduced with stylet in place with a boring motion (clockwise and counterclockwise) in the direction of anterior superior iliac spine until there is a decrease in resistance. Stylet is removed and the needle is further advanced till 2 to 3 cm of marrow is obtained. Marrow specimen is removed with the distal cutting edge of the needle. The instrument containing the specimen is withdrawn by rotation along its axis with quick full twists. Smear must be made immediately and stained with eosin and hematoxylin after decalcification.

A part of the biopsy material can be utilised for Leishman's stain. In trephine biopsy, histology is well delineated and myelofibrosis can be confirmed.

Liver Biopsy

Indications

1. Unexplained hepatomegaly/hepatosplenomegaly
2. Infiltrative disorders (sarcoid, malignancy, granulomatous lesions, lymphomas, storage disorders like haemochromatosis and Wilson's disease)
3. Pyrexia of unknown origin
4. Carcinoma (suspected hepatoma or metastasis)
5. Cholestasis of uncertain origin
6. Persistent abnormal liver function tests
7. Cirrhosis

8. Chronic hepatitis (chronic active hepatitis, chronic persistent hepatitis, chronic lobular hepatitis)
9. Alcoholic liver disease.

Contraindications

1. Bleeding disorder
2. Known hepatocellular malignancy
3. Unwilling or uncooperative patients.
4. Presence of tense ascites (may lead to continuous leak)
5. Dilated biliary radicle (may lead to bile peritonitis)
6. Vascular tumours
7. Infected right pleural space or septic cholangitis.

Liver Biopsy Needles

1. Menghini's needle (aspiration needle)
2. Vim Silverman's or Klatskin needle (cutting needle)
3. Trucut biopsy needle.

Procedure

The patient should be adequately prepared before performing liver biopsy.

Injection vitamin K one ampoule is given intramuscularly daily for 3 consecutive days before the procedure.

Blood grouping and cross matching of the patient's blood must be done and a bottle of compatible blood should be kept in readiness at the time of procedure.

Caution

The procedure should not be performed when
1. Prothrombin time is prolonged > 3 sec. above the control.
2. Platelet count < 50,000/cmm
3. Bleeding time, clotting time or partial thromboplastin time is prolonged.

1. Menghini's Needle

- The tip of the needle is not bevelled. A separate track making needle is present. A small guard with a head and flattened stalk which fits in with the barrel of the base of the needle. Since it is flattened and not circular, it can allow free flow of blood and saline and not the biopsied material.
- The patient lies along the edge of the bed in the supine posture.
- The biopsy may be performed in the 8th or 9th intercostal space in the mid axillary line, or one intercostal space below that of liver dullness obtained in full expiration in the mid axillary line.

- The procedure is carried out under strict aseptic precautions.
- The procedure is performed under local anaesthesia.
- A track is made in the subcutaneous tissue upto the liver (not in the liver) with the track making needle. The patient is asked to hold his breath in expiration and the Menghini's needle with the guard on and with a saline filled syringe is passed through the readymade track. Before entering into the liver, the unwanted tissue that would have entered the needle, should be syringed off by pushing saline. With suction on, the needle must be pushed into the liver and withdrawn immediately like a bonnet drill.
- Now the liver tissue is inside the biopsy needle and the same can be pushed into a bottle with formalin by injecting saline in the syringe. A cord like liver tissue can be obtained if the liver is not cirrhotic.
- The success rate of the procedure using this needle is approximately 75%.

2. Vim Silverman's Needle

This is a larger needle and has a stylet, barrel and biforked biopsy blade which is longer than the needle and which has to be rotated to 180° to get a good biopsy material. The advantage of this needle is that it has a success rate of approximately 95%. The disadvantage is that it is more traumatic.

3. Trucut Needle

It has a trocar and cannula. The trocar is longer than the cannula.

The skin is nicked with a scalpel blade and the biopsy needle is advanced slowly with the patient breathing quietly. The needle is advanced till it begins to swing with respiration. The needle is then slightly withdrawn until it stops swinging. The patient is then instructed to hold his breath in expiration and the needle is thrust for about 2 to 3 cm into the liver. The inner trocar is advanced holding the outer cannula with the cutting sheath still. The outer cutting sheath is then advanced over the inner trocar to cut the liver in the biopsy notch. The needle (trocar and cannula) is then quickly withdrawn after completing the procedure.

Aftercare

The patient is instructed in to lie on the right side for four hours and to remain in bed for 24 hours.

Pulse rate and blood pressure are recorded hourly.

Complications

1. Shock is usually caused by rapid loss of blood from a large vessel or vascular tumour

2. Severe pain may be caused by bleeding or leakage of bile. Pain may be referred to the shoulder tip
3. Septicaemia may result from needling an infected bile duct or liver abscess
4. Pneumothorax
5. Biliary peritonitis (injury to gallbladder)
6. Bacterial peritonitis (injury to hepatic flexure of colon).

Kidney Biopsy

Patients with renal glomerular disease may present with similar clinical features yet have conditions ranging from trivial to life threatening. Their prognosis and treatment depend on the renal pathology, and histological examination of the kidney is often the only way to make the diagnosis.

Needle biopsy provides a sample of about 20–30 of the 2,000,000 glomeruli and so is unhelpful and may give misleading results in patchy conditions such as reflux nephropathy. It is most valuable in assessing and, in particular, indicating the prognosis of patients with diffuse glomerular disease.

Contraindications

Laceration of the kidney may cause haemorrhage, which may lead to nephrectomy. The risk is small and biopsy should be done only if the other kidney is normal.

A single kidney or major abnormality of the contralateral kidney are contraindications, in the presence of any haemorrhagic tendency, including advanced uraemia. The platelet count should be over 1,00,000/mL and the prothrombin time must be normal.

Biopsy should not be done on shrunken kidneys because they are difficult to locate, the histological findings are often non-specific, and the results are unlikely to provide information of any therapeutic relevance.

Procedure

Before starting the procedure, grouping and cross matching of the patient's blood must be done and a bottle of compatible blood should be kept ready.

The procedure should be explained to the patient, and patient should practice holding his breath in inspiration. Biopsy is unsafe if patient cannot cooperate. Informed consent may be obtained in writing.

Renal biopsy is potentially hazardous.

Premedication with intravenous diazepam makes the procedure less unpleasant for the patient; general anaesthesia is required only for infants and young children.

Indications

Clinical syndrome	Indications for biopsy
Asymptomatic proteinuria	Protein excretion more than 1 g/24 h Red blood cells in urine Impaired renal function
Haematuria-macroscopic and microscopic	Urography and cystoscopy do not show source of bleed
Acute nephritic syndrome	Persisting oliguria
Nephrotic syndrome	*Adults:* Unless cause is apparent from extrarenal manifestations. *Children:* Only if haematuria also present, or if proteinuria persists after trial of corticosteroid
Acute renal failure	No obvious precipitating cause; Obstruction of the renal tract excluded
Chronic renal failure	Radiographically and ultrasonographically normal kidneys
Renal allograft	To differentiate rejection from cyclosporine toxicity and to diagnose recurrence of original disease

The patient is placed in the prone position. Biopsy may be done under ultrasound guidance. The site of choice is the edge of the lower pole of the left kidney. This avoids major renal vessels and is likely to contain more cortex than medulla. The radiologist marks the surface anatomy on the skin and information of the depth of the kidney from the skin is given.

The skin is prepared and the skin and subcutaneous tissues are anaesthetised. An exploring needle is then inserted into the lumbar muscles and then advanced 5 mm at a time until a definite swing with respiration show that the point is within the kidney. The patient is asked to hold his breath in inspiration each time the needle is advanced. After locating the kidney the local anaesthetic is injected along the track formed, while withdrawing the needle.

A 11.4 cm trucut needle is used for obtaining the biopsy specimen. A nick is made in the skin with the point of a scalpel blade and then the biopsy needle is advanced towards the kidney.

The cannula of the biopsy needle is closed over the obturator. The obturator is longer than the cannula and has a bevelled edge. After introduction of the biopsy needle, the appearance of a large arc of swing of the needle indicates that the kidney has been located. With the tip of the needle just within the kidney, the patient is asked to hold his breath in inspiration. The obturator is pushed in and the cannula is then pushed over the length of the obturator, to cut the specimen. The obturator handle is kept firmly fixed with one hand while the cannula is pushed in with the other hand. The obturator and the cannula are withdrawn after completing this procedure.

A successful biopsy produces a strip of kidney upto 20 mm long. The specimen is divided into three portions.

One portion is sent for light microscopy examination, the second portion for electron microscopy examination and the third for immunofluorescent microscopy.

Aftercare and Complications

- The patient should remain in bed for 24 hours.
- Pulse and blood pressure are checked every hour for four hours and thereafter for every four hours.
- The most important complications of renal biopsy is haemorrhage, which may be perirenal, causing loin pain and sometimes a palpable mass as well as signs of blood loss.
- There may be persistent heavy haematuria and sometimes clot retention.
- Minor haematuria is common and usually settles quickly. Continuing haemorrhage should be treated by blood transfusion.

Setting up a Drip

Indications

1. Replacement of fluids (blood products, colloids or electrolyte solutions).
2. To provide a route for administering intravenous medication or nutrition.
3. Monitoring of central venous pressure.

Precautions

1. No absolute contraindications exist, but particular care is needed in some circumstances: In presence of incipient heart failure an extra circulating fluid load may result in severe pulmonary oedema. If a blood transfusion or intravenous infusion is essential this problem may be alleviated by giving diuretics simultaneously.

2. In presence of renal failure it is important that the fluid and electrolyte loads, as well as the amount of drugs given, do not exceed the excretory capacity of the kidney.
3. In patients with impaired immune responses or damaged heart valve, a drip site is an important portal for the entry of potentially fatal infection.
4. If small veins with inadequate blood flow are cannulated, inflammation may occur at the venepuncture site.

Procedure

Choice of Vein

The most convenient site for peripheral cannulation is the non-dominant forearm (left forearm in a right handed individual and vice versa). This permits comfortable mobility of the dominant arm and allows the dominant arm to carry out activities like writing, eating, etc.

Veins of the elbow should be avoided if possible, as the cannula is difficult to fix firmly, and uncomfortable immobilisation of the joint is required. The dorsum of the hand is a convenient site. Veins near the ankle may be used in a restless patient as the leg is often easier to immobilise. Other sites of cannulation are the jugular, subclavian, or saphenous veins.

Venepuncture

Clothing is removed from the limb and a tourniquet is applied to occlude venous return. A suitable superficial vein is selected and the area around the chosen site should be cleaned well with an alcohol swab.

The needle is pierced through the skin parallel to the vein chosen to be cannulated, with the bevelled edge facing upwards.

The vein is then pierced by moving the needle in the direction of the vein and continued for a distance in the lumen of the vein.

The tourniquet is then released and the IV fluid set is connected and allowed to flow into the vein. The rate of flow of the fluid is controlled by use of an adjustable valve attached to the IV set.

The fluid or blood is usually present in a collapsible plastic bag. If the fluid is present in a rigid bottle, an air inlet tube will be required to prevent the formation of a vacuum when fluid flows out of the bottle into the IV set.

The site of cannulation is firmly fixed with adhesive plaster. A segment of the tube of the IV set close to the needle is folded upon itself into a loop and fixed so as to allow free movement of the limb cannulated.

Problems

When no veins are visible or palpable, a 'blind' cannulation of the jugular or subclavian vein may be performed.

Alternatively, a 'cut down' procedure may be employed.

A small incision is made at the elbow or ankle and, with a tourniquet on the limb, a vein is displayed by blunt dissection of subcutaneous tissue and is under direct vision.

Appearance of inflammation at the site of cannulation is an indication for prompt removal of the cannula. The local infection will not clear or respond to treatment as long as the foreign material is present. Persistent infection may lead to bacteremia.

An unexplained fever in a patient with a drip is often due to inflammation at the venepuncture site.

Administration of Intravenous Cytotoxics

The administration and management of intravenous cytotoxic drugs is a specialist's task, requiring extensive knowledge and practical experience about the pharmacology, toxicology, and effectiveness of these drugs.

Procedure

Patient should be adequately informed about the procedure to be adopted and also of the side effects that may be expected as a result of cytotoxic drug administration.

The needle is introduced into the vein as explained above. The patency of the vein and the needle is confirmed by injecting about 5–10 ml of isotonic saline and watching the vein carefully. A large vein, preferably on the dorsum of the hand is selected. Cytotoxic drugs should never be injected into the veins of the leg.

After injecting the drug, flushing with isotonic saline is done to prevent the drug from leaking from the puncture site.

Contraindications for Cytotoxic Therapy

1. Low RBC, WBC or platelet count. A fresh blood count should always be obtained before administering cytotoxic drugs.
2. Dysfunction of an organ which may be worsened by the cytotoxics to be used or which is the organ of excretion for that drug. For instance, cisplatin, a renal toxic drug, should be avoided in renal failure.

3. Known hypersensitivity to the cytotoxic drug.
4. Presence of infection, whereby administration of the cytotoxic drug may be postponed.

Problems

Extravasation

Many cytotoxics are very vesicant and if they extravasate they may cause severe tissue damage. If, despite careful administration, extravasation does occur, the injection is stopped immediately and the following procedure is adopted.

a. Withdraw any remaining drug by aspirating through the needle.
b. Instillation of 50 mg hydrocortisone into the site of cannulation via the IV needle.
c. Removal of the IV needle and instillation of a further 50 mg of hydrocortisone subcutaneously into the swollen area.
d. Analgesics may be administered in the presence of severe pain.

Local Reactions

Redness and irritation sometimes develop along the vein being injected as a local reaction to the drug, especially when small veins are used. This may be reduced by further dilution, achieved, for example, by injecting the drug into a fast flowing infusion or injecting it more slowly. Intravenous hydrocortisone may be used at the end of the procedure.

Pain on Administration

Some drugs (especially dacarbazine, vinblastine, and mustine) cause muscular and venous pain on administration. This pain is felt along the vein and not just at the site of the needle, and so is different from that caused by extravasation. Further dilution or injection into a fast running infusion often alleviates the problem.

Complications

Many cytotoxic drugs cause severe emesis. It is therefore mandatory to ensure a good antiemetic cover prior to administration of the cytotoxic drug.

Cytotoxic therapy may culminate in bone marrow depression causing infection and fever. Patients with a suspected potential infection should have an immediate blood count performed. Sepsis in presence of neutropenia is an emergency and urgent measures should be adopted for its treatment.

Patients may develop severe stomatitis and should be advised on proper oral hygiene.

Metabolites of some cytotoxic drugs like ifosfamide and cyclophosphamide may cause a chemical cystitis and patients should therefore be advised on adequate fluid intake.

Percutaneous Central Venous Cannulation

Central venous pressure is the resultant of venous blood volume, right ventricular function and venous tone. Rapid changes in blood volume, especially associated with impaired right heart function, is the most common reason for monitoring central venous pressure.

Infusion of antibiotics, chemotherapeutic agents, and other substances irritant to veins and tissues are best administered through a line whose tip lies in a central vein.

Drugs used in resuscitation of cardiac arrest should be given through a central line if one is available.

This route is also widely used for long-term intravenous alimentation.

It is also used for insertion of a Swan-Ganz catheter to monitor the pulmonary artery and left atrial pressure and also for introduction of intracardiac pacing devices.

Venepuncture should be avoided at any site in which there is sepsis.

Apical emphysema or bullae contraindicate infraclavicular or supraclavicular approaches to the subclavian vein.

A carotid artery aneurysm precludes using the internal jugular vein on the same side.

Procedure

Strict aseptic precautions should be observed during the insertion of the cannula.

Equipments

One of the following equipments may be used.
1. *Catheter through cannula:* Cannula on the outside of a needle is placed in the vein and the needle is withdrawn. A catheter is then inserted into the vein. When the catheter is in position the cannula is withdrawn.
2. *Catheter over needle:* The needle and the catheter are placed in a arm vein. The needle (which is attached to a wire) is withdrawn, and the catheter advanced into position.
3. *Catheter over guide wire:* A flexible guide wire is inserted into the vein through a needle. After removal of the needle the catheter is inserted over the wire, which guides it into the central vein.

Index

A

Abdomen 254
    clinical examination 255
        signs and symptoms 255
    general examination 257
Abdominal pain 33
    pain due to disorders of GIT 33
        abdominal wall pain 35
        acute pancreatitis 34
        biliary colic 35
        colonic obstruction 34
        esophageal pain 33
        mechanical small bowel obstruction 33
        metabolic causes of abdominal pain 35
        neurogenic abdominal pain 35
        pain in acute appendicitis 34
        pain of peritonitis 35
        pain referred to abdomen 35
        peptic ulcer pain 33
        psychogenic abdominal pain 35
        superior mesenteric artery occlusion 35
    renal pain 35
Absent breath sounds 207
Absolute reticulocyte count 322
Acanthosis nigricans 6
Achalasia cardia 270
    complications 270
    investigations 271
    treatment 271
Acid-base balance and its disorders 390
Acute coronary syndromes 172
Acute lymphoblastic leukaemia 349
    classification 349
    clinical features 350
    investigations 350
    management 350
Acute pancreatitis 312
    causes 312
    clinical features 312
    complications 314
    differential diagnosis 314
    investigations 313
    management 314
Acute renal failure 381
    causes 381
    clinical features 382
    complications 382

    management 382
    recovery 382
Acute respiratory distress syndrome 247
    clinical features 248
    investigations 248
    management 248
Acute transverse myelitis 542
    clinical features 542
Added sounds 207
Adenoma sebaceum 5
Adipsic hypernatraemia 574
Administration of intravenous cytotoxics 752
Agnosia 404
Airway obstruction 690
Alcohol and drug interactions 718
Alcohol 714
Alcohol and central nervous system (CNS) 716
Alcohol and lymphatic system 718
Alcoholic cirrhosis 300
    clinical features 300
    investigations 300
    treatment 300
Amoebic abscess 298
    complications 298
    treatment 299
Amyotrophic lateral sclerosis 511
Anaemia 324
    causes 324
    classification 324
    symptoms and signs 324
Anaemia of chronic disease 330
    causes 330
    clinical features 330
    investigations 330
    management 330
Angina pectoris 77
    anginal equivalent 77
        nocturnal angina 77
        prinzmetal angina 77
        unstable angina 77
    characteristics of anginal pain 77
        levine test 77
    second wind angina 78
    causes of angina pectoris 78
        aortic regurgitation 78
        aortic stenosis 78
        coronary artery disease 78
        hypertrophic obstructive cardiomyopathy 78
        systemic hypertension 78

Angiography 732
Anomalous origin of a coronary artery from the pulmonary artery 143
    clinical features 143
    treatment 143
Anomalous pulmonary venous connection 137
    clinical features 137
    PAPVC 137
    TAPVC 137
Anorexia nervosa 73
Aortic regurgitation 152
    causes 152
        aortic valve involvement 152
        aortic wall involvement 152
    management 153
    other signs 153
    severity 153
    symptoms 152
Aortic stenosis 150
    common causes 150
    complications 151
    investigations 151
    management 152
    prognosis 152
    severity 151
    signs 151
    symptoms 151
Aplastic anaemia 336
    clinical features 336
    investigations 336
    management 337
Approach to acid-base disorders 393
Approach to bleeding disorders 358
Apraxia 404
Arterial blood gas analysis 216
Arterial pulse 80
    collapsing pulse 81
    pulse character 81
        anacrotic pulse 81
        hyperkinetic pulse 81
        hypokinetic pulse 81
    pulse rate 80
    pulse volume 81
    rhythm 81
Arterial puncture 757
Arteriovenous malformation 502
    clinical features 502
    investigations 502
    treatment 502
    types 502

Arthritis 649
  classification 649
    axial arthritis 649
    monoarthritis 649
    polyarthritis 649
Ascites 305
  causes of 305
  pathogenesis 305
Ascitic fluid aspiration (paracentesis) 747
Ataxia telangiectasia 485
Ataxic disorders 515
  hereditary ataxia 515
    ataxic disorders of unknown
      aetiology of early onset 518
    ataxic disorders of unknown
      aetiology of late onset 519
    ataxic disorders with known
      metabolic or other causes 517
    congenital ataxias 515
Atrial septal defect 125
  clinical features 126
    differential diagnosis 126
    treatment 126
Auscultation 94, 206, 267
  auscultatory areas 206
  general principles of auscultation 206
  importance of auscultation 206
  technique of auscultation 206
Austin-Flint murmur 154
Autoimmune diseases 51
  non-organ specific disorders 51
  organ specific disorders 51
Autonomic nervous system 527

B

Barber's chair sign or Lhermitte's sign 474
Behcet's syndrome 670
Bell's palsy 435
Benign intracranial hypertension 505
Biliary cirrhosis 301
Biliary obstruction 691
Biotin 63
  clinical features 63
  management 63
Blood pressure 85
  blood pressure in the basal condition 85
  classification of hypertension 86
    accelerated hypertension 86
    episodic or paroxysmal hypertension
      87
    hypertensive emergency 86
    hypertensive urgency 86
    isolated systolic hypertension 86
    labile hypertension 87
    malignant hypertension 86
    paradoxical hypertension 87
    pseudohypertension 87
    transient hypertension 87
    white coat hypertension 87
  korotkoff sounds 85
  normal blood pressure 86
Bone marrow aspiration 747

Bone marrow transplantation 363
Brain death 502
Bronchial asthma 217
  clinical features 218
    acute severe asthma 218
    chronic asthma 218
    episodic asthma 218
    exercise-induced asthma 218
    gastric asthma 218
    nocturnal asthma 218
  factors precipitating asthma 217
  investigations 219
  management 219
  mechanism 218
  types 217
    extrinsic asthma 217
    intrinsic asthma 217
Bronchiectasis 224
  clinical features 224
    dry bronchiectasis 224
    middle lobe bronchiectasis (Brock's
      syndrome) 224
    pseudo (reversible) bronchiectasis
      225
    sequestration of lung 224
    upper lobe bronchiectasis 224
  complications 225
  factors predisposing to bronchiectasis
    224
    acquired 224
    congenital 224
  investigations 225
  management 225
  types 224
Bronchogenic carcinoma 244
  clinical features 244
    extrathoracic manifestations 244
    thoracic manifestations 244
  investigations 245
  management 245
Bronchoscopy 217
  fibreoptic bronchoscope 217
  rigid bronchoscope 217
Bulimia 73

C

Calcium 67
  daily requirements 67
  dietary sources 67
Carcinoid tumours 286
  clinical features 286
  investigations 286
  management 286
Cardiac arrest 187
  causes 187
    anatomical/mechanical 187
    electrical 187
Cardiac cirrhosis 301
  aetiology 301
  clinical features 301
  investigations 302
  pathogenesis 301
  treatment 302

Cardiac failure 158
  afterload 158
  classification of cardiac failure 159
    high output and low output failure
      159
    right and left sided heart failure 159
  investigations 159
  preload 158
  treatment 160
Cardiac tamponade 186
  causes 186
  clinical features 186
  management 186
Cardiac transplantation 188
Cardiomyopathies 182
  dilated (congestive) cardiomyopathy 182
    clinical features 182
    differential diagnosis 183
    management 183
  hypertrophic obstructive cardiomyo-
    pathy 183
    differential diagnosis 183
    signs 183
    symptoms 183
  primary cardiomyopathies 184
  restrictive (obliterative) cardiomyopathy
    183
    clinical features 183
    differential diagnosis 183
  secondary cardiomyopathies 184
    causes 184
Cardiopulmonary resuscitation 187
Cardioversion (DC shock) 188
Causes of hepatomegaly 267
Causes of hepatosplenomegaly 268
Causes of hepatosplenomegaly lymphadeno-
  pathy 269
Causes of painful hepatomegaly 268
Causes of pulsatile liver 268
Causes of right ventricular enlargement 93
  pressure overload 93
  volume overload 93
Causes of splenomegaly 268
Causes of tubulointerstitial disease 380
Cell biology of cancer 673
Cerebellum 466
  causes of cerebellar lesions 468
  clinical manifestations of cerebellar
    dysfunction 467
    abnormalities of the gait 467
    dysdiadochokinesia 467
    dysmetria 467
    dyssynergia 467
    hypotonia 467
    intention tremor 468
    nystagmus 468
    pendular knee jerk 468
    rebound phenomenon 467
    speech disturbances 467
    titubation 468
  localisation of cerebellar lesions 468
  morphological and functional divisions
    of the cerebellum 466

nuclei of the cerebellum 466
treatable cerebellar lesions 468
Cerebral palsy 542
  causes 542
  clinical features 542
Cerebral tumours 507
  clinical features 507
  investigations 507
  management 508
Cerebrovascular disorders 485
  stroke 485
    causes 485
    clinical classification 486
    pathophysiology 486
    risk factors 486
Cervical spondylosis 537
  symptoms and signs 537
Characteristic types of facies 12
  acromegalic facies 12
  Bell's palsy 14
  cirrhotic facies 14
  congenital pulmonary stenosis 14
  cretinoid face 14
  Cushing's syndrome 12
  face in COPD 14
  face in nephrotic/nephritic syndrome 14
  face in pneumonia 14
  face in Sjögren's syndrome 14
  face in SLE 14
  hyperthyroid face 12
  hypothyroid face 12
  leonine facies 12
  myasthenic facies 14
  myotonic dystrophy 14
  Parkinsonian face 14
Charcot-Marie-Tooth disease 558
Chemotherapy 705
Chest deformities 199
  barrel chest 199
  flat chest 199
  Harrison's sulcus 199
  pectus excavatum (funnel chest, cobbler's chest) 199
  pigeon chest (pectus carinatum) 199
  rickety rosary 199
  scorbutic rosary 199
Chest film 724
Chest pain 195
  general examination 195
  mid or lower retrosternal pain 195
  pancoast syndrome 195
  pleural pain 195
  upper retrosternal pain 195
Chromium 69
Chromosomal abnormalities 42
  numerical chromosome aberrations 42
    autosomal aneuploidy 42
    sex chromosome aneuploidy 42
  single gene disorders 43
    autosomal dominant inheritance 43
    autosomal recessive inheritance 43
    X-linked dominant inheritance 44

X-linked recessive inheritance 43
    Y-linked or holandric inheritance 44
  structural aberration of chromosome 42
Chronic hepatitis (CH) 295
  causes 295
  classification 295
  management of chronic hepatitis B 296
  management of chronic hepatitis C 297
  prevention of hepatitis 297
Chronic inflammatory demyelinating polyneuropathy 557
  clinical features 557
  diagnostic criteria 557
  investigations 557
  treatment 557
Chronic kidney disease 383
Chronic lymphocytic leukaemia 351
  clinical features 351
  complications 352
  investigations 351
  management 352
Chronic myeloid leukaemia 347
  clinical features 347
  investigations 348
  management 348
Chronic obstructive pulmonary disease (COPD) 221
  complications 223
  investigations 223
  management 223
  pathogenesis 222
  predisposing factors for COPD 221
Chronic pancreatitis 314
  clinical features 314
  investigations 314
  treatment 315
Chronic renal failure 383
Churg-Strauss disease 668
Chylous ascites 307
Cirrhosis of liver 299
  aetiopathological classification 299
  causes of 299
  morphological classification 299
Clinical features of cancer 677
  general features 677
    breathlessness 678
    cachexia 677
    extreme anaemia 678
    metabolic syndromes 678
    nausea and vomiting 677
    pain 677
    pruritus 677
  specific features 678
    anal cancer 678
    colorectal cancer 678
    esophageal cancer 678
    gastric cancer 678
    head and neck cancer 679
    small bowel cancer 678
Closed mitral valvotomy/commissurotomy 147
Clubbing 195
  causes of clubbing 196

grading of clubbing 195
  theories of clubbing 196
Coarctation of the aorta 135
  clinical features 136
  complications 136
  treatment 137
Cobalt 69
Common chromosomal disorders 45
Complete transposition of the great vessels 139
  clinical features 139
  treatment 139
Complications of cancers 682
Complications of hypertension 172
Complications of sternal puncture 749
Complications of therapy 703
Computerized tomography 737
Confirmation of apical impulse 202
Congenital abnormalities of the coronary arteries 142
  complications 142
  coronary arteriovenous fistula 142
  treatment 143
Congenital aortic stenosis 134
  clinical features 135
  treatment 135
  types 134
    congenital AS associated syndrome 135
    subvalvular aortic stenosis 135
    supravalvular aortic stenosis 134
    valvular aortic stenosis 134
Congenital complete heart block 141
  aetiology 141
  complications 141
  treatment 142
Congenital heart diseases 121
  cardiac malposition 122
  classification 121
    aortic root to right heart shunt 121
    aortopulmonary level shunt 121
    gross anomalies 121
    lesions without shunts 121
    multiple level shunts 121
    shunt lesions—left to right 121
    shunt lesions—right to left 121
    ventricular level shunt 121
Congenital jaundice 291
    treatment 292
Congenitally corrected transposition of the great vessels 140
  clinical features 140
  treatment 140
Connective tissue disorders 648
Coordination of the limbs 452
Copper (Cu) 69
  daily requirement 69
  source 69
Cor pulmonale 251
  clinical features 251
  investigations 251
  management 251

Cortical sensations 474
Cortical venous thrombosis 497
  causes 497
    clinical features 497
    investigations 497
    treatment 498
Crack pot resonance 205
Craniopharyngioma 573
Craniovertebral junction anomalies 549
Creutzfeldt-Jakob disease 527
Crigler-Najjar syndrome 292
Cryptogenic cirrhosis 301
Cushing's syndrome 593, 685
Cyanosis 79
  causes 79
  types 79
Cystic fibrosis 226
  clinical features 226
  complications 227
  investigations 227
  management 227

D

Diabetes mellitus 603
Diabetic foot 629
Diabetic nephropathy 630
Diabetic neuropathy 626
  classification 626
  management 628
Diagnosis of cancers 681
Dialysis 386
  continuous ambulatory peritoneal dialysis 386
  haemodialysis 386
  haemofiltration 386
  intermittent peritoneal dialysis 386
Diarrhoea 277
  clinical classification 277
    acute diarrhoea 277
    chronic diarrhoea 278
    osmotic diarrhoea 277
    secretory diarrhoea 277
Disorder of the neurohypophysis 573
Disorders of parathyroid gland and calcium and phosphorus metabolism 586
Disorders of the white cells 37
  basophils 338
  eosinophils 338
    causes 338
  lymphocytes 337
    causes 338
  monocytes 338
    causes 338
  neutrophils 337
    causes 337
Dubin-Johnson syndrome 292
Dyspnoea 194
  clinical aspects of dyspnoea 194
  grading of dyspnoea 194
  receptors involved in mechanism of dyspnoea 194

E

Eaton-Lambert syndrome 565
Ebstein's anomaly 138
  clinical features 138
  diagnosis 138
ECG changes with drug intoxication 111
  causes of pathological Q-wave 112
  causes of shortened Q-Tc interval 112
  digoxin effect 111
  ECG features of COPD 112
  ECG features of hypothermia 112
  ECG in acute pulmonary embolism 112
  quinidine effect 111
ECG in coronary artery disease 108
  myocardial injury 108
  myocardial ischaemia 109
    right ventricular infarct 109
    subendocardial infarct 109
    true posterior wall infarct 109
  myocardial necrosis 108
ECG in electrolyte imbalance 110
  hypercalcaemia 111
  hyperkalaemia 110
  hypermagnesemia 111
  hypocalcaemia 111
  hypokalaemia 111
  hypomagnesemia 111
  uraemia 111
ECG in various arrhythmias 113
  bradyarrhythmias 120
    heart block 120
    indications for permanent pacemakers 120
    second degree heart block 120
    sick sinus syndrome 120
  tachyarrhythmias 113
    analysis of ECG 113
    atrial fibrillation 115
    atrial flutter 115
    AV node 117
    broad complex tachycardia 118
    management of narrow complex tachycardia 116
    paroxysmal AV nodal tachycardia 117
    paroxysmal supraventricular tachycardia 114
    radiofrequency ablation 116
    rule of hundreds for tachycardias 113
    specific management 116
    ventricular 117
Ectopic acromegaly 685
Ectopic ACTH syndrome 685
Edema 36
  characteristic features of edema of various etiologies 37
    cardiac edema 37
    cyclical or premenstrual edema 38
    edema of nutritional origin 38
    edema seen in liver disease 37
    idiopathic edema 38
    less common causes of facial edema 38
    other causes of edema 38
    renal edema 37
  etiology and types of edema 36
    fast edema 36
    generalised edema 36
    localised edema 36
    slow edema 36
  pathophysiology of edema 36
Effect of alcohol on liver 714
Eisenmenger syndrome 129
  clinical features 130
Electrocardiogram 104
  biventricular hypertrophy 106
  electrical axis 104
  left atrial enlargement 105
  left bundle branch block 106
    complete LBBB 106
    incomplete LBBB 107
  left ventricular hypertrophy 105
  right atrial enlargement 105
  right bundle branch block 106
    complete RBBB 106
    incomplete RBBB 106
    significance 106
  right ventricular hypertrophy 106
    significance 107
Emphysema 221
  special varieties of emphysema 222
    compensatory emphysema 222
    mediastinal emphysema 222
  types of 222
    centriacinar emphysema 222
    irregular 222
    panacinar emphysema 222
    paraseptal emphysema 222
Empty sella syndrome 573
  treatment 573
  types 573
    primary 573
    secondary 573
Encephalitis 525
Endoscopy 275
Endotracheal intubation 758
Epidural abscess 536
Epidural haemorrhage and haematomyelia 536
  causes 536
  clinical features 536
  investigations 536
Epilepsy 478
  causes 478
  classification 478
    generalized seizures 478
    partial (focal, local) seizures 478
    reflexly induced seizures 478
    status epilepticus 478
    unclassified epileptic seizures 478
  clinical features 479
  investigations 479
  management 481
Erythema nodosum 6
Essential thrombocythaemia 341
  clinical features 341

diagnostic criteria 341
management 341
Examination of higher mental functions 398
Examination of neck veins 87
jugular venous pressure 87
jugular venous pulse 88
Examination of the cranial nerves 414
abducent (sixth) 423
cranial nerves 423
eighth cranial nerve 436
eleventh cranial nerve 441
accessory nerve 441
fifth cranial nerve (trigeminal nerve) 431
first cranial nerve (olfactory nerve) 414
glossopharyngeal and vagus nerves 441
hypoglossal nerve 442
ninth and tenth cranial nerves 441
oculomotor (third) 423
second cranial nerve (optic nerve) 415
seventh cranial nerve (facial nerve) 433
trochlear (fourth) 423
twelfth cranial nerve 442
vestibulocochlear nerve 436
Examination of the neck 197
Examination of the respiratory system 198
External features of cardiac disease 90

F

Face 8
forehead 8
absence of wrinkling of forehead 9
prominent forehead 8
wrinkling of forehead 8
Feet and toes 21
clawed toes 22
genu valgum 21
genu varum 21
large feet 21
pes cavus 21
rocker bottom feet 21
short and broad feet 21
Fibrosis 211
investigations 211
lung function tests 211
types 211
Fingers 20
absence of digits 21
arachnodactyly 21
polydactyly 20
sausage fingers 21
syndactyly 20
Fluid and electrolyte imbalance 387
Fluorine 68
source 68
Folate deficiency 328
causes of 328
clinical features 328
investigations 328
management 329
metabolism of folate 328
Frontal lobe lesions 412
Fulminant hepatic failure 307
causes 307

clinical features 308
treatment 308
Functions of occipital lobe 413
Functions of parietal lobe 412
Functions of temporal lobe 413
Fundamentals in genetics 41
Fundus in cardiology 90

G

Gait 457
Gastroesophageal reflux disease 271
complications 271
diagnosis 271
treatment 271
Gastrointestinal bleeding 275
Gastrointestinal system 269
dysphagia 269
causes of dysphagia 269
diagnostic approach to dysphagia 270
treatment 270
Genes and cancer 673
Geriatric medicine 706
Giants of geriatric medicine 709
Gilbert's syndrome 292
Glomerulonephritis 377
Glomerulopathies 374
Goodpasture's syndrome 378
Grading of ascites 266
Guillain-Barre syndrome 555
Gynaecomastia 602

H

Haematologic syndromes 686
Haematological malignancies 342
Haematopoietic growth factors 319
Haematopoietic stem cell differentiation 319
Haematopoietic stem cells 319
Haemochromatosis 311
Haemolytic anaemia 331
causes 331
acquired 331
congenital 331
investigations 331
Haemoptysis 193
causes 193
severity 193
types 193
Haemoptysis 690
Hair 6
causes of hypertrichosis 8
colour of hair 8
phases of hair growth 7
anagen phase 7
catagen phase 7
telogen phase 7
stages of hair follicle growth 7
types of alopecia 7
cicatricial 7
noncicatricial 7
Hamman's mediastinal crunch 210
Handedness 403

Hands 19
acromegalic hand 19
cretinism 19
Down's syndrome 19
Dupuytren's contracture 20
eunuchoidal hand 19
Holt-Oram syndrome 19
pseudohypoparathyroidism 19
Heart murmurs 99
continuous murmurs 101
approach to continuous murmurs 102
classification of 101
diastolic murmurs 100
early diastolic murmurs 100
late diastolic murmurs 101
functional murmurs 103
innocent murmurs 102
systolic murmurs 99
early systolic murmurs 99
late systolic murmurs 99
mid systolic murmurs 99
pansystolic murmurs 100
systolico-diastolic murmur 102
causes 102
Heart sounds 95
first heart sound (S1) 95
abnormalities of S1 95
splitting of S1 95
fourth heart sound (S4) 97
second heart sound (S2) 95
third heart sound (S3) 97
Hemiblocks 107
left anterior hemiblock 107
causes 107
ECG features 107
left posterior hemiblock 107
ECG features 107
Henoch-Schönlein purpura 378
Hepatic coma 308
classification 308
clinical features 308
diagnosis 309
pathogenesis 308
treatment 309
Hepatocellular carcinoma (hepatoma) 309
aetiology 309
clinical features 310
investigations 310
management 310
pathology 310
Hepatology and pancreas 288
Hepatorenal syndrome 309
management 309
pathogenesis 309
Hereditary sensory motor neuropathy 558
Hereditary spherocytosis 332
clinical features 332
investigations 332
management 332
Hirsutism and virilism 602
Histocompatibility antigens 50
class I antigens 50